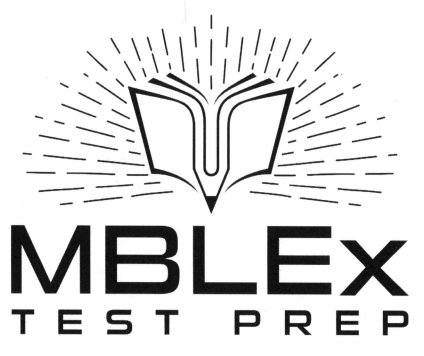

MBLEx
TEST PREP

Comprehensive Study Guide
and Workbook

David Merlino, LMT

Table of Contents

Introduction

Hello! My name is David Merlino, and I am the author of this study guide.

A lot of time and energy has gone in to the creation of this guide. I am extremely proud to share this guide with you, and I am honored that you have chosen my study guide to help prepare you for the MBLEx. You have a tall task ahead of you, but it isn't something you can't overcome. Trust me, I've taken, and passed, the MBLEx! My score was 797, for the record. Beat my score!

I've been a Licensed Massage Therapist for over 11 years, and I've learned so much, and experienced so much. However, it all began with passing my licensing exam. I understood how to take tests, how to study, and how to give myself the best chance possible to advance into my career. I hope to share this knowledge with you.

In 2011, I began my new career, preparing students to take their massage licensing exams at a career college in beautiful Reno, Nevada. It was here where I honed my craft, helping students achieve a near-90% pass rate on the licensing exam. How did I do this? It's quite simple. I emphasize efficient studying and information over excessive studying and information. Simply put, it's called the minimum effective dose for the MBLEx. I review the information most likely to be seen on the exam, and don't review information I feel isn't necessary, or is unlikely to be seen on the exam. As pole vaulter Henk Kraaijenhof once said, "Do as little as needed, not as much as possible." This approach makes preparing for the MBLEx much easier to manage.

With this view, my students achieved amazing success. You can too. Before you begin, however, I need to remind you of something: you will be tested on information that isn't present in this study guide. You will be tested on information you have never even seen before. This happened to all of my students. It even happened to me, someone who had been teaching this information for five years. It's all the luck of the draw. Despite not seeing this information before, you can still do extremely well on these questions. Make sure you check out the Study Skills, Test-Taking Techniques, and Reducing Test Anxiety sections immediately following this page.

I've poured months of my life into the production and creation of this study guide. You are now my student. I believe in you, and I know you will do great.

If you have any questions, I am here to help. Please don't hesitate to send me an email with any questions you may have in regards to the study guide, practice tests, or the MBLEx in general. My personal email address is: david@massagetestprep.com. Just note, I am very much willing to help, but if your email is rude or disrespectful in any way, there will be no response from me. Just be cool!

Thank you again. I am honored that you have entrusted me with helping you pass the MBLEx. So let's dominate this test!

Your Instructor,

David Merlino, LMT

How To Use This Study Guide

This study guide is designed to not just TELL information, but to help you, the student, LEARN information. This is achieved in many different ways, including standard study guides, fill-in-the-blanks, assignments, and practice exams.

To get the complete, most effective and efficient experience from this study guide, I recommend doing the following:

Before starting, figure out the area you need to study most: Massage Therapy, Kinesiology, Pathology, or Anatomy and Physiology. Most people tend to choose Kinesiology first. A common study routine I've helped many students implement is the following(you can change the subjects as you see fit, depending on how comfortable you are with each), with an average of one month of study time before the exam. For this example, we'll say the study order is Kinesiology, Pathology, Anatomy and Physiology, and then Massage Therapy:

Week 1: Study nothing but Medical Terminology and Kinesiology, depending on schedule, for up to 10 hours.
Week 2: Study Pathology for 80% of the time, and study Medical Terminology and Kinesiology the other 20% of the time. So, if you're studying for 10 hours, 8 hours will be dedicated to Pathology, and 2 hours will be dedicated to Medical Terminology and Kinesiology.
Week 3: Study Anatomy and Physiology for 80% of the time, and study Pathology, Medical Terminology, and Kinesiology for the remaining 20% of the time.
Week 4: Study Massage Therapy for 80% of the time, and study Anatomy and Physiology, Pathology, Medical Terminology, and Kinesiology for the remaining 20% of the time.
Final Week: Study every subject an equal amount.

This way of studying, I've found, is great for long-term memory growth in these subjects, as there is a consistent review of information every week.

While studying, especially in the final week before the exam, I highly recommend taking as many practice tests as possible. Go to the following website to take unlimited online practice exams: **http://www.mblextestprep.com/resources.html**

Watch video lectures I have created, which puts you in a class-like study session with me as your instructor. Go to the following website to view all available video lectures and follow along while studying: **http://www.mblextestprep.com/resources.html**

Utilize pre-made flashcards I've created for you, which cover the most important information you need to study. Go to the following website to utilize flashcards:
http://www.mblextestprep.com/resources.html

While studying, be sure to finish the assignments and practice exams in the book. These are great for assessing your knowledge on the subjects you will have just covered, and help you figure out what you still need to study, and what you've learned.

Study Skills

➤ Do not do all of your studying the night before or day of the test. Study consistently, up to several times per week. Cramming is good for short-term learning, but does not help with long-term learning. The more you study, the more likely you are to retain the information.

➤ Use all of your class and home work as study materials. The information in these assignments is information that might be on your exam.

➤ Take many short breaks as you study. Memory retention is higher at the beginning and end of study sessions than it is in the middle. This is called the Serial Position Effect. Study for no longer than ten minutes, then take a short break.

➤ Focus on one subject at a time while studying. You don't want to confuse yourself by mixing information.

➤ Study the subject you have the most difficulty with more than subjects you are comfortable with. Studying what you aren't weak in doesn't help. If you need work on a specific subject, focus the majority of your time learning that information, even if it means taking away study time from other areas. You're better off being 80% proficient in every subject than 100% in four subjects and only 50% in the last. Not studying this information could prevent you from passing the exam.

➤ While studying, take notes on important information, especially if it's information you don't recognize or remember. Use this information to study with.

➤ Assign yourself tests, reports, assignments and projects to complete. You are more likely to remember information if you write a report on it than if you just read the information.

➤ Teach information you are studying to another person. If you are responsible for someone learning something, you have to know and understand the material, and be able to put that information into the simplest terms possible, so someone else can understand it. This will only help you. Trust me, from personal experience, this really works.

➤ Understand the material you are studying. Do not just try to memorize certain answers you think may be on the test. Certain "key words" might not be on the test. Learn everything about a subject, and you'll never get any question on that subject wrong.

Serial Position Effect: http://www.simplypsychology.org/primacy-recency.html

Test-Taking Tips

➤ Go to the restroom before taking the exam. Using the restroom beforehand ensures that you are 100% focused on the exam, and not on your bladder.

➤ Read the entire question slowly and carefully. Never make assumptions about what a question is asking. Assuming you know what a question is asking may lead to you missing key words in the question that tell you exactly what the question is asking. Read every single word in every single question, multiple times if necessary.

Understand what the question is asking before you try answering it.

➢ Identify key words in each question. Key words are words that tell you exactly what the question is asking. Identify these words easily by reading questions aloud to yourself. The words you find yourself emphasizing while reading aloud are likely the key words.

Here is an example. Read this question:
Q: Which of the following statements is true regarding Swedish massage?
In this question, there are two key words, which are telling you exactly what the question is asking. Now read the question aloud. Which words did you put emphasis on? Most likely, you read the question like this: "Which of the following statements is TRUE regarding SWEDISH massage?" These are the key words.

➢ Do not change your answers, unless you misread the question. Changing your answers puts doubt into your mind, and leads to more changing of answers. The answer you put first is usually correct. Do not change your answers!

➢ Match key words in the answers with key words in the questions. Sometimes it's as simple as matching terms, if you've exhausted all other avenues.

➢ Eliminate answers you know aren't correct and justify the reason they aren't correct. If you can eliminate one answer from each question, that brings your odds of getting that question right up to 33%. If you can eliminate two answers that can't be right, that brings it up to 50%. Then it's just a coin flip!

Here's an example. Read this question, and the answers:
Q: Of the following, which is not contagious?
A. Athlete's Foot
B. Herpes Simplex
C. Influenza
D. Osgood-Schlatter Disease

Have you ever heard of Osgood-Schlatter Disease? Even if you haven't, you can still get this question right by eliminating the other answers. Athlete's Foot is caused by a fungus, and is contagious. That leaves us with three possible answers. Herpes Simplex is caused by a virus, and is contagious. That leaves us with two possible answers. So even if you're guessing at this point, it's only a 50/50 chance you get it right! Influenza is caused by a virus, and is contagious. This process of elimination just gave us the answer: D, Osgood-Schlatter Disease.

➢ Read the entire question before looking at the answers. Again, never make assumptions about what the question is asking.

➢ Come up with the answer in your head before looking at the answers. If the same answer you come up with is in the list of answers, that's most likely the right answer.

➢ Read every answer given to make sure you are picking the most correct answer. Some questions have multiple right answers, and you need to make sure you're picking the most correct answer.

➢ Make sure you are properly hydrated before the test. Studies have been done on the effects of proper hydration on those taking tests. People who are properly hydrated tend to score higher than those who are not.

> Exercise for twenty minutes before the exam. Exercise has also been shown to increase test scores.

Exercise and Test-Taking: http://lifehacker.com/20-minutes-of-exercise-before-an-exam-may-boost-your-pe-1541773646

Reducing Test Anxiety

> Study consistently. If you understand the material, you won't be as stressed out about the test. There are ways you can study without this book or your class notes as well. An example, whenever you take a bite of food, think about every structure the food passes through in the alimentary canal and what each of the organs do. Another example, whenever you are massaging someone, tell yourself everything about every muscle you work on, like origin, insertion, and action.

> Keep a positive attitude while preparing for the test and during the test. If you think you're going to fail, you will not be as motivated to study, you won't adhere to your test-taking techniques, you'll become stressed out during the exam much more easily, and you'll be more likely to fail.

> Try to stay relaxed. Utilize deep breathing techniques to calm down if you start feeling nervous or stressed. You will have two hours to finish the exam. You can afford one or two minutes to calm yourself down if you need to.

> Exercise consistently up until the day of the test to reduce anxiety. Exercise has been shown to significantly reduce stress, and also helps with memory retention. Try utilizing flash cards while riding an exercise bike.

> Take your time on the test. If you find yourself rushing, slow down. Again, you have two hours to finish the exam. Do not rush through it. You may miss important information in the exam and answer questions incorrectly because of this.

Massage Therapy

The MBLEx is a test designed with the massage therapist in mind. There are numerous topics covered on the MBLEx that fall under the general category of Massage Therapy.

In this section, we will discuss many subjects, covering a wide range of information.

Information covered in this section includes:

History of Massage
People of Importance
Massage Technique
Joint Movements
Stretching
Assessment
Precautions
Draping
Bolsters
Body Mechanics
Massage Modalities
Business
Liability Insurance
SOAP Notes
Ethics
Communication
Psychology
Types of Employment
Tax Forms

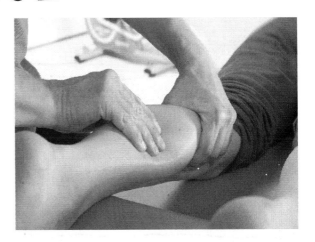

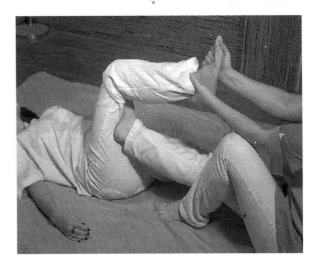

This information is followed by three assignments:

Massage Therapy Matching
Massage Therapy Crossword
Massage Therapy Fill-In-The-Blank

The end of the section has a 50 question practice exam on Massage Therapy. These questions ARE NOT the exact same questions will you see on the MBLEx. They are meant to test information that MAY be seen on the MBLEx.

While taking the practice exam, make sure to utilize your test-taking strategies(page 3) to optimize your test scores.

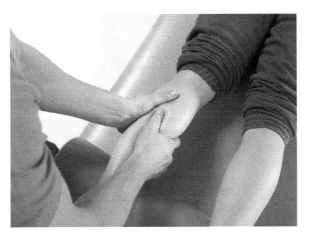

Massage Therapy

History of Massage

Massage Therapy has been practiced for thousands of years, in many different countries and cultures. In **China**, massage has been practiced as early as **3000 BC**. The first massage technique created by the Chinese was known as **Amma**. Amma consisted of rubbing, vibration, and pressing movements. Modern Chinese massage techniques are known as **Tuina**.

Around 500 AD, massage entered **Japan** from China. Amma was adopted by the Japanese, and renamed **Tsubo**, despite the manipulation areas remaining the same. Tsubo, much like Amma, involves pressing specific points on the body to increase to flow of **fluids** and **Ki**(energy, life force). Tsubo eventually evolved into another treatment known as **Shiatsu**.

In **India**, a book was written that details health and personal hygiene, know as **The Ayurveda**, or "Art of Life". This book primarily focuses on medicine, including massage, the use of herbs, diet, and other holistic means of well-being.

People of Importance

Numerous people have had some influence over the development of massage therapy over the past thousands of years. Some of these people include:

Celsus, a Roman physicist, wrote a series of books called **De Medicina**(Italian: Of Medicine), one of, if not the first, printed medical books. These books detailed subjects such as diet, exercise, personal hygiene, disease management, medicines, and the use of massage.

Per Henrik Ling, a Swedish physiologist, developed a system of active and passive movements, used to improve physical conditions. This system became known as **Medical Gymnastics**. This system of movements evolved into what we know today as physical therapy and massage therapy. Per Henrik Ling is considered the father of physical therapy and massage therapy as a result.

In the mid-1850's, **Charles Taylor** learned Medical Gymnastics. Eventually, he introduced Medical Gymnastics to the United States, where it became known as Swedish Gymnastics, or the Swedish Movement Cure. This was the precursor to the development of Swedish Massage.

Johann Mezger, a Dutch physician, helped to simplify the movements involved in Medical Gymnastics, categorizing them to make them easier to understand. He developed the **terms** for the **massage strokes**: effleurage, petrissage, friction, and tapotement.

Emil Vodder, along with his wife Estrid, developed the technique known as **Lymphatic Drainage**, which aids in increasing lymph flow and decreasing swelling caused by excessive lymph in an area.

John Harvey Kellogg, aside from co-founding Kellogg's Cereal, was deeply involved in massage therapy. He wrote a book titled **The Art of Massage**, which details the **physiological** effects of massage therapy, or the effects that massage therapy has on the body.

Dolores Krieger, along with Dora Kunz, developed a technique known as **Therapeutic Touch**, an energy-based modality similar to Reiki.

James Cyriax, a British physician, is considered the **father of orthopedic medicine**. He developed a technique known as **deep transverse friction**, which is used to promote the formation of healthy scar tissue.

Massage Technique

In western massage, there are **six** main massage strokes, which have been in a constant state of evolution since being developed.

Effleurage is the most common stroke in western massage, consisting of long, **gliding** strokes that are directed **towards the heart**. Effleurage is used to increase circulation of blood and lymph, remove waste from tissues, introduce the therapist's touch to the client, transition between strokes, and apply massage lubricant. Effleurage may be used throughout the massage, but is the main stroke used at the beginning of the treatment. The majority of the time, effleurage is performed by the therapist in the **archer(bow) stance**.

Petrissage utilizes **kneading** movements, lifting and squeezing tissue, to increase circulation, loosen adhesions that may be present in the tissue, and release metabolic waste from tissues. Petrissage is an important stroke to use in post-event sports massage, as it helps flush waste from the muscles and bring fresh oxygen-rich blood into them.

Friction consists of strokes that move **across** tissue. Friction is especially useful in breaking up adhesions and scar tissue, increasing circulation, and stretching muscles. There are many different forms of friction, such as superficial friction(rubbing the surface of the skin), parallel friction, circular friction, and cross-fiber friction.

Tapotement consists of **percussion** strokes, rhythmically affecting the tissues of the body in many different ways. Tapotement increases spindle cell activity in the muscles, which helps activate them and get them ready for use, which makes tapotement a very important stroke to use in pre-event sports massage. Tapotement may also help loosen any phlegm, or mucous, in the respiratory tract, and is very helpful in conditions such as asthma or chronic bronchitis. There are many different forms of tapotement, including hacking, cupping, tapping, and beating.

Vibration is performed by **shaking** a part of the body, using **trembling** actions. Vibration can have different effects on the body, depending on how fine the vibration is. Slow vibration is used to sedate an area(think of massage chairs that vibrate, numbing the area). Fast vibration is used to stimulate an area.

A **nerve stroke** is an **extremely light** form of **effleurage**. Like effleurage, nerve strokes, also called feather strokes, are directed towards the heart. These strokes are primarily used at the end of a massage, or at the end of work on a specific body part, to separate the therapist from the client(ending the massage session), or to transition from one part of the body to another.

Joint Movements

Joint movements describe how a joint is, well, moved! There are four main types of joint movements, performed by the therapist on the client, the therapist and the client working together, the therapist and the client working against one another, or the client performing the action by themselves.

An **active joint movement** involves the client actively performing a movement **without assistance** from the massage therapist. An example would be a massage therapist asking a client to perform a range-of-motion as part of assessment. The therapist does not help with the action, as they would want to see how much movement the client can perform by themselves, and to see where any restrictions may be.

An **active assistive joint movement** involves the client performing a movement **with assistance** from the massage therapist. Active assistive joint movements are very helpful in rehabilitative settings, allowing the client to move the joint, but making sure someone is there to help move and support the joint to prevent further injury.

Passive joint movements involve the massage therapist moving the joint, with the **client completely relaxed**, not helping at all. Passive joint movements are helpful for performing stretches, feeling for restrictions in movements, and for assisting the client to further relax.

Resistive joint movements are when the client and massage therapist are moving a joint in **opposite directions** at the same time. This creates an isometric contraction(muscle tension increases, length doesn't change), which is extremely helpful in a specific type of stretch known as Proprioceptive Neuromuscular Facilitation.

Stretching

Stretching is an exercise that is performed by **elongating**, or lengthening, a muscle. Stretching is extremely beneficial to a person's health.

An **unassisted stretch** is performed by the client stretching into resistance, **without any help** from the massage therapist. It is similar to an active joint mobilization, but instead of just moving the joint through its normal range-of-motion, it moves past that point and into a stretch.

An **assisted stretch** is performed by the client, **with assistance** from the massage therapist. Again, this is similar to an active assistive joint movement, where the massage therapist's role is to help the client move the joint into a stretch while stabilizing the joint to ensure there is no damage to the joint.

Proprioceptive Neuromuscular Facilitation(PNF) is a stretch that is very useful in loosening adhesions and scar tissue in muscles, and is very beneficial in athletes. To perform PNF, a massage therapist moves a client's joint into a stretch. Once resistance is met, the client will actively resist the movement being performed by the massage therapist. This puts the muscle into an **isometric contraction**. After holding this resisted movement for 5-10 seconds, the client **relaxes**, and the massage therapist is able to move the stretch further, until resistance is met again. The process is then repeated. PNF allows a highly noticeable increase in the amount of range-of-motion in a joint.

During stretching and joint mobilizations, we experience **end feels**. An end feel is what causes a joint movement or stretch to not move any further.

A **soft end feel** is the result of **soft tissues**, such as muscles and tendons, pulling back on the joint, preventing any further movement. An example is when stretching the hamstrings. The hip joint is moved into flexion until resistance is met. The resistance is due to the hamstrings pulling back on the joint. If the hamstrings are loosened, the joint will move further. This is a soft end feel.

A **hard end feel** is the result of structures, primarily **bone**, preventing a joint from moving further. An example is extension of the knee or elbow. Straightening these joints can only go to a certain point. Bones will prevent these joints from extending any further. That's why hyperextension of these joints may result in broken bones. This is a hard end feel.

An **empty end feel** is caused by neither muscles nor bones interfering with movement. Empty end feels are the result of **trauma** to an area, which prevents movement. An example could be a sprained ankle. With a sprained ankle, inflammation may be present, which immobilizes a joint to prevent further injury. This is an empty end feel.

➤ *Easy to Remember: A soft end feel is caused by soft tissues; a hard end feel is caused by hard tissues!*

Assessment

Assessments are a vital component of any massage treatment. Assessments are **evaluations** of the client primarily done before a massage, but the therapist is constantly assessing, even during and after a treatment.

Assessments have many different uses, from determining any contraindications the client may have, to tailoring a massage session specifically for that client and what they need. An example could be, if a client complains of low back pain, the therapist could then do visual assessment, range-of-motion exercises, and palpation to determine what the possible cause of the low back pain could be. Then, after the assessment is complete, the therapist may tailor the session to work specifically on the areas of concern(possibly the hamstrings, quadratus lumborum, psoas major, or rectus femoris).

Assessments may be performed in many different ways:
- **Listening** to the client and their complaints is the most effective way to determine issues a client may be experiencing.
- **Visual assessment** may be performed, focusing on alignment of specific bony landmarks to determine areas of concern. Some of these areas to compare bilaterally include the ears(possible neck tension), acromion processes(shoulder/back/chest tension), iliac crests(back/hip/thigh tension), anterior superior iliac spines(back/hip/thigh tension), and head of fibulae(back/hip/thigh tension).
- **Gait analysis** may help determine hypertonic muscles unilaterally, and injuries.
- **Palpation** is useful in feeling for adhesions or restrictions in muscles,

localized ischemia, and inflammation.
- **Intake forms** are extremely helpful in determining contraindications via medical history, medications, any hobbies or jobs that may lead to issues physically or mentally(an example could be the hobby of gardening, which may strain the back or hamstrings).

Precautions

During a massage, certain precautions need to be adhered to, to prevent injury or complications to the client.

Endangerment sites are areas of the body that, while massage may be performed on, need to be treated with **extra caution**. These are commonly due to insufficient tissues in the area to support, cushion, and protect important structures like blood vessels and nerves. Endangerment sites include the anterior triangle of the neck, the axilla, the anterior elbow, and the popliteal region.

Local contraindications are areas of the body that must be **avoided** when performing a massage. While endangerment sites allow for massage to be performed, local contraindications do not permit massage on localized areas. Reasons for a part of the body to be considered a local contraindication vary, from inflammation and trauma to infections(such as athlete's foot). The rest of the body may receive massage, but these specific areas must be avoided.

Absolute contraindications prohibit the use of massage. Massage on a person with an absolute contraindication, such as when a person is infected by a virus like influenza, can worsen the condition for the client, cause damage to the body, or even spread an infection or condition to the massage therapists. Do not perform a massage on a client with an absolute contraindication!

Draping

Draping is the use of **linens** to keep a client covered during a massage session. There are many different types of linens that may be used to cover a client. Most commonly, sheets are used. Blankets and towels are other common forms of linens. Draping is a very important step in establishing **boundaries** between the massage therapist and the client. Draping the client tells the client what part of the body the therapist is, and isn't, going to work on, increasing the professionalism required of a massage therapist. Draping also helps the clients establish boundaries, telling the therapist where the client may not want massage to be performed. Communication is key in establishing boundaries. If there is any question about a client's boundaries with regards to draping, just ask!

Top cover draping refers to the linen placed **atop** the client, which acts as the drape. As previously stated, the most common form is a sheet.

Bolsters

Bolsters are used to place the client into a comfortable position during a massage session. There are many different positions a client may be placed in during a massage, which requires the bolster to be placed in different locations to optimize comfort.

When a client is positioned **supine(face up)** on the massage table, the client may experience low back pain. A bolster should be placed **under the knees** in this case. Low back pain is likely caused by a tight psoas major, iliacus, or rectus femoris. A bolster under the knees produces slight flexion of the hip, which takes pressure off all these muscles.

When a client is positioned **prone(face down)** on the massage table, the client may experience low back pain. A bolster should be placed **under the ankles** in this case. Low back pain is likely caused by tight hamstrings. A bolster under the ankles produces slight flexion of the knee, which takes pressure off the hamstrings.

Side-lying position should be used for pregnant clients, or clients who have difficulty lying prone, such as people with kyphosis. Bolstering for side-lying clients includes placing a bolster between the **knees** to relieve pressure on the hips, under the **arms**, and under the **head**.

Certain clients may need to be placed in a **semi-reclined position**, such as pregnant clients who experience dizziness from lying supine(caused by the fetus placing pressure on the abdominal aorta). When a client is semi-reclined, a bolster should be placed **under the knees**, and behind the **head**.

Body Mechanics

Body mechanics are extremely important for massage therapists. Proper body mechanics prevent the therapist from **injuring** themselves during a massage, which increases the longevity of their career. It makes performing a massage less physically strenuous, and allows the therapist to perform a **better** massage by utilizing pressure and leverage more efficiently.

While performing a massage, the massage therapist's **back** should remain **straight**. Knees should be in a **slightly flexed** position. While performing compression, **joints** should be **stacked** to relieve pressure on one specific joint. An important factor in body mechanics that often is overlooked, however, is the **height**

of a **massage table**. The table should be at the proper height for the therapist, based on the type of massage being performed. Deep tissue massages require the table to be slightly lower than Swedish massages.

Body stances are very important while performing massage strokes, making them easier to perform, and makes the strokes flow and transition more smoothly.

The **bow** stance, also called the **archer** stance, is performed with the therapist's **feet** placed **parallel** to the massage table. This allows the therapist to perform long, gliding strokes, such as those seen in effleurage.

The **horse** stance, also called the **warrior** stance, is performed with the therapist's **feet** placed **perpendicular** to the massage table. The feet will face the table, the knees will be slightly flexed. This allows short, powerful strokes to be performed, such as compression and friction.

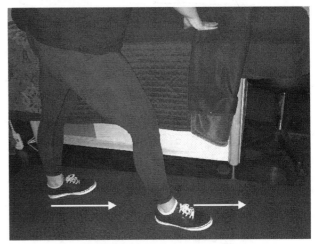

Bow/Archer Stance

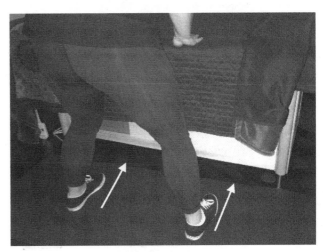

Horse/Warrior Stance

Massage Modalities

There are many different forms of massage, and many different modalities(specialties) that may be performed by massage therapists. Some require training and certification to perform, and others do not. Check with your local licensing board to determine requirements to perform specific modalities.

Aromatherapy is any treatment utilizing **essential oils**, which may affect the brain's **limbic** system. Essential oils have many different effects on the body, depending on the type of oil used, and how it is administered. Examples include oils having a stimulating effect, such as lemon and grapefruit, having a sedative effect, such as eucalyptus on the respiratory tract, having antiseptic properties, such as tea tree on insect bites, or having calming effects on the brain, such as lavender. Always check with a client for any allergies before using essential oils in a treatment.

Craniosacral Therapy, developed by **John Upledger**, is a very light massage technique that helps to release **blockages** in the flow of **cerebrospinal fluid**, which runs from the **cranium** to the **sacrum**. Blockages in these fluids may cause numerous side effects, including headaches, dizziness, and difficulty processing and understanding information.

Deep Tissue massage is performed by working the **deeper** layers of tissue in the body, including muscles and fascia. Deep tissue may require deeper pressure to be used by the massage therapist to reach deeper structures(an example could be working deeper through the rectus femoris to reach the vastus intermedius).

Hot Stone massage is a treatment that utilizes **heated stones**. The stones may be **placed** on certain parts of the body(hands, feet, lumbar, abdomen), may be used to physically massage a client, or both. Temperature of the stones should be checked by the massage therapist on their own skin(anterior forearm) before attempting to place on the client, to ensure the client does not suffer any burns. Hot stone is used to increase circulation into muscles and tissues, and aids in relaxation.

Hydrotherapy is the use of **water** in any treatment. There are several different types of hydrotherapy, utilizing water in solid(ice), liquid(water), or vapor(steam). **Contrast baths** utilize both a **heated** bath and a **cold** bath. Contrast baths are used to decrease systemic inflammation and increase circulation. A typical contrast bath treatment sees the client use cold water, then hot, then cold, then hot, and end with cold for inflammation relief. A **Vichy shower** is a piece of equipment that hangs over a **water-proof table**. This equipment has seven shower heads attached to it, which can pin-point specific areas of the body to be sprayed.

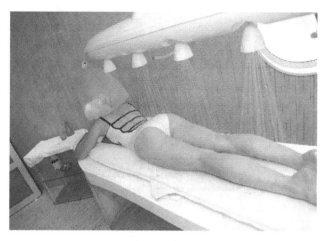

Vichy Shower

Lomi Lomi(Hawaiian "lomi": massage) is a **Hawaiian** massage, similar to a Swedish massage, which utilizes rhythmic gliding strokes. These strokes are used on the entire body, and can move from the feet up to the head in only fluid motion. This requires minimal draping, usually nothing more than a hand towel covering the gluteal cleft, exposing the glutes.

Lymphatic Drainage, developed by **Emil Vodder**, is a technique designed to increase the circulation of **lymph** utilizing very light strokes directed towards the heart. Increasing lymph circulation may help reduce swelling in areas such as the limbs or face.

Myofascial Release, popularized by **John Barnes**, is a type of treatment aimed at releasing **restrictions** in **muscles** and **fascia**. Myofascial Release utilizes light strokes that move in the direction of the restriction, helping the muscle "unwind" on its own.

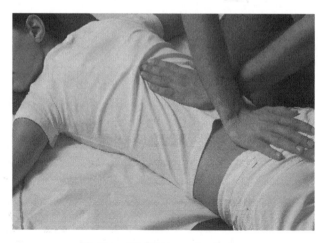

Myofascial Release technique

11

Pregnancy massage is, well, massage for pregnant clients. As discussed earlier, pregnant clients may need to be placed into side-lying or semi-reclined position. Endangerment sites for pregnant clients include the **abdomen** and around the **ankles**.

Reflexology is used to treat **reflex points** on the hands, feet, and ears that correspond to other tissues inside the body, such as **organs**. A map of these locations can be found on page 286.

Reiki is a form of **energy work**, similar to Therapeutic Touch, discussed earlier. In reiki, the therapist primarily(but not always) holds their hands an inch or two **above the client**, and manipulate the client's energy to promote relaxation or other benefits.

blood into the muscles to aid in recovery.

Swedish massage, the most common massage technique in western massage therapy, is mainly focused on **relaxation**. Effleurage is a stroke commonly utilized in Swedish massage, with strokes aimed towards the heart to increase circulation.

Thai massage, originating in Thailand, isn't necessarily what we consider a normal massage. Thai massage is performed with the client wearing loose-fitting clothes, on a mat, on the floor. The therapist's main goal during a Thai massage is to **stretch** the client. Massage may be incorporated into these stretching techniques.

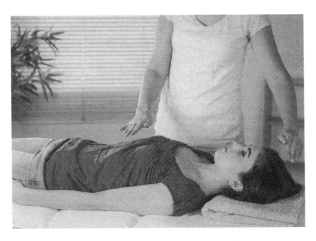

Aura strokes seen with Reiki

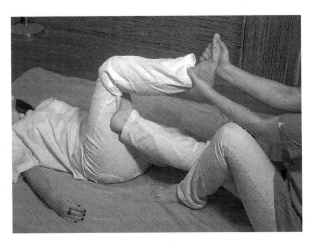

Thai Massage

Rolfing, developed by **Ida Rolf**, is known as a **structural realignment** technique. The basic principles of Rolfing involve the body being placed back into proper vertical alignment. The Rolfer works on the **fascia** of the body. Loosening the fascia helps the body return to its natural position. Rolfing typically takes place over ten sessions, with a different part of the body worked on during each session.

Sports massage is a massage designed for **athletes**. Sports massage may be performed in many different ways, depending on the needs of the athlete. **Pre-event** sports massage, which may be performed up to 15 minutes before an event, will typically be **stimulating**, increasing circulation into the muscles, and using tapotement to activate spindle cells. Inter-event massage will look to achieve the same results as pre-event massage, but does not utilize tapotement. Using tapotement may result in cramping. **Post-event** massage will be much slower, rhythmic, and relaxing. The primary goal of a post-event massage is to **calm the body** down, remove metabolic waste from tissues, and increase the flow of oxygen-rich

Tuina, as discussed earlier, is the name of **modern Chinese** massage. It is used to balance the eight principles of Chinese medicine. Tuina incorporates rhythmic strokes focused on specific areas of the body.

Business

Even if you aren't planning on becoming a business owner, understanding how businesses operate is knowledge everyone should have. It can help in retaining clientele, business relationships, and even keep you out of trouble from things like HIPAA violations.

Business for a massage therapist, in most locations, begins with a **certification**. A certification is a credential obtained by completing a certification course, usually in a **school** setting. It also may involve completing a certification exam. Certifications show that you have gained enough knowledge in a given subject to be able to perform that task. In this case, you gain a certificate after completing massage school.

A **license** is a jurisdictional requirement, which is used to **regulate** the practice of massage therapy. Licensing boards set rules and laws that a person is required to follow if they wish to be a licensed massage therapist. Licenses, in most jurisdictions, allow a massage therapist to practice massage therapy and receive money as compensation.

Reciprocity refers to the ability for a massage license in one jurisdiction to be recognized as **valid** in another jurisdiction. Some jurisdictions may require a new license to be obtained, but no more schooling required. Others may require more schooling in addition to paying for a new license.

Liability Insurance

When operating a business at a physical location where there is customer exposure, liability insurance is often required. There are two types of liability insurance: General liability insurance, and Professional liability insurance.

General liability insurance protects the massage therapist in cases such as **accidental falls** by the client that result in bodily injury. **Professional liability insurance** is similar, but instead of protecting the therapist from workplace accidents, it protects the therapist from lawsuits regarding **malpractice** or **negligence**. If a massage therapist knowingly performs a service or treatment they are not authorized, licensed, or certified to perform, this is known as malpractice. If a client tells a therapist not to work on a specific part of the body(say, the feet), and the therapist forgets and works on that area, and injury results, this is considered negligence.

SOAP Notes

SOAP notes are the most common form of post-massage documentation. SOAP notes help a massage therapist **document** everything that happened or was said during a massage session. Documenting this information can be helpful in many different ways, from tailoring future massage treatments to protecting the therapist from any malpractice or negligence lawsuits that may arise.

The "**S**" of SOAP stands for "**Subjective**". Under this section of SOAP notes, a massage therapist documents anything the client details about themselves. This can include where they experience pain, their job or hobbies, etc.

The "**O**" of SOAP stands for "**Objective**" or "**Observation**". Under this section of SOAP notes, a massage therapist documents the type of massage or techniques being performed(objective), and anything about the client the therapist can physically see(observe). This can include bruising, inflammation, visual assessments, and gait analysis.

The "**A**" of SOAP stands for "**Assessment**". Under this section of SOAP notes, a massage therapist documents any changes in the client as a result of the massage treatment. An example could be "Pre-massage, right shoulder elevated. Post-massage, right shoulder less elevated".

The "**P**" of SOAP stands for "**Plan**". Under this section of SOAP notes, a massage therapist documents any recommendations for future treatments, or exercises suggested for the client between sessions(such as increase stretching in a specific muscle or area, or increase water intake).

Client files, including intake forms, SOAP notes, and receipts, should be kept by the massage therapist for a minimum of **six** years, per the IRS. This allows for audits to take place by the IRS. Having all documentation stored can help prevent any possible penalties issued by the IRS.

Ethics

Ethics are **guiding moral principles**. These guiding moral principles are used to direct a massage therapist in proper course of action in ethical dilemmas. There are many different ethical dilemmas that may arise in the practice of massage therapy. Examples include becoming sexually attracted to a client(refer the client to another therapist) and attempting to sell products or merchandise to a client outside the scope of massage(don't do it).

Scope of practice is performing treatments and techniques you are **qualified to perform**. Working outside of the scope of practice can lead to malpractice lawsuits. Examples of working outside of the scope of practice include performing treatments such as acupuncture or chiropractic work without proper licensing. Stay within your scope of practice at all times!

Boundaries, as discussed earlier, are **limitations** that can be set by the massage therapist and the client. They can be verbally set, such as a client asking a massage therapist to avoid working on a specific part of the body, or non-verbal, such as a client leaving an article of clothing on, which typically means they might not want to have that part of the body worked on. The best way to identify boundaries is to communicate with the client. Ask questions, reinforce the boundaries you or the client have set.

Confidentiality, quite simply, is keeping client information **private and protected**. Client information includes anything that happens or is said during a massage session, client files, intake forms, SOAP notes, and even something as simple as names. This information needs to be kept private. Releasing this information is a violation of HIPAA.

HIPAA(Health Insurance Portability and Accountability Act of 1996) was created by the US Department of Health and Human Services. Inside HIPAA lies the **Privacy Rule**, which is used to **protect** all individually identifiable health information. The Privacy Rule ensures client/patient information is kept private. It does, however, allow this information to be transferred between health care providers when necessary, which allows high-quality health care. Assessments and diagnoses do not need to be re-done, as the information is already present.

Communication

Communication, as we've discussed, is extremely important in the client/therapist relationship. One of the main ways we communicate with clients is by asking questions.

An **open-ended question** is a question used when asking for **feedback** from clients. Often, open-ended questions are meant to extract more detail, more information. It allows the answer to be more open and abstract.

A **close-ended question** is a question used when asking for a **yes-or-no response** only. These questions are used to extract important pieces of information in a short amount of time. During the pre-massage interview, when time is a factor, close-ended questions are primarily used to gather the important information without sacrificing too much time.

Transference and counter-transference occur when one person in the therapeutic relationship begins viewing the other as more than just their client or therapist. **Transference** is when the **client** begins viewing the massage therapist **similarly to a person** in their own personal life. They develop an emotional attachment to the massage therapist. **Counter-transference** is the opposite: a **massage therapist** develops an **emotional attachment** to a client. If either of these occur, it's best to refer the client to another massage therapist, separating the massage therapist from any possible ethical dilemmas.

Self disclosure is when the **client** shares information about **themselves** during a massage session. This information, which may be documented if relevant, needs to be kept confidential.

Psychology

A massage may leave a client in a psychologically vulnerable place, and they may exhibit defense mechanisms to help cope with their internal struggles.

Denial, a common defense mechanism, is a **refusal** to acknowledge a given situation, or acting as if something didn't happen.

Displacement is often negative. Displacement is satisfying an impulse by **substitution**. An example could be, you have a very bad day at work or school, you go home, and instead of being upset at school or work, you lash out at a significant other. Releasing your pent-up emotions at something other than what is causing the emotions.

Projection is placing one's own internal feelings onto **someone else**. An example could be my wife: when she gets hungry, she becomes easily agitated She'll then accuse me of being in a bad mood, even though I'm feeling great. This is projection. For the record, this happens a lot.

Regression is taking a **step back** psychologically when faced with stress. An example could be quitting smoking. A person doesn't smoke for a few days, and then they are presented with a stressful situation, which causes them to regress and smoke again.

Repression is subconsciously **blocking out** unwanted emotions. Not even knowing you have something to be upset about. Your mind can erase certain memories to help protect you from stress.

Types of Employment

There are many different types of employment you may encounter as a massage therapist. These are among the most common.

An **independent contractor** is a massage therapist that works independently, for themselves, but **contracts** with another person or company to perform work. Independent contractors are not beholden to the same limitations as employees, however. Independent contractors may work whatever schedule they want, charge their own prices, wear their own uniform. Independent contractors do not receive benefits from an employer, however.

Sole proprietors are often categorized similarly to independent contractors. Sole proprietorships are businesses owned by **one person**. Sole proprietors may differ from independent contractors in licensing requirements.

A **partnership** is a business owned by **two or more** people. Ownership may be split differently depending on variables such as money entering into a business relationship, assets, etc.

S Corporations are corporations that pass income and taxes onto the **shareholders**. This requires the shareholders to shoulder the responsibility of reporting income and taxes to the IRS.

Tax Forms

Along with different types of employment, there are many different types of tax forms required to be filed, depending on the type of employment.

A **1099** is issued to an **independent contractor** by the company they contract with. This statement details the amount of income accrued by the independent contractor through the year.

A **Schedule C** is filed to the IRS by **sole proprietors**, detailing the amount of money the business made during the previous year.

A **Schedule K-1** is a form filed by individual **partnership members**. It is similar to a W-2, detailing the amount of money each partnership member made during the previous year.

Profit and Loss(income and expense) statements are forms filed by businesses that show how much money was made(**profit**) and how much money was expended(**loss**) during the year.

Gift taxes may be used as deductions on taxes. If a business buys a gift for a customer, no more than **$25** may be claimed as a deduction for that specific client. Other gifts for different clients may also be reported, but each gift reported cannot exceed $25.

Massage Therapy Matching

_____: Limitations set by the client or massage therapist

_____: Author of "The Art of Massage"

_____: Stoppage of range-of-motion due to tight muscles

_____: Guiding moral principles.

_____: Stance with feet placed perpendicular to the table

_____: Area of the body that warrants extra caution while massaging

_____: Gliding strokes directed towards the heart

_____: Modern Chinese massage

_____: Massage therapist moving a joint without assistance from the client

_____: Protects a massage therapist from malpractice lawsuits

_____: Developed Lymphatic Drainage

_____: Kneading strokes

_____: Stance with feet placed parallel to the table

_____: Jurisdictional requirement used to regulate the practice of massage therapy

_____: Client moving a joint without assistance from the massage therapist

_____: Stoppage of range-of-motion due to bone

_____: Massage involving stretching performed on a mat on the floor

_____: Developed Therapeutic Touch

_____: Author of "De Medicina"

_____: Credential obtained by completing a course in a school setting

A: Tuina

B: Celsus

C: Thai Massage

D: Effleurage

E: Ethics

F: Dolores Krieger

G: Emil Vodder

H: John Harvey Kellogg

I: Petrissage

J: Professional Liability Insurance

K: Boundaries

L: Endangerment Site

M: Soft End Feel

N: Active Joint Movement

O: Bow Stance

P: Certification

Q: Passive Joint Movement

R: Horse Stance

S: Hard End Feel

T: License

Massage Therapy

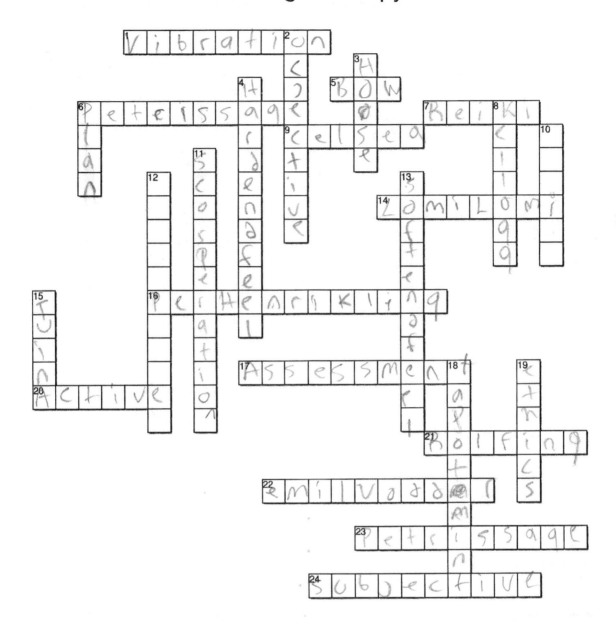

Across

1. Shaking or trembling movements
5. Stance in which one foot is placed in front of another, feet parallel to the table
6. Kneading massage strokes
7. Modality working with universal energy
9. Wrote De Medicina
14. Hawaiian massage technique
16. Developed Medical Gymnastics
17. Changes in the client due to a massage session, SOAP notes
20. Client performing a movement without help from the Massage Therapist
21. Structural realignment therapy
22. Developed Lymphatic Drainage
23. Long, gliding massage stroke directed towards the heart
24. Information the client shares about themselves, SOAP notes

Down

2. Any measurable information the Massage Therapist can see, SOAP notes
3. Stance in which the feet are placed perpendicular to the table
4. Stoppage of range-of-motion due to bones
6. Recommendations for future treatments, SOAP notes
8. Wrote The Art of Massage, which deals with physiology
10. Father of Orthopedic medicine, developed deep transverse friction
11. Business that passes income and taxes to its shareholders
12. Developed chair massage
13. Stoppage of range-of-motion due to tight muscles
15. Modern Chinese massage
18. Percussion strokes
19. Guiding moral principles

Massage Therapy Fill-In-The-Blank

History of Massage

In China, massage has been practiced as early as _3000_. First Chinese technique was known as _Amma_. Modern Chinese massage is known as _Tuina_.

Massage from China entered Japan and was renamed _Tusbo_, which increases the flow of _fluid_ and _Ki_.

A book was written in India called The _Ayurveda_, focusing on medicine, massage, and other holistic means of well-being.

People of Importance

Celsus, a Roman physicist, wrote a series of books known as _De mediana_.

Per Henrik Ling, a Swedish physiologist, developed _Medical_ Gymnastics. He is considered the father of _physical_ therapy and _Massage_ therapy.

Charles Taylor introduced _Medial_ Gymnastics to the United States, where it evolved into _Swedish_ Massage.

Johann Mezger developed _4 movements_ for the massage strokes, based in French.

Emil Vodder, along with his wife Estrid, developed _Lymphacic_.

John Harvey Kellogg wrote the book The _Art of massage_, which details the _psycological_ effects of massage therapy.

Dolores Krieger developed _Theraputic touch_, an energy-based modality similar to Reiki.

James Cyriax, considered the father of _orthic_ medicine, developed a technique known as _Deep_ transverse friction to help promote healthy scar tissue formation.

Massage Technique

Effleurage consists of _gliding_ strokes directed towards the _heart_.

Petrissage consists of _kneading_ strokes.

Friction consists of strokes that move _across_ tissue.

Tapotement consists of _tapping_ strokes such as hacking and cupping.

Vibration is performed by _shaking_ a part of the body.

Nerve strokes are extremely light forms of _effleurage_.

Joint Movements

An active joint movement is performed by the _client_ without _help_ from the massage therapist.

An active assistive joint movement is performed by the _client_ with _help_ from the massage therapist.

A passive joint movement is performed by the _therapist_ without _help_ from the client.

A resistive joint movement is performed by the _therapist_ and _client_ moving the body part in opposite directions, creating an _muscle_ contraction.

Stretching

To perform a stretch, a muscle must be _pulled_.

An unassisted stretch is performed by the _client_, without assistance from the _therapist_.

An assisted stretch is performed by the _therapist_, with assistance from the _client_.

Proprioceptive Neuromuscular Facilitation is a stretch involving moving the body part into resistance, then having the client _repeat_ the action, which performs an _isometric_ contraction. The client then relaxes, and the stretch is moved further.

An end feel is what causes a joint movement or stretch to stop moving.

A soft end feel is the result of _muscle_ tissues pulling back on the part of the body being stretched, preventing further movement.

A hard end feel is the result of _Bone_ tissues preventing a joint from moving further.

An empty end feel is caused by _Trama_ to a joint, limiting range-of-motion.

Assessment

An assessment is a preliminary _evulation_ of the client.

Precautions

An endangerment site is an area of the body that needs to be treated with extra _caution_ while being massaged.

A local contraindication is an area of the body that must be _skipped_ when performing a massage, but allows the rest of the body to be massaged.

An absolute contraindication _No massage_ the use of massage in any way.

Draping

Draping is the use of _linen_ to keep a client covered during a massage. Draping helps establish _boundaries_ between the therapist and client.

Top cover draping is using a linen to _cover_ the client during the massage.

Bolsters

When a client is placed into a supine position, a bolster should be placed under the _knees_.

When a client is placed into a prone position, a bolster should be placed under the _ankles_.

When a client is placed into a side-lying position, a bolster should be placed between the _knees_, and under the _arm_ and _head_.

When a client is placed into a semi-reclined position, a bolster should be placed under the _knees_ and behind the _head_.

Body Mechanics

Body mechanics are important to prevent _injury_ to the massage therapist, and to provide a _balanced_ massage for the client.

The archer/bow stance is used while performing effleurage, and requires the feet to be placed _parrell_ to the massage table.

The horse/warrior stance is used while performing short powerful strokes like petrissage or friction, and requires the feet to be placed _towards_ to the massage table.

Massage Modalities

Aromatherapy is any treatment that utilizes _ess oil_, which affects the brain's _nervous_ system.

Craniosacral Therapy, developed by John Upledger, releases blockages in the flow of cerebrospinal fluid from the _cranial_ to the _sacrum_.

Deep Tissue is performed by working the _deep_ layers of tissue in the body.

Hot Stone massage is a treatment that utilizes _hot_ stones, that may be _placed_ on the body or physically massage the client.

Hydrotherapy is the use of _water_ in any treatment. Contrasts baths utilize both _cold_ baths and _hot_ baths, and should always end with cold to reduce inflammation. A Vichy shower is a piece of equipment with seven shower heads, placed over a _massage_ table.

Lomi Lomi is a _hawiian_ massage, similar to Swedish, with large gliding movements that work the entire body with minimal draping.

Lymphatic Drainage, developed by _emil vodder_, increases the circulation of _fluid_.

Myofascial Release treats restrictions in the _muscles_ and _fasia_, utilizing light strokes.

Pregnancy massage is massage for pregnant clients. Client may need to be placed in semi-reclined position to take pressure off the _____ aorta, which may cause _____.

Reflexology is used to treat _trigger_ points on the hands, feet, and ears that correspond to other tissues in the body, such as _organs_.

Reiki is a form of _energy_ work, typically performed by the therapist holding their hands _above_ the client.

Rolfing, developed by Ida Rolf, is known as a _structure realignment_ technique, working on the fascia of the body to bring the body back to a vertical axis.

Sports massage is a massage designed for _athletes_. Pre-event sports massage should be invigorating, while post-event sports massage should be relaxing, focusing on releasing metabolic waste from tissues.

Swedish massage, the most common massage technique in western massage, is primarily focused on _relaxation_.

Thai massage, originating in Thailand, is a technique mainly focused on _stretching_ the client, on a mat, on the floor, with the client wearing loose-fitting clothing.

Tuina, which is _modern_ Chinese massage, focuses on balancing the eight principles of Chinese medicine.

Business

A certification is a credential obtained by completing a certificate program, usually in a __School__ setting.

A license is a jurisdictional requirement, used to __regulate__ the practice of massage therapy.

Reciprocity refers to the ability for a massage license in one jurisdiction to be recognized as __therapist__ in another jurisdiction.

Liability Insurance

General Liability Insurance protects the massage therapist in cases such as __malpractice__ by the client that result in bodily injury.

Professional Liability Insurance protects the massage therapist in cases such as __lawsuits__ or __malpractica__.

SOAP Notes

The "S" in SOAP stands for __Subjective__. Under this section, the massage therapist should document anything the __client__ details about themselves during a massage session.

The "O" in SOAP stands for __objective__ or __observation__. Under this section, the massage therapist should document anything the massage therapist can __see__, and the type of __technic__ being performed.

The "A" in SOAP stands for __Assessment__. Under this section, the massage therapist should document any __changes__ seen in the client after the massage session.

The "P" in SOAP stands for __Plan__. Under this section, the massage therapist should document any __plans__ for future treatments, or __health__ suggested to the client between sessions.

Client files should be kept and maintained by the massage therapist for __6__ years, per the IRS.

Ethics

Ethics are guiding __moral__ principles, used to direct a massage therapist in proper course of action in __ethical__ dilemmas.

Scope of practice is performing treatments and techniques you are __trained__ to perform.

Boundaries are __limitation__ set by the client or massage therapist.

Confidentiality is keeping client information __safe__ and __private__.

HIPAA(Health Insurance Portability and Accountability Act of 1996) was created by the US Department of Health and Human Services. The Privacy Rule is used to __protect__ all individually identifiable health information.

Communication

An open-ended question is a question used when asking for __information__ from clients.

A close-ended question is a question used when asking for a __yes/no__ response only.

Transference is when the __client__ views a __therapist__ similarly to a person in their early life.

Counter-transference is when the __therapist__ develops an emotional attachment to the __client__.

Psychology

Denial is a __refusal__ to acknowledge a given situation.

Displacement is satisfying an impulse by __substitution__, often negatively.

Projection is placing one's own internal feelings onto __a spouse__.

Regression is taking a __step back__ psychologically when faced with stress.

Repression is subconsciously __forgetting__ unwanted emotions.

Types of Employment

An independent contractor is a person who works independently, but __sub contract__ with another person or company to perform work.

Sole proprietorships are businesses owned by __one__ person.

A partnership is a business owned by __2__ or more people.

S Corporations are corporations that pass income and taxes onto the __spouses__.

Tax Forms

A 1099 is issued to an __independent contractor__ by the company they contract with.

A Schedule C is filed to the IRS by
Sole propietor.

A Schedule K-1 is a form filed by individual
partnyship members.

Profit and Loss statements detail _profit_
and _los_ for a business.

Gift taxes may be used as deductions on taxes.
No more than _25_ may be deducted per
client per year.

Massage Therapy Matching

K   G
H   I
M   O
E   T
R   N
L   S
D   C
A   F
Q   B
J   P

Massage Therapy Answers

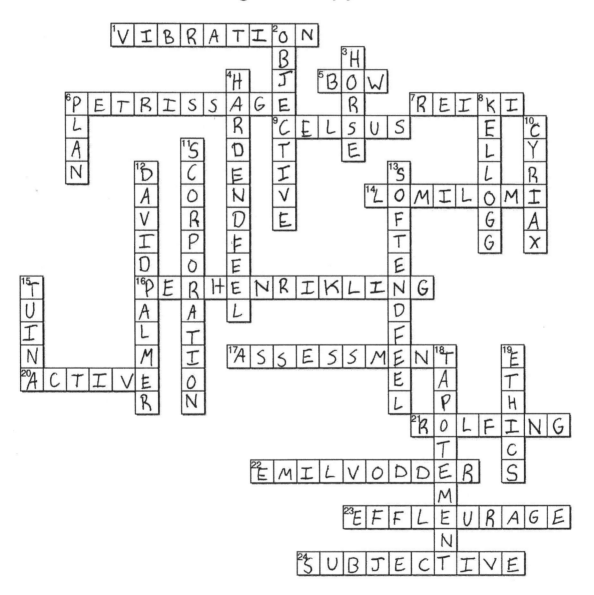

Massage Therapy Practice Exam

1. Essential oil commonly used to aid in treatment of insomnia and chronic fatigue syndrome
A. Eucalyptus
B. Sweet orange
C. Lavender
D. Rosemary

2. A massage table that is able to be folded and transported easily from one location to another
A. Hydraulic
B. Adjustable
C. Pressurized
D. Portable

3. Counter-transference
A. The client viewing a massage therapist as a significant person in their early life
B. The massage therapist bringing their own unresolved issues into the therapeutic relationship
C. Keeping a client's information private and protected
D. Relocating from one office to another

4. A client performing an action with the help of the massage therapist is an example of which joint movement
A. Active
B. Resistive
C. Passive
D. Assistive

5. Stoppage of a range of motion due to muscle and other soft tissues
A. Soft end feel
B. Hard end feel
C. Empty end feel
D. Nervous end feel

6. Gentle rhythmic massage designed to increase lymph circulation, developed by Emil Vodder
A. Lymphatic drainage
B. Swedish massage
C. Sports massage
D. Orthobionomy

7. Lomi Lomi, Craniosacral Therapy, and Rolfing are all forms of
A. Energy techniques
B. Movement techniques
C. Manipulative techniques
D. Kinesiology techniques

8. A massage room should contain all of the following except
A. A music source
B. A bathroom
C. Subdued lighting
D. Comfortable temperature

9. Stance in which the feet run perpendicular to the massage table
A. Bow
B. Archer
C. Horse
D. Swimmer

10. Petrissage
A. Light gliding strokes towards the heart, used to increase circulation and apply lubricant
B. Strokes that move across tissue, used to break up adhesions
C. Kneading strokes, used to release adhesions and increase circulation
D. Percussion strokes, used to stimulate muscle spindle cells

11. Universal precautions should be followed with
A. Clients with allergies
B. Only clients with contagious conditions
C. Every client
D. Clients with no previous medical conditions

12. Questions asked in a pre-massage interview should be
A. Forced
B. Open-ended
C. Abrupt
D. Closed-ended

13. The "A" of "SOAP" stands for
A. Alleviate
B. Assessment
C. Arrangement
D. Alignment

14. A sole proprietorship is a business that has how many owners
A. More than ten
B. Two
C. Four
D. One

15 The most common substance used in body scrubs
A. Salt
B. Sugar
C. Ground coffee
D. Powdered milk

16. A certification is obtained via
A. Passing a jurisprudence exam
B. Paying a fee to a jurisdiction licensing agency
C. Obtaining liability insurance to protect against malpractice
D. Completing educational requirements in a school setting

17. Structural realignment therapy working on muscles and fascia over the course of ten sessions
A. Rolfing
B. Trager method
C. Feldenkrais
D. Myofascial release

18. Massage results in increased production of
A. Cortisol
B. Blood cells
C. Pathogens
D. Water retention

19. Information the client shares about themselves is documented under which section of SOAP notes
A. Objective
B. Subjective
C. Assessment
D. Plan

20. Percussion strokes, used to loosen phlegm in the respiratory tract and activate muscle spindle cells
A. Petrissage
B. Effleurage
C. Friction
D. Tapotement

21. Massage may have all of the following psychological effects except
A. Increased relaxation
B. Decreased stress
C. Increased stress
D. Increased energy

22. After a massage, the massage therapist notifies the client of stretches that the therapist thinks might help with a client's range-of-motion. This information would be documented under which section of SOAP notes
A. Subjective
B. Objective
C. Assessment
D. Plan

23. The primary goal of a massage performed after a sporting event is
A. Move metabolic waste out of tissues
B. Increase circulation
C. Stimulate muscle fibers
D. Break up adhesions between tissues

24. Technique used to treat adhesions found between fascia and muscles
A. Rolfing
B. Myofascial release
C. Deep tissue
D. Osteosymmetry

25. Celsus wrote the following book, which details the importance of massage, bathing, and exercise
A. The Ayur-Veda
B. De Medicina
C. The San-Tsai-Tou-Hoei
D. The Cong Fou

26. Business expenses include all of the following except
A. Massages
B. Advertising
C. Electricity
D. Credit card fees

27. Slightly bent knees, straight back, and limp wrists are all examples of
A. Proper massage modalities
B. Improper body mechanics
C. Proper body mechanics
D. Improper massage modalities

28. If a client is unable to withstand any amount of pressure during a massage, a treatment the therapist might recommend would be
A. Reiki
B. Rolfing
C. Myofascial release
D. Lymphatic drainage

29. A massage license from one jurisdiction being recognized as valid in another jurisdiction
A. Reciprocity
B. Certification
C. Liability
D. Malpractice

30. A bolster is placed between the legs and arms and under the head in which position
A. Slightly elevated
B. Supine
C. Prone
D. Side-lying

31. Swedish massage is based on the Western principals of
A. Anatomy and physiology
B. Energy
C. Life force
D. Chi

32. Stretch technique in which a muscle is stretched to resistance, followed by an isometric contraction by the client, then the muscle stretched further after the contraction
A. Active static stretch
B. Proprioceptive neuromuscular facilitation
C. Strain counter-strain
D. Myofascial release

33. A set of guiding moral principles is known as
A. Regulations
B. Scope of practice
C. Ethics
D. Reputation

34. If a Massage Therapist begins to feel sexual attraction towards a client, what should the Massage Therapist do
A. Act upon these urges
B. Do nothing
C. Tell the client
D. Recommend the client see another therapist

35. Goals are
A. Measurable or attainable accomplishments
B. A generalized statement about the purpose of a business
C. The theme of a business
D. Business plans detailing projected income

36. Technique primarily used to work on trigger points
A. Wringing
B. Ischemic compression
C. Cross-fiber friction
D. Myofascial release

37. Areas of the body in which caution is advised during massage of a pregnant client include all of the following except
A. Face
B. Abdomen
C. Ankles
D. Lumbar

38. Massage stroke directed toward the heart used to increase circulation, transition between strokes, and apply massage lubricant
A. Friction
B. Petrissage
C. Effleurage
D. Vibration

39. A pre-event sports massage requires the following kinds of strokes to be performed
A. Relaxing
B. Invigorating
C. Slow
D. Sedative

40. An aura stroke is a massage stroke in which
A. The hands are pressed firmly into the body
B. The hands are touching the body very lightly
C. The hands are held just above the body
D. The hands are placed on the body without substantial pressure

41. A resistive joint movement
A. Client moves the joint without the assistance of a massage therapist
B. A client moves the joint with the assistance of a massage therapist
C. A client resists a movement being performed by a massage therapist
D. A massage therapist moves a client's joint without the help of the client

42. Essential oil commonly used to aid in relaxation of smooth muscles in the respiratory tract
A. Eucalyptus
B. Lavender
C. Lemongrass
D. Peppermint

43. Protection from malpractice lawsuits is gained by obtaining
A. Limited Liability Corporation
B. Massage certification
C. Licensure
D. Professional liability insurance

44. With a client lying supine, a bolster should be placed
A. Between the legs and arms, and under the head
B. Under the ankles and neck
C. Under the knees
D. Under the head only

45. Ability to perform services legally according to occupational standards and licensing
A. Certification
B. Scope of practice
C. Reciprocity
D. Regulations

46. Gait analysis is observation and interpretation of a person's
A. Walking pattern
B. Somatic holding pattern
C. Sitting pattern
D. Range of motion

47. Which of the following massage strokes is best in aiding lung decongestion
A. Tapotement
B. Effleurage
C. Friction
D. Petrissage

48. A client demonstrating range of motion is an example of which joint movement
A. Active
B. Assistive
C. Passive
D. Resistive

49. Johann Mezger was responsible for
A. Popularizing the word "massage" in America
B. Developing Swedish Gymnastics
C. Introducing Swedish massage to the US
D. Developing the terms for the massage strokes, based in French

50. A Massage Therapist solicits a product to a client not related to a massage session or treatment. This could be a violation of
A. Ethics
B. Scope of Practice
C. Licensure
D. Reciprocity

Massage Therapy Practice Exam Answer Key

01. C		26. A	
02. D		27. C	
03. B		28. A	
04. D		29. A	
05. A		30. D	
06. A		31. A	
07. C		32. B	
08. B		33. C	
09. C		34. D	
10. C		35. A	
11. C		36. B	
12. D		37. A	
13. B		38. C	
14. D		39. B	
15. A		40. C	
16. D		41. C	
17. A		42. A	
18. B		43. D	
19. B		44. C	
20. D		45. B	
21. C		46. A	
22. D		47. A	
23. A		48. A	
24. B		49. D	
25. B		50. A	

For detailed answer explanations, watch the
video at mblextestprep.com/resources.html

Medical Terminology

Medical Terminology can be divided into three primary components: Word Roots, Prefixes, and Suffixes.

The Word Root of a medical term is the primary structure involved. It gives us a starting point when breaking down a word. An example is the Word Root "hepat/o", which means "liver".

A Prefix is used to modify a Word Root. An example is "a-", which means "without". A pathology that uses "a-" is "arrhythmia", which means "without rhythm".

A Suffix is used to add description to, or alter, a Word Root. An example is "-itis", which means "inflammation". A pathology that uses "-itis" is "hepatitis". As stated before, the word root "hepat/o" means liver. If we attach "-itis", it becomes "inflammation of the liver".

Many medical terms, prefixes, suffixes, and word roots, have the same meaning. The reason for different terms having the same meaning can be traced back to the origin languages. Modern medical terminology originated in both Latin and Greek, with the majority of words being Greek. When people like Celsus, a Roman physician, began creating medical terminology, they often used Greek terms, but conformed them to be Latin in origin. This is the reason for many terms sharing the same definition.

Medical Terminology

Cardiovascular Word Roots

angi/o:	vessel
aort/o:	aorta
arteriol/o:	arteriole
arteri/o:	artery
ather/o:	fatty plaque
atri/o:	atrium
bas/o:	alkaline
cardi/o:	heart
chrom/o:	color
eosin/o:	rose colored
granul/o:	granule
hemangi/o:	blood vessel
hem/o:	blood
kary/o:	nucleus
leuk/o:	white
nucle/o:	nucleus
lymph/o:	lymph
morph/o:	form
myel/o:	canal
phag/o:	eat
phleb/o:	vein
poikil/o:	irregular
reticul/o:	mesh
scler/o:	hard
sider/o:	iron
sphygm/o:	pulse
thromb/o:	clot
vascul/o:	vessel
ven/o:	vein
ventricul/o:	ventricle

Digestive Word Roots

append/o:	appendix
appendic/o:	appendix
bucc/o:	cheek
cheil/o:	lip
chol/e:	bile
cholangi/o:	bile vessel
cholecyst/o:	gallbladder
choledoch/o:	bile duct
col/o:	large intestine
colon/o:	large intestine
dont/o:	teeth
duoden/o:	duodenum
enter/o:	small intestine
esophag/o:	esophagus
gastr/o:	stomach
gingiv/o:	gums
gloss/o:	tongue
hepat/o:	liver
ile/o:	ileum
jejun/o:	jejunum
labi/o:	lip
lingu/o:	tongue
odont/o:	teeth
or/o:	mouth
pancreat/o:	pancreas
pharyng/o:	pharynx
proct/o:	anus
pylor/o:	pylorus
rect/o:	rectum

sial/o:	saliva
sigmoid/o:	sigmoid colon
stomat/o:	mouth

Endocrine Word Roots

aden/o:	gland
adren/o:	adrenal glands
adrenal/o:	adreanl glands
calc/o:	calcium
gluc/o:	sugar
glyc/o:	sugar
gonad/o:	gonads
home/o:	same
kal/i:	potassium
pancreat/o:	pancreas
thym/o:	thymus gland
thyr/o:	thyroid
thyroid/o:	thyroid
toxic/o:	poison
thalam/o:	thalamus

Integumentary Word Roots

adip/o:	fat
albin/o:	white
carcin/o:	cancer
cirrh/o:	yellow
cutane/o:	skin
cyan/o:	blue
derm/o:	skin
dermat/o:	skin
erythem/o:	red
erythemat/o:	red
erythr/o:	red
hidr/o:	sweat
histi/o:	tissue
hist/o:	tissue
ichthy/o:	scaly
jaund/o:	yellow
kerat/o:	hard
leuk/o:	white
lip/o:	fat
melan/o:	black
myc/o:	fungi
onych/o:	nail
pil/o:	hair
scler/o:	hard
seb/o:	sebum
squam/o:	scale
sudor/o:	sweat
trich/o:	hair
ungu/o:	nail
xanth/o:	yellow
xer/o:	dry

Lymphatic Word Roots

aden/o:	gland
adenoid/o:	adenoids
immun/o:	immune
leuk/o:	white
lymph/o:	lymph
lymphaden/o:	lymph gland

lymphangi/o:	lymph vessel
myel/o:	canal
phag/o:	eat
splen/o:	spleen
tonsill/o:	tonsils
thym/o:	thymus

Muscular Word Roots

adhes/o:	stick to
aponeur/o:	aponeurosis
duct/o:	carry
erg/o:	work
fasci/o:	fascia
fibr/o:	fiber
fibros/o:	fiber
flex/o:	bend
is/o:	same
kinesi/o:	movement
lei/o:	smooth
lev/o:	lift
levat/o:	lift
metr/o:	length
quadr/i:	four
quadr/o:	four
rect/o:	straight
rhabd/o:	rod-shaped
ten/o:	tendon
tend/o:	tendon
tendin/o:	tendon
tens/o:	strain
ton/o:	tension
tort/i:	twisted

Nervous Word Roots

astr/o:	star
ax/o:	axon
cephal/o:	head
cerebell/o:	cerebellum
clon/o:	clonus
cortic/o:	cortex
crani/o:	skull
dendr/o:	tree
dur/o:	dura mater
encephal/o:	brain
esthesi/o:	sensation
gangli/o:	ganglion
gli/o:	glue
kinesi/o:	movement
lex/o:	word
lob/o:	lobe
medull/o:	medulla
mening/o:	meninges
ment/o:	mind
mot/o:	move
myel/o:	canal
narc/o:	stupor
neur/o:	nerve
olig/o:	few
phas/o:	speech
phren/o:	mind
psych/o:	mind
spin/o:	spine

synapt/o:	point of contact
tax/o:	order
thalam/o:	thalamus
thec/o:	sheath

Reproductive Word Roots

amni/o:	amnion
andr/o:	male
cervic/o:	neck
colp/o:	vagina
vagin/o:	vagina
embry/o:	embryo
epididym/o:	epididymis
episi/o:	vulva
fet/o:	fetus
galact/o:	milk
genti/o:	genitalia
gynec/o:	woman
hyster/o:	uterus
hymen/o:	hymen
lact/o:	milk
leiomy/o:	smooth muscle
mamm/o:	breast
mast/o:	breast
men/o:	menstruation
metr/o:	uterus
nat/o:	birth
o/o:	egg
oophor/o:	ovary
orch/o:	testicle
ovari/o:	ovary
pen/o:	penis
perine/o:	perineum
prostat/o:	prostate
salping/o:	fallopian tube
sperm/o:	sperm
spermat/o:	sperm
test/o:	testicle
uter/o:	uterus
vagin/o:	vagina
vas/o:	vessel
vesicul/o:	seminal vesicle
vulv/o:	vulva

Respiratory Word Roots

alveol/o:	alveolus
anthrac/o:	black
atel/o:	incomplete
bronch/o:	bronchus
bronchi/o:	bronchus
coni/o:	dust
cyan/o:	blue
embol/o:	plug
emphys/o:	inflate
epiglott/o:	epiglottis
hem/o:	blood
laryng/o:	larynx
lob/o:	lobe
muc/o:	mucous
nas/o:	nose
or/o:	mouth
orth/o:	straight
ox/o:	oxygen
pector/o:	chest
pharyng/o:	pharynx

phon/o:	sound
phren/o:	diaphragm
pleur/o:	pleura
pneum/o:	lung
pneumon/o:	lung
pulm/o:	lung
rhin/o:	nose
sinus/o:	sinus
spir/o:	breathe
steth/o:	chest
thorac/o:	chest
trache/o:	trachea

Skeletal Word Roots

acr/o:	extremity
acromi/o:	acromion
ankyl/o:	crooked
arthr/o:	joint
brachi/o:	arm
calcane/o:	calcaneus
carp/o:	carpals
cephal/o:	head
cervic/o:	neck
chondr/o:	cartilage
clavicul/o:	clavicle
cleid/o:	clavicle
condyl/o:	condyle
cost/o:	ribs
crani/o:	cranium
dactyl/o:	fingers/toes
femor/o:	femur
fibul/o:	fibula
humer/o:	humerus
ili/o:	ilium
ischi/o:	ischium
kyph/o:	hill
lamin/o:	lamina
lord/o:	curve
metacarp/o:	metacarpals
metatars/o:	metatarsals
myel/o:	canal
orth/o:	straight
oste/o:	bone
patell/o:	patella
ped/i:	foot
pelv/i:	pelvis
pelv/o:	pelvis
phalang/o:	phalanges
pod/o:	foot
pub/o:	pubis
rachi/o:	spine
radi/o:	radius
sacr/o:	sacrum
scapul/o:	scapula
scoli/o:	crooked
spondyl/o:	vertebrae
synov/o:	synovium
tal/o:	talus
tars/o:	tarsals
thorac/o:	chest
uln/o:	ulna
vertebr/o:	vertebrae

Urinary Word Roots

| albumin/o: | albumin |

azot/o:	nitrogenous
cyst/o:	bladder
glomerul/o:	glomerulus
kal/i:	potassium
ket/o:	ketone bodies
meat/o:	opening
nephr/o:	kidney
pyel/o:	renal pelvis
ren/o:	kidney
trigon/o:	trigone
ur/o:	urine
ureter/o:	ureter
urethr/o:	urethra
urin/o:	urine
vesic/o:	bladder

Oncology Word Roots

aden/o:	gland
blast/o:	germ cell
carcin/o:	cancer
cauter/o:	burn
chem/o:	chemical
cry/o:	cold
hist/o:	tissue
immun/o:	immunity
leiomy/o:	smooth muscle
leuk/o:	white
mut/a:	genetic change
myel/o:	canal
onc/o:	tumor
rhabdomy/o:	skeletal muscle
sarc/o:	connective tissue

Miscellaneous Word Roots

aur/i:	ear
bi/o:	life
burs/o:	bursa
cerat/o:	horn
chir/o:	hand
corac/o:	crow-like
coron/o:	crown
dextr/o:	right
dors/o:	back
dynam/o:	power
ect/o:	outside
faci/o:	face
glauc/o:	gray
hydr/o:	water
irid/o:	iris
kerat/o:	cornea
lacrim/o:	tear
lapar/o:	abdominal wall
myring/o:	eardrum
omphal/o:	navel
opthalam/o:	eye
phot/o:	light
py/o:	pus
pyr/o:	heat
therm/o:	heat
tympan/o:	eardrum
viscer/o:	internal organs
zo/o:	animal
zym/o:	fermentation

Prefixes

a-:	without	primi-:	first
ab-:	away	pro-:	before
ad-:	towards	pseudo-:	false
af-:	towards	quadri-:	four
allo-:	other	retro-:	behind
an-:	without	semi-:	half
ana-:	against	sub-:	under
aniso-:	unequal	super-:	above
ante-:	before	supra-:	above
anti-:	against	sym-:	together
auto-:	self	syn-:	together
bi-:	two	tachy-:	rapid
brady-:	slow	trans-:	through
cine-:	movement	tri-:	three
circum-:	around	ultra-:	excessive
contra-:	against	uni-:	one
de-:	cessation		
di-:	double		
dia-:	through		
dipl-:	double		
dys-:	difficult		
ec-:	out		
echo-:	repeated sound		
ecto-:	outside		
ef-:	away		
en-:	within		
end-:	within		
endo-:	within		
epi-:	above		
eso-:	inward		
eu-:	good		
ex-:	outside		
exo-:	outside		
extra-:	outside		
hemi-:	half		
hetero-:	different		
homo-:	same		
hyper-:	excessive		
hypo-:	below		
im-:	not		
in-:	in		
infra-:	below		
inter-:	between		
intra-:	inside		
iso-:	same		
macro-:	large		
mal-:	bad		
meso-:	middle		
meta-:	change		
micro-:	small		
mono-:	one		
multi-:	many		
neo-:	new		
nulli-:	none		
oxy-:	sharp		
pan-:	all		
para-:	beside		
per-:	through		
peri-:	around		
poly-:	many		
post-:	after		
pre-:	before		

Suffixes

-ac:	referring to	-ile:	referring to
-acusis:	hearing	-ine:	referring to
-al:	referring to	-ism:	condition
-algia:	pain	-ist:	specialist
-ar:	referring to	-itis:	inflammation
-ary:	referring to	-kinesia:	movement
-ate:	form of	-lalia:	speech
-ation:	process	-lampsia:	shine
-asthenia:	weakness	-lepsy:	seizure
-blast:	germ cell	-lith:	stone
-capnia:	carbon dioxide	-logist:	specializing in
-cele:	hernia	-logy:	study of
-centesis:	puncture	-lucent:	clear
-clasis:	break	-lysis:	dissolve
-clast:	break	-malacia:	soften
-crine:	secrete	-mania:	frenzy
-cusis:	hearing	-megaly:	enlargement
-cyte:	cell	-meter:	measuring tool
-desis:	binding	-metry:	measuring
-derma:	skin	-oid:	resembling
-duction:	bringing	-oma:	tumor
-dynia:	pain	-orexia:	appetite
-eal:	referring to	-ory:	referring to
-ectasis:	dilation	-ose:	referring to
-ectomy:	removal	-osis:	condition
-edema:	swelling	-ous:	referring to
-emesis:	vomiting	-paresis:	partial paralysis
-emia:	blood	-pathy:	disease
-esis:	condition	-penia:	deficiency
-esthesia:	sensation	-pexy:	fixation
-ferent:	to carry	-phasia:	speech
-gen:	produce	-philia:	attraction
-genesis:	produce	-phobia:	fear
-globin:	protein	-phoria:	feeling
-gnosis:	knowing	-phylaxis:	protection
-gram:	record	-physis:	growth
-graph:	recording	-plasia:	formation
-graphy:	recording	-plasm:	growth
-ia:	condition	-plasty:	repair
-iasis:	abnormal condition	-plegia:	paralysis
-iatry:	medicine	-pnea:	breathing
-ic:	referring to	-poiesis:	formation
-ical:	referring to	-porosis:	porous
-ician:	specialist	-rrhage:	bursting forth
-icle:	small	-rrhaphy:	suture
		-rrhea:	discharge
		-rrhexis:	rupture
		-scope:	examining
		-spasm:	twitch
		-scopy:	visual exam
		-stenosis:	narrowing
		-stomy:	opening
		-tension:	stretch
		-thorax:	chest
		-thymia:	emotion
		-tic:	referring to
		-tomy:	incision
		-toxic:	poison
		-tripsy:	crushing
		-trophy:	nourishment
		-uria:	urine
		-y:	condition

Anatomy and Physiology

Anatomy and Physiology is a large part of the MBLEx, with so many body systems and body parts that may be covered during the test.

In this section, we will discuss many subjects, covering a wide range of information.

Information covered in this section includes:

Homeostasis
Regional Anatomy
Body Planes
Body Regions
Tissue
The Cardiovascular System
The Digestive System
The Endocrine System
The Integumentary System
The Lymphatic System
The Muscular System
The Nervous System
The Respiratory System
The Skeletal System
The Urinary System

This information is followed by three assignments:

Anatomy and Physiology Matching
Anatomy and Physiology Crossword
Anatomy and Physiology Fill-In-The-Blank

The end of the section has a 50 question practice exam on Anatomy and Physiology. These questions ARE NOT the exact same questions will you see on the MBLEx. They are meant to test information that MAY be seen on the MBLEx.

While taking the practice exam, make sure to utilize your test-taking strategies(page 3) to optimize your test scores.

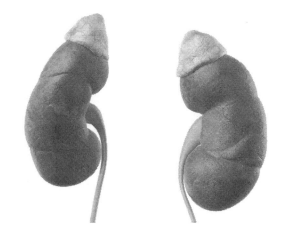

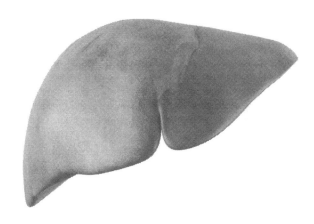

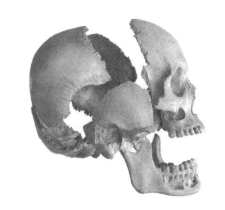

Anatomy and Physiology

Anatomy and Physiology, two extremely important aspects of the human body. **Anatomy**, simply put, is the study of the **structure** of the human body. All of the parts that make up the body constitute anatomy, from bones, muscles, and nerves, to cells, tendons, ligaments, and everything in between.

Physiology is the study of the **function** of the body. How do the parts of the body that make up the body's anatomy function? What do they do? This is physiology. Anatomy and Physiology go hand-in-hand.

Homeostasis

Homeostasis is the existence and maintenance of a **constant internal environment**. The body's internal environment is constantly changing and responding to various stimuli. Examples of stimuli are temperature, hormones, diet, and the body's pH level. These stimuli that change the body's internal environment in some way are known as **homeostatic variables**. As the variables change, so too does the internal environment.

How does the body respond to these changes? Using **homeostatic mechanisms**, such as sweating and shivering. An example, when your body temperature gets too high, your body mechanically(physically) responds by sweating. Sweat evaporates off the skin, which cools the body down, lowering body temperature. When the body becomes too cold, the body responds by mechanically increasing the amount of twitching in the skeletal muscles. This increased twitching, which is normally undetectable, results in shivering, which produces body heat, raising body temperature.

The body's internal environment is constantly changing, and the body constantly adjusts certain aspects of itself to respond to these changes. If temperature is an example, the **set point**(normal range) of a body's temperature is 98.6 degrees Fahrenheit. The internal body temperature is never set right at 98.6 degrees. It is constantly fluctuating around it, maintaining a normal range of optimal body function.

Regional Anatomy

Regional Anatomy is the study of the structures of the body, broken down into different parts. When describing the position of one structure in the body in relation to another structure or structures, we use **directional terms**. An example, using the term "medial condyle" instead of just "condyle" lets us communicate effectively which condyle is being discussed.

The main directional terms are:

- **Superior**: Above.
- **Inferior**: Below.
- **Anterior**: Front.
- **Posterior**: Back.
- **Proximal**: Closer to the midline.
- **Distal**: Further from the midline.
- **Medial**: Middle.
- **Lateral**: Side.
- **Deep**: More internal.
- **Superficial**: Towards the surface.

Body Planes

Body planes are important for viewing structures from different aspects. These can be used when doing simple visual assessment, or in instances such as surgery or cadaver dissection.

There are four main body planes: A **midsagittal**, or **median** plane, runs down the **midline** of the body, splitting the body into **equal left and right sides**. This is the only location for a midsagittal plane.

A **sagittal** plane also splits the body into left or right sides, but **not equally**. It can be located anywhere along the body except down the midline.

A **transverse**, or **horizontal** plane, splits the body into **superior and inferior** portions. It does not have to be at the waist. It can split the body into superior and inferior at any point along the body.

A **frontal**, or **coronal** plane, as the name suggests, splits the body into front and back, or **anterior and posterior**. If a person wanted to dissect the heart and make all four chambers visible, they would cut the heart into a frontal or coronal plane. See photo on page 36.

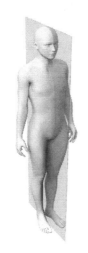

Midsagittal Plane

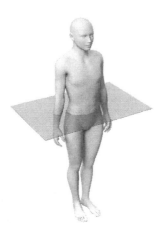

Transverse Plane

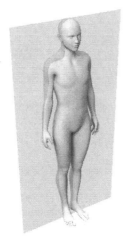

Frontal Plane

Body Regions

The body, as stated earlier, can be broken down into different parts, or regions. There are three main body regions: the **central** body region, the **upper limb**, and the **lower limb**.

The **central** body region contains all of the structures located in the center of the body: the **head**, the **neck**, and the **trunk**. Take away the arms and legs, and you're left with the central body region.

The **trunk** can be further divided into three regions: the **thorax**, or chest, the **abdomen**, and the **pelvis**. The thorax contains the heart, lungs, esophagus, thymus, and major blood vessels connecting to the heart. The abdomen contains the majority of our digestive organs, including the stomach, liver, gallbladder, pancreas, small intestine, and large intestine. It also contains the kidneys and ureters. The pelvis contains the urinary bladder, urethra, and reproductive organs.

The **upper limb** can be broken down into four regions: the **arm**, **forearm**, **wrist**, and **hand**. The arm contains the humerus. The forearm contains the radius and ulna. The wrist contains the carpals. The hand contains the metacarpals and phalanges.

The **lower limb** can also be broken down into four regions: the **thigh**, **leg**, **ankle**, and **foot**. The thigh contains the femur. The leg contains the tibia and fibula. The wrist contains the tarsals. The foot contains the metatarsals and phalanges.

Tissue

The body is constructed by smaller parts making bigger parts, until we have an organism. The organization of the body is: cells > tissues > organ > organ system > organism. A **tissue** is made of a group of **cells** with **similar function and structure**. When these cells, all formed roughly the same way, which perform the same action, come together, they form a tissue. There are **four** types of tissue in the human body: **epithelial**, **muscular**, **nervous**, and **connective**.

- **Epithelial** tissue forms most **glands**, the **digestive tract**, the **respiratory tract**, and the **epidermis**. Anywhere there is a mucous membrane, there is epithelium. Epithelial tissue is responsible for **protection**(the epidermis protects the body from pathogens and trauma), **secretion**(glands secrete substances, from hormones to mucous), and **absorption** of nutrients(the linings of the small intestine are made of epithelium, which allows nutrients to be absorbed into the blood stream). Epithelial tissue is also **avascular**, which means there is no direct blood supply to the tissue. This is what allows layers of the epidermis to be peeled

33

away without any bleeding.

- **Muscular** tissue creates **muscles**. There are three types of muscles: **skeletal** muscles, so named because they connect to the skeleton, **cardiac** muscles, which create the heart, and **smooth** muscles, which are abundant in several locations in the body.

    Skeletal muscle(also known as **striated** muscle) connects to the **skeleton**, and is under **voluntary** control. When skeletal muscle contracts, **movement** takes place at a joint. Skeletal muscle, as discussed in homeostasis, is responsible for creation of **heat**.

    Cardiac muscle(also known as **branching** muscle) is the muscle of the **heart**, and is responsible for **pumping blood** throughout the body. It is under **involuntary** control.

    Smooth muscle(also known as **non-striated** muscle) is found all over the body in places such as the **walls of hollow organs**(like the digestive and respiratory tracts), the **skin**, and the **eyes**. It is under **involuntary** control. In the digestive tract, it helps push food through the body by using **rhythmic** contractions, known as **peristalsis**.

- **Nervous** tissue forms the **brain**, **spinal cord**, and **nerves**. The primary cell of nervous tissue is known as a **neuron**. Neurons process nervous impulses, sending these impulses to other tissues, such as muscles, or between other neurons.

    Neurons receive **action potentials**(electric impulses), which are brought into the cell by **dendrites**, branch-like projections coming off the cell body of the neuron. Once the nucleus processes the information coming into the cell, it sends the impulse out of the cell to its destination by way of the **axon**, a long projection coming off the cell body. The axons terminate at other neurons, or help innervate muscles.

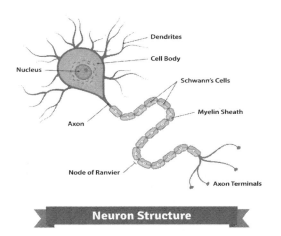

Neuron Structure

- **Connective** tissue is the most abundant form of tissue in the body. There are several different structures made by connective tissue, including **tendons**, **ligaments**, **fascia**, **bones**, **lymph**, **cartilage**, and **blood**. Connective tissue, as the name suggests, is responsible for **connecting** tissues. In addition to connecting tissues, it helps to **separate** tissues, as seen in serous membranes and cartilage.

Connective tissue contains two specific types of cells known as **blast** cells and **clast** cells. These cells play a very important role in the health of connective tissue. Blast cells are germ cells that are responsible for **building** connective tissue. Blast cells divide and build tissue until the structure is complete. Once the structure is complete, the blast cells mature, and stop dividing. Clast cells are responsible for **breaking down** tissue, which is very important in keeping the tissue healthy. If a person suffers a fracture, clast cells will enter the area and destroy the dead tissue, cleaning the area, which allows blast cells a clean surface to build new tissue on.

Blood is the most **abundant** form of connective tissue in the body. Blood is mainly a mode of **transportation** for blood cells, hormones, nutrients, and waste products. There are four parts of blood: **erythrocytes**, **leukocytes**, **thrombocytes**, and **plasma**.

Erythrocytes, also known as red blood cells, are responsible for **transporting oxygen** and **carbon dioxide** throughout the body. The cytoplasm of erythrocytes is made of a protein known as **hemoglobin**, which is primarily made of iron. Hemoglobin is what oxygen and carbon dioxide attach to. In the lungs, when the erythrocytes are exposed to the alveoli, carbon dioxide detaches from the erythrocytes, and oxygen then attaches in its place. This is how gas exchange occurs in erythrocytes.

Leukocytes, also known as white blood cells, are the body's primary **defense** against **pathogens**. There are several different types of leukocytes, ranging from T-cells to basophils. These cells eat pathogens(such as bacteria), dead cells, and debris floating in the blood stream.

Thrombocytes, also known as **platelets**, have one function: to **clot the blood**. This is vitally important when a person is bleeding. If the blood does not clot, the person could continue bleeding until they lose too much blood.

Plasma is the **fluid** portion of blood. The majority of blood, around 56%, is made of plasma. Plasma is what allows all of the blood cells, hormones, nutrients, and waste to move throughout the body. Without plasma, these substances would go nowhere!

Serous membranes are forms of connective

tissue that are used to **separate** organs from one another, preventing friction. They accomplish this by **surrounding** the organ or body cavity.

Inside the thorax, there are two serous membranes: the **pericardium**, which surrounds the **heart**, and the **pleural** membranes, which surround the **lungs**. These membranes help protect these organs from injury.

Inside the abdomen and pelvis, there is one serous membrane: the **peritoneum**. This membrane keeps the organs inside the abdomen and pelvis from being injured, and provides a pathway for many blood vessels, lymph vessels, and nerves to travel.

Inside of a serous membrane is a thick fluid, known as serous fluid. This fluid helps the membranes absorb shock. Holding the fluid in place are two walls. The inner wall, which comes into contact with the organs, is known as the **visceral serous membrane**. The outer wall, which comes into contact with other structures such as bones or other organs, is known as the **parietal serous membrane**.

➤ *Test It Out!: To get a visual of a serous membrane, find a balloon, and fill it about halfway with some sort of oil, tying it off. Gently push a finger into the balloon, so it wraps around your finger. The part of the balloon that is pressed up against your finger would be the visceral serous membrane. Inside the balloon is the serous fluid. The outside of the balloon would be the parietal serous membrane. NOTE: Do this over a sink, in case the balloon accidentally breaks!*

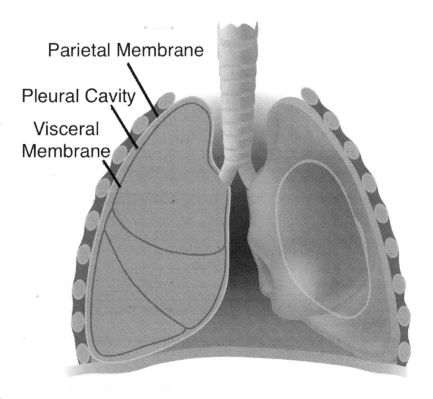

Serous Membrane

Cardiovascular System

- The Cardiovascular System is one of the most important organ systems in the body, responsible for **transportation** of nutrients such as oxygen and hormones to tissues. It also allows for waste to be moved to areas of the body where it can be eliminated, such as the lungs, liver, and kidneys. Wastes include carbon dioxide and urea.

The primary organ of the Cardiovascular System is the **heart**. The heart, a large, powerful muscle, has one function: to **pump blood** throughout the body.

- When blood first enters the heart, it is deoxygenated, and enters into the **right atrium**. It then passes through the **tricuspid valve**(which separates the right atrium from the right ventricle), into the **right ventricle**. The cardiac muscle in the right ventricle contracts, and it sends the deoxygenated blood out of the heart to the lungs through the **pulmonary arteries**. Despite carrying deoxygenated blood, these vessels are still called arteries because they carry blood away from the heart. After blood cycles through the lungs, exchanging oxygen and carbon dioxide, the blood returns back to the heart through the **pulmonary veins**.

Again, despite carrying oxygenated blood, these vessels are called veins because they carry blood towards the heart. The blood re-enters the heart into the **left atrium**. It passes through the **bicuspid/mitral valve**(which separates the left atrium and left ventricle), into the **left ventricle**. An extremely powerful contraction occurs in the left ventricle, which shoots blood out of the heart to the rest of the body through the **aorta**, the **largest artery** in the body.

Blood vessels are the main mode of transportation for not only blood, but other substances, such as hormones. These substances are carried throughout the body in blood vessels. The largest types of blood vessels are known as **arteries**. Arteries primarily carry oxygenated blood away from the heart, to tissues. **Veins** are blood vessels that primarily carry deoxygenated blood towards the heart, where it can replace carbon dioxide with oxygen. **Capillaries** are microscopic arteries, and are where gas exchange takes place between blood vessels and tissues.

The pathway of blood flow through the heart

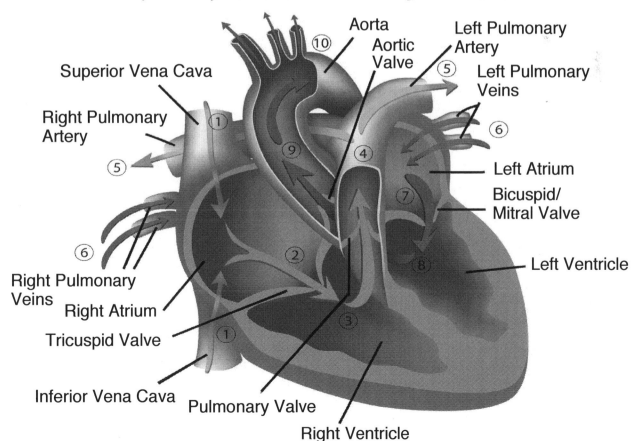

36

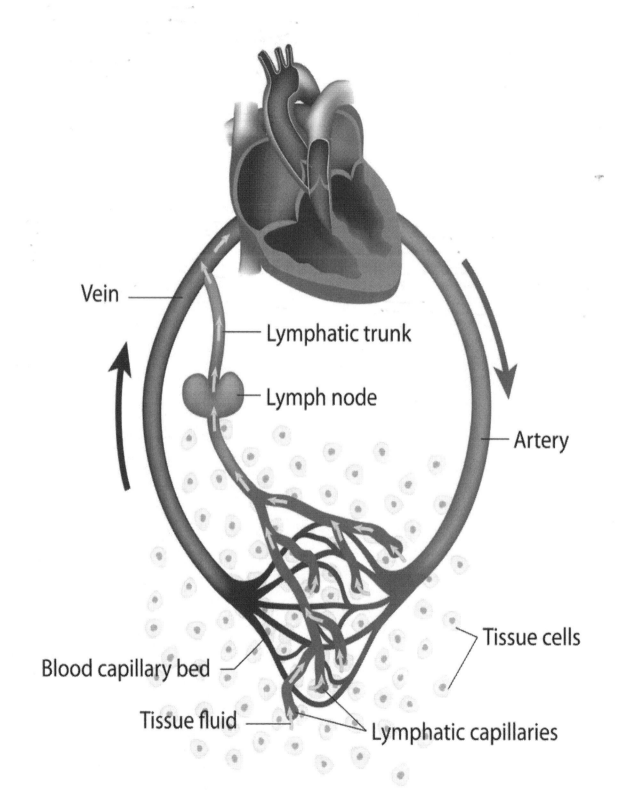

Vein

Lymphatic trunk

Lymph node

Artery

Tissue cells

Blood capillary bed

Tissue fluid

Lymphatic capillaries

Digestive System

- The Digestive System has many structures, organs, and functions. It is one of the most important systems in the body, responsible for bringing nutrients **into** the body, **digestion** of food, **absorption** of nutrients into the body's tissues, and **elimination** of waste products.

Structures of the Digestive System include the **mouth**, **pharynx**, **esophagus**, **stomach**, **liver**, **gallbladder**, **pancreas**, **small intestine**, and **large intestine**.

Digestion

- The **mouth**, also known as the **oral cavity**, is the first place digestion begins taking place. The **teeth** manually break down food by **chewing**. The food mixes with **saliva**, which contains digestive enzymes such as **amylase**, that help to break down carbohydrates. The **tongue** assists with mastication(chewing) by pressing food against the teeth. Once food has been properly chewed, it is swallowed.

- After food is swallowed, it moves from the mouth into the **pharynx**, also known as the **throat**. The pharynx is simply a passage-way for food, water, and air on the way to their respective destinations. Food leaves the pharynx and enters the esophagus.

- The **esophagus** is a long tube that runs from the pharynx inferiorly, passes through the diaphragm, and connects to the **stomach**. The esophagus, much like the pharynx, has one function: transporting food. The esophagus, and every hollow organ of the Digestive System, are lined with smooth muscle. When the smooth muscle rhythmically contracts, it forces food further along in the organ. This is known as **peristalsis**.

- Once food reaches the **stomach**, both ends of the stomach close off, and the stomach begins **digesting** the food. Powerfully, it churns the food, breaking it down manually. Stomach acids like hydrochloric acid and pepsin mix with the food inside the stomach and further help to break down the food. Once food is properly digested, the stomach opens at the pylorus, and food exits the stomach and enters into the small intestine.

- The **small intestine** is where the majority of **absorption** of nutrients occurs. **Accessory organs** produce substances that help aid the small intestine in digestion. These accessory organs are the liver, gallbladder, and pancreas.

- The **liver**, the heaviest internal organ, mainly acts as a **blood detoxifier**. It filters harmful substances from the blood. However, it aids in digestion by producing **bile**, a yellowish substance that aids in the emulsification of fats. Connecting to the liver is the gallbladder. Once the liver produces bile, it empties the bile into the gallbladder, where it is stored until it is needed.

- The **gallbladder** simply has one function: to **store bile** and empty bile into the small intestine through the bile duct, which connects to the duodenum, the first section of the small intestine.

- The **pancreas** is an extremely important organ, and is vital in the processing and breaking down of glucose in the body. The pancreas produces **glucagon**(created by alpha cells), which aids in increasing glucose concentration in the blood. It also produces **insulin**(created by beta cells), which aids in lowering glucose concentration in the blood. These substances empty into the small intestine through the same path as bile, the bile duct.

Liver, Gallbladder, Pancreas and Bile Passage

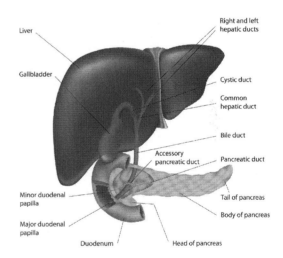

- Food moves from the stomach into the **small intestine**. The first section of the small intestine is known as the **duodenum**. The duodenum is the last section of the Digestive System that digestion of food takes place. Bile, glucagon, and insulin all mix with food in the duodenum and further break down substances. Peristalsis forces the food from the duodenum further into the small intestine, into the middle portion, known as the **jejunum**. The jejunum is where the majority of nutrient absorption takes place in the small intestine. As the food is forced through the small intestine, it moves into the final section, known as the **ileum**. Final absorption occurs in the ileum. Food moves through the ileum and into the large intestine.

- The **large intestine** has two primary functions: **absorption** of **water**, and **elimination** of **waste**. As feces moves through the large intestine, water is absorbed. If too much water is absorbed, constipation may result. If not enough water is absorbed, diarrhea may result. The large intestine has four sections: the **ascending colon**, the **transverse colon**, the **descending colon**, and the **sigmoid colon**. As the feces leaves the sigmoid colon, it enters the rectum, where it is ready to be eliminated from the body.

Sphincters

In the Digestive System, there are **ring-like** bands of **muscle** between digestive organs, known as **sphincters**. Sphincters function to allow food to enter into an organ, or to keep food from moving backwards.
There are four primary sphincters in the Digestive System:

- The **esophageal** sphincter is located between the **pharynx** and the **esophagus**. It opens and allows food to move down into the esophagus.

- The **cardiac** sphincter is located between the **esophagus** and the **stomach**. It is named after the region of the stomach it connects to, which is known as the cardia. When food enters the stomach, the cardiac sphincter closes, preventing food and stomach acid from ascending into the esophagus.

- The **pyloric** sphincter is located between the **stomach** and the **small intestine**. It is named after the region of the stomach it connects to, which is known as the pylorus. When food enters the stomach, the pyloric sphincter closes, preventing food from leaving the stomach before digestion has taken place. When food has been properly digested, the pyloric sphincter opens, and food leaves the stomach.

- The **ileocecal** sphincter is located between the **small intestine** and the **large intestine**. It is named after the parts of the two organs that come together, the ileum(small intestine) and cecum(large intestine).

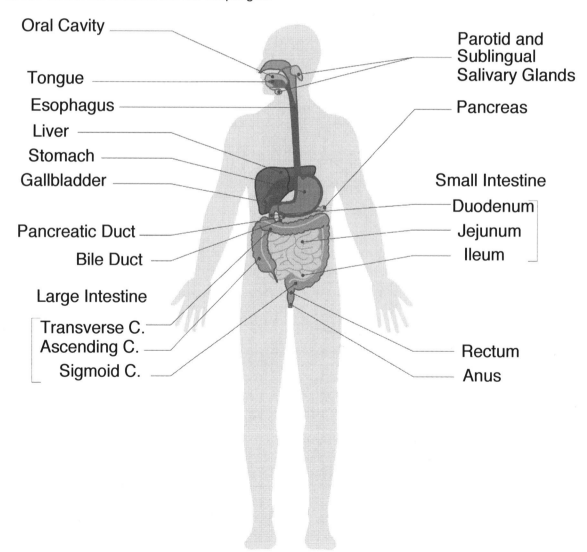

Oral Cavity

Tongue

Esophagus

Liver

Stomach

Gallbladder

Pancreatic Duct

Bile Duct

Large Intestine

Transverse C.
Ascending C.
Sigmoid C.

Parotid and Sublingual Salivary Glands

Pancreas

Small Intestine

Duodenum

Jejunum

Ileum

Rectum

Anus

Endocrine System

- The Endocrine System is responsible for coordinating specific activities of cells and tissues by releasing **hormones** into the body. Endocrine glands differ from exocrine glands in two specific ways: endocrine glands create and secrete hormones, while exocrine glands create and secrete things like sweat, saliva, and oil. Endocrine glands secrete hormones directly into the **blood stream**, while exocrine glands secrete their substances onto a **surface**(such as the surface of the mouth or skin).

Endocrine glands have many different functions that help regulate body function and homeostasis.

Glands

The **adrenal** glands, located atop the kidneys(ad-: towards; renal: kidney), secrete **epinephrine** and **norepinephrine**. These hormones help to elevate blood pressure, heart rate, and blood sugar. They are considered stress hormones, and are secreted when the body is under stress, or in the sympathetic nervous response.

The **hypothalamus** produces **dopamine**, an important hormone that increases blood pressure and heart rate. It is considered the reward center hormone. If you win at a game or contest, your hypothalamus may release dopamine, which gives a sensation of excitement.

The **ovaries** are the female gonads. They create **estrogen** and **progesterone**, two hormones important to female development and bone growth.

Pancreatic Islets are the parts of the pancreas that create **glucagon**, which increases blood sugar levels, and **insulin**, which decreases blood sugar levels.

The **pituitary** gland, which many consider the "master gland", secretes **growth hormone**, which regulates the amount of growth a person may experience. It also secretes **prolactin**, which stimulates milk production, and **follicle-stimulating hormone**, which influences production of female egg cells and male sperm cells.

The **testes** are the male gonads. The testes secrete **testosterone**, the primary male hormone, responsible for increasing bone and muscle mass.

The **thyroid** is a gland in the neck that produces **calcitonin**, which aids in decreasing the levels of calcium in the blood stream. Too much calcium in the blood may weaken the bones and cause kidney stones.

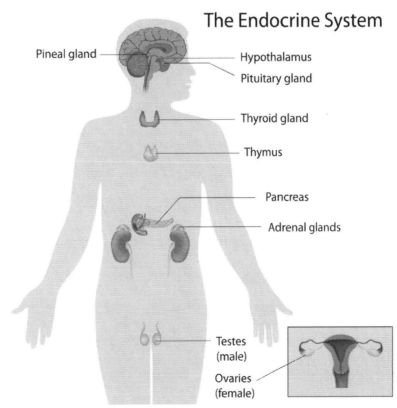

The Endocrine System

Pineal gland

Hypothalamus

Pituitary gland

Thyroid gland

Thymus

Pancreas

Adrenal glands

Testes (male)

Ovaries (female)

Integumentary System

- The Integumentary System is the body's first line of defense against pathogens and trauma. It's primary function is to protect the body. It also secretes substances, may absorb certain substances, and even eliminates waste.

Skin

The **skin**, which is the body's largest organ, is the main structure of the Integumentary System. The skin **protects** the body by creating a thick barrier that prevents pathogens from entering, and helps to cushion the body from blunt trauma.

Aiding the skin in protection are the **nails**. Finger and toe nails are made of **keratin**, the same cells that create thick layers in the skin called calluses. The nails prevent damage to the distal phalanges.

Hair also aids in protection, but in a different way. Hair is used to regulate temperature. When body temperature drops, smooth muscle that attaches to each hair, known as **arrector pili**, contract, forcing the hair to stand up. This creates an insulating layer, which is meant to trap warmth underneath the hair, much like a blanket. This does little for humans, but is utilized by animals to retain heat in cold environments.

Glands

Inside the skin are glands, which also aid in protection. **Sudoriferous** glands emerge from deep in the skin to the surface directly through tubes. Sudoriferous glands create and secrete **sweat**. Sweat is mostly made of water, but may also contain salt and waste products such as ammonia. Sweat is used to lower body temperature by evaporating off the surface of the skin. The evaporation cools the skin, which helps lower the internal body temperature.

Sebaceous glands are glands that connect to hair, and produce **oil(sebum)**. Oil helps to protect the body from pathogens and debris in the air. Blockage of a sebaceous gland, however, may lead to a bacterial infection, and acne.

Sensory Receptors

Inside the skin, there are many types of receptors that detect certain sensations, relaying the information to the brain. Sensory receptors aren't exclusive to the skin, but there are an abundance of them in the skin.

Nociceptors are a type of sensory receptor that detects the sensation of **pain**. Pain, while unpleasant, is actually vital in protection of the

body. The term "noci-" is Latin for "hurt".

Meissner's Corpuscles are sensory receptors that are very superficial in the skin, and detect **light pressure**. Massage strokes such as effleurage and feather strokes are detected by Meissner's Corpuscles.

Pacinian Corpuscles are sensory receptors that are very deep in the skin, and detect **deep pressure**. Deep massage strokes, such as compression, are detected by Pacinian Corpuscles.

➢ *Easy to Remember: Nociceptors detect pain. Remember the old saying "No pain, No gain".*

➢ *Easy to Remember: Pacinian Corpuscles detect deep pressure. Match up "Paci" of Pacinian with "Paci" of Pacific Ocean. The Pacific Ocean is deep.*

Human Skin Anatomy

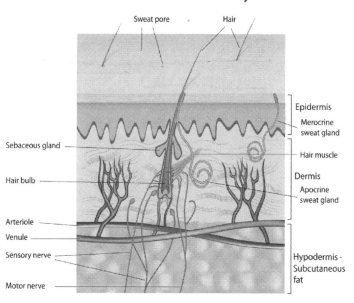

Lymphatic System

The Lymphatic System is vital in the body's **defense** against pathogens and disease. Not only are leukocytes abundant in lymph, but antibodies are created in the Lymphatic System. The Lymphatic System contains **lymph**, **lymph nodes**, **lymph vessels**, and **lymph organs**.

Lymph, the primary structure of the Lymphatic System, is a fluid composed of **water**, protein, leukocytes, urea, salts, and glucose. Lymph allows **transport** of all of these substances through the body, ultimately dumping into the blood stream. Lymph is made of **interstitial fluid**, fluid found between cells.

Lymph travels throughout the body through **lymph vessels**. Lymph vessels are similar to blood vessels, but only flow in one direction, towards the heart. Lymph vessels absorb foreign bodies and nutrients from tissues, bringing them into the lymph to be transported to the blood stream or lymph nodes. The **largest lymph vessel** in the body is located in the trunk. It is known as the **Thoracic Duct**. The Thoracic Duct drains lymph into the **left subclavian vein**, where it joins with blood.

Lymph nodes are large **masses** of lymphatic tissue. They are responsible for production of **antibodies**, and help destroy any foreign objects that enter the lymph. During an infection, lymph nodes may become tender and swollen.

The **thymus**, located in the chest, is responsible for production of **T-lymphocytes**, or T-cells. T-cells are vital in regulation of the body's immune system. If a person contracts HIV, the virus destroys the T-cells, which essentially disables the immune system.

The **spleen** is an organ of the Lymphatic System that is responsible for **destroying** dead or dying **red blood cells** from the blood stream, in addition to destroying pathogens and debris.

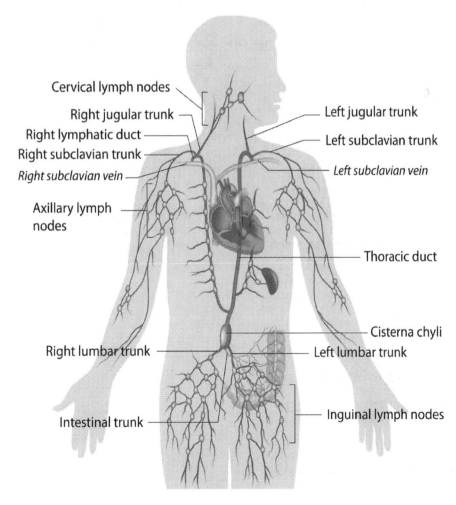

Cervical lymph nodes
Right jugular trunk
Right lymphatic duct
Right subclavian trunk
Right subclavian vein
Axillary lymph nodes
Right lumbar trunk
Intestinal trunk

Left jugular trunk
Left subclavian trunk
Left subclavian vein
Thoracic duct
Cisterna chyli
Left lumbar trunk
Inguinal lymph nodes

Muscular System

- Muscles have numerous actions in the body, primarily **producing body heat**, contracting to allow **movements**, and constricting **organs** and **blood vessels**.

Muscles can all be categorized under three main types: **Skeletal**, **Cardiac**, and **Smooth**.

Skeletal muscles, as the name implies, attach to the **skeleton**. Another name for Skeletal muscle is "**striated**" muscle, due to its appearance under a microscope. These muscles are **voluntary**, meaning you can control them. When these muscles contract, they pull on the bones they attach to, which allows **movement**.

Skeletal muscles are always in a state of **twitching**, even if you can't feel it. It's this twitching, very fine contractions, that produces **body heat**. When body temperature drops, the Skeletal muscles increase the amount of contraction, which produces high body temperature, with the twitching of the muscles becoming more apparent. This is what happens when you shiver!

Cardiac muscle is the muscle that makes the **heart**. Another name for Cardiac muscle is "**branching**" muscle, due to its appearance under a microscope. Cardiac muscle is **involuntary**, meaning you can't control it. Cardiac muscle is powerful, sending **blood** shooting out of the heart with each contraction. The only function of Cardiac muscle is to send blood from one place to another.

Smooth muscle is found in several locations throughout the body. Another name for Smooth muscle is "**non-striated**" muscle, due to its appearance under a microscope. Smooth muscle is **involuntary**, meaning you can't control it. Smooth muscle, because it is found in several different regions of the body, has several different functions. Smooth muscle can be found in the **walls** of **hollow organs** such as the stomach and intestines. When these muscles contract, they force food through the digestive system, which is known as **peristalsis**.

Other locations Smooth muscle can be found are in the **skin**, and in the **eyes**. In the skin, Smooth muscle attaches to hair. When these muscles contract, they stand hair up, producing goosebumps. These muscles are known as the **arrector pili** muscles. In the eyes, Smooth muscles help to **dilate** the **iris** and **pupil**.

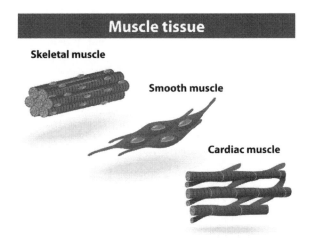

Muscle Shapes

- Muscles have numerous different shapes. These include:
Circular: Circular muscles are arranged in a **circular** manner. Examples include Orbicularis Oris and Orbicularis Oculi.
Convergent: Convergent muscles are **spread out** on one end and **merge** together at another end. An example is Pectoralis Major.
Parallel: Parallel muscles have muscle fibers that all run in the **same direction**. Examples include Sartorius and Coracobrachialis.
Pennate: Pennate muscles have an appearance resembling a **feather**. These muscles can be **unipennate**(one feather), **bipennate**(two feathers), or **multipennate**(multiple feathers). Examples include Flexor Pollicis Longus(unipennate), Rectus Femoris(bipennate), and Deltoid(multipennate).

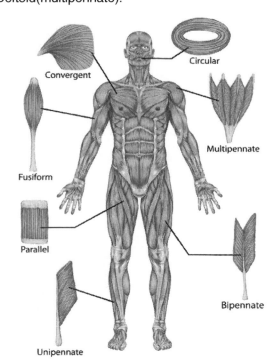

Muscle Contractions

- When there is **tension** in a muscle, it is **contracting**. A muscle can contract without moving, though. There are four types of muscle contractions.

    Isometric Contraction: Iso means "**Same**" or "**Equal**". Metric means "**Length**". When an isometric contraction occurs, as the name implies, the length of the muscle **stays the same**, but tension in the muscle **changes**. An example: imagine trying to lift something that is too heavy for you to lift. The muscles required to lift the object increase in tension, but because the muscle isn't strong enough, the length of the muscle doesn't change.

    Isotonic Contraction: Iso means "**Same**" or "**Equal**". Tonic means "**Tension**". When an isotonic contraction occurs, as the name implies, the tension in the muscle **stays the same**, but the muscle length **changes**. There are two separate types of isotonic contractions:

    Concentric Contraction: When a concentric contraction occurs, several things take place. The tension in the muscle **initially increases** until the amount of tension required to perform the action is reached, then the tension **remains constant**. While the tension remains constant, the muscle **length decreases**. An example is performing a Biceps curl.

    Eccentric Contraction: When an eccentric contraction occurs, several things take place. The tension in the muscle **initially decreases** until the amount of tension required to perform the action is reached, then the tension **remains constant**. While the tension remains constant, the muscle length **increases**. An example is extending the elbow and lowering the weight down after the Biceps curl in a concentric contraction.

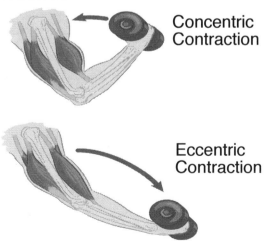

Concentric Contraction

Eccentric Contraction

- > *General Rule of Thumb: With concentric contractions, the muscle length decreases. With eccentric contractions, the muscle length increases.*

Muscle Actions

- Muscles perform numerous actions on the body, depending on which muscle is contracting. Muscle actions include the following:

    Flexion: **Decreasing** the **angle** of a joint.
    Extension: **Increasing** the **angle** of a joint.
    Adduction: Moving a structure **towards** the **midline**.
    Abduction: Moving a structure **away** from the **midline**.
    Protraction: Moving a structure **anteriorly**.
    Retraction: Moving a structure **posteriorly**.
    Inversion: Turning the **sole** of the foot **in** towards the **midline**.
    Eversion: Turning the **sole** of the foot **out** away from the **midline**.
    Elevation: Moving a structure **superiorly**.
    Depression: Moving a structure **inferiorly**.
    Supination: Rotating the **palm** so it is facing **upwards**.
    Pronation: Rotating the **palm** so it is facing **downwards**.
    Rotation: **Turning** a structure around its **long axis**.
    Circumduction: **Turning** a structure around the **circumference** of a joint.
    Opposition: Moving structures in **opposite** directions.
    Lateral Deviation: Moving a structure from **side-to-side**.
    Plantarflexion: Pointing toes **down**.
    Dorsiflexion: Pointing toes **up**.

    When a muscle performs an action, other muscles associate with the muscle in different ways.

    A **Prime Mover/Agonist** is the muscle that primarily performs a specific action. An example: when plantarflexion is performed, the **strongest** muscle performing it is the Gastrocnemius. That means Gastrocnemius is the prime mover/agonist.

    A **Synergist** is the muscle that **assists** the prime mover/agonist in performing the action. Synergists are not as strong as prime movers. An example: when plantarflexion is performed, Soleus contracts to allow more strength, assisting Gastrocnemius in performing the action. That means Soleus is the synergist.

    An **Antagonist** is a muscle that performs the **opposite** action of the prime mover/agonist. Every muscle has an antagonist. An example: Gastrocnemius contracts, performing plantarflexion. To return the foot to the starting position, Gastrocnemius relaxes, and Tibialis Anterior contracts, which performs dorsiflexion. This makes Tibialis Anterior the antagonist to Gastrocnemius.

    A **Fixator** is a muscle that **stabilizes** an area or joint while an action is being performed.

Stabilizing the joint prevents things like injury and allows optimal movement to occur. An example: Supraspinatus stabilizes the head of the humerus in the glenoid fossa, keeping the joint together during the numerous movements the glenohumeral joint performs.

➢ *Easy to Remember: Just think of it like this: Batman is the Agonist, the main character. Robin is the Synergist, the helper. The Joker is the Antagonist, who does the opposite of Batman. Alfred is the Fixator, who helps hold Batman together.*

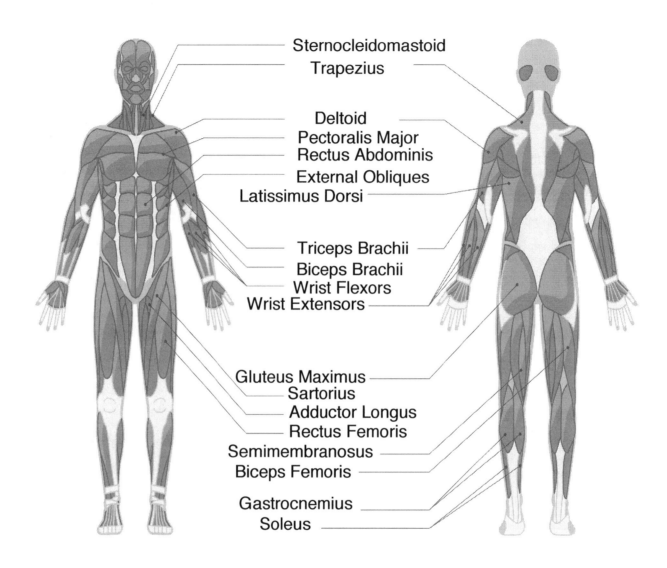

Sternocleidomastoid
Trapezius

Deltoid
Pectoralis Major
Rectus Abdominis
External Obliques
Latissimus Dorsi

Triceps Brachii
Biceps Brachii
Wrist Flexors
Wrist Extensors

Gluteus Maximus
Sartorius
Adductor Longus
Rectus Femoris
Semimembranosus
Biceps Femoris

Gastrocnemius
Soleus

Nervous System

- Nerves are structures in the **Nervous System**, made of Nervous Tissue. Nerves have many functions, from regulating vital functions within the body, to controlling muscles.

There are two divisions of the Nervous System: the **Central Nervous System**, and the **Peripheral Nervous System**. The Central Nervous System consists of the **brain** and **spinal cord**. The Central Nervous System is under involuntary control, responsible for interpretation of sensations and mental activity.

Central Nervous System

The brain consists of three parts: the **cerebrum**, which is the largest part of the brain and split into left and right hemispheres, the **cerebellum**, located at the back and bottom of the brain, and the **brain stem**, which connects the brain to the spinal cord.

Each side of the **cerebrum** is divided into **lobes**, named after the bones atop them: **frontal** lobe(processes motivation, aggression, mood), **temporal** lobe(processes memory, hearing, and smell), **parietal** lobe(processes most sensory information), and **occipital** lobe(processes vision).

The **cerebellum** is responsible for regulation of **muscle tone**, **balance**, **coordination**, and control of **general body movements**.

The **brain stem**, which consists of(in descending order) the **midbrain**, the **pons**, and the **medulla oblongata**, controls the **vital functions** of the body, such as breathing, heart rate, coughing, sneezing, vomiting, and blood vessel diameter.

Median section of the brain

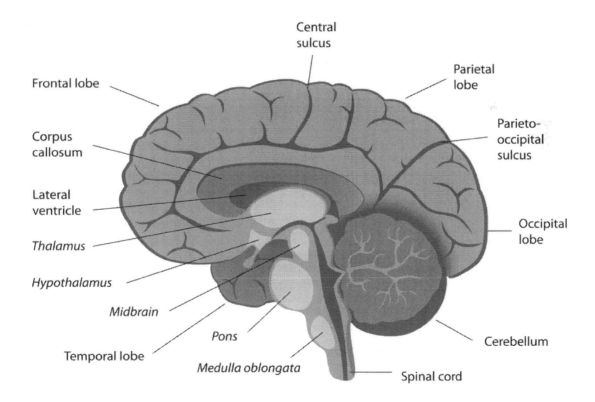

46

Peripheral Nervous System

The Peripheral Nervous System consists of the body's **nerves**. There are two divisions of the Peripheral Nervous System: **Cranial Nerves** and **Spinal Nerves**. Cranial Nerves, as the name suggests, emerge from the brain, and help to regulate the functions of the head and face. There are **twelve pairs** of Cranial Nerves, each numbered in Roman Numerals:

- Olfactory(I)
- Optic(II)
- Oculomotor(III)
- Trochlear(IV)
- Trigeminal(V)
- Abducens(VI)
- Facial(VII)
- Vestibulocochlear(VIII)
- Glossopharyngeal(IX)
- Vagus(X)
- Accessory(XI)
- Hypoglossal(XII)

Spinal Nerves are much more numerous than Cranial Nerves. There are **31 pairs** of Spinal Nerves. The Spinal Nerves, as the name suggests, emerge from the spinal cord, and are responsible for controlling skeletal muscle.

A bundle of Spinal Nerves that emerge from the spinal cord is known as a **Plexus**. There are three plexi in the body: **Cervical Plexus**, **Brachial Plexus**, **Lumbosacral Plexus**. The Cervical Plexus emerges from the spinal cord in the range of **C1-C4**. The primary nerve of the Cervical Plexus is known as the **Phrenic Nerve**.

The Phrenic Nerve descends inferiorly from the Cervical vertebrae and innervates(provides nervous stimulation to) the **Diaphragm**.

The Brachial Plexus emerges from the spinal cord at **C5-T1**. As the name suggests, the nerves of the Brachial Plexus move distally, controlling the muscles of the **upper limb**. There are five primary nerves of the Brachial Plexus:

- Radial
- Musculocutaneous
- Axillary
- Median
- Ulnar

The **Radial Nerve** is located on the posterior arm and forearm, and innervates the Triceps Brachii, Anconeus, Brachioradialis, and Wrist Extensors.

The **Musculocutaneous Nerve** is located in the anterior arm, and innervates the Biceps Brachii, Brachialis, and Coracobrachialis.

The **Axillary Nerve** is primarily located in the armpit, and innervates the Teres Minor and Deltoid.

The **Median Nerve** is located in the anterior arm, forearm, and hand, and innervates the Wrist Flexors, and most muscles on the lateral side of the hand.

The **Ulnar Nerve** is located on the anterior arm, medial forearm, and medial hand, and innervates the Wrist Flexors and most muscles on the medial side of the hand.

The Lumbosacral Plexus, as the name suggests, emerges from the **entire span** of the Lumbar and Sacral vertebrae. The major nerves of the Lumbosacral Plexus include:

- Sciatic
- Femoral
- Obturator
- Tibial
- Common Peroneal
- Deep Peroneal
- Superficial Peroneal

The **Sciatic Nerve** is a large nerve located on the posterior thigh. The Sciatic Nerve is actually both the Tibial Nerve and the Common Peroneal Nerve bundled together. Once the Sciatic Nerve reaches the back of the knee, it branches off into two separate nerves. The Sciatic Nerve innervates the Hamstring muscle group.

The **Femoral Nerve** is located on the anterior thigh, and innervates the Quadriceps muscle group, Iliacus, Sartorius, and Pectineus.

The **Obturator Nerve** is located on the medial portion of the thigh, and innervates the Adductor muscle group.

The **Tibial Nerve**, after branching off the Sciatic nerve, runs down the posterior leg, and innervates the Gastrocnemius, Soleus, Tibialis Posterior, and Plantaris.

The **Common Peroneal Nerve**, after branching off the Sciatic Nerve, actually branches off into two other nerves of its own: The Deep Peroneal and Superficial Peroneal Nerves.

The **Deep Peroneal Nerve** is located on the anterior leg, and innervates the Tibialis Anterior.

The **Superficial Peroneal Nerve** is located on the lateral portion of the leg, running along the fibula, and innervates the Peroneus Longus and Peroneus Brevis.

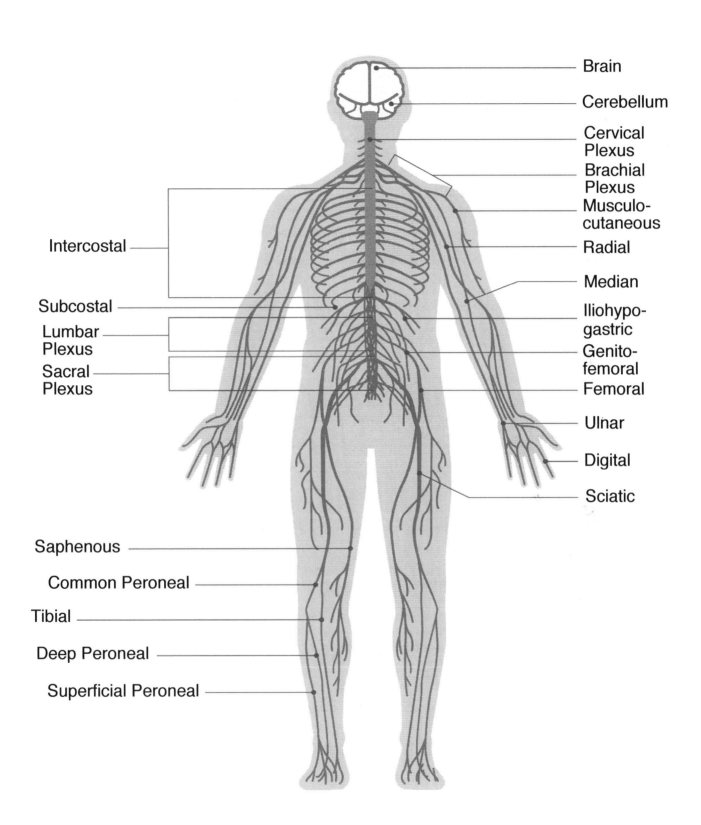

Brain

Cerebellum

Cervical
Plexus

Brachial
Plexus

Musculo-
cutaneous

Radial

Median

Iliohypo-
gastric

Genito-
femoral

Femoral

Ulnar

Digital

Sciatic

Intercostal

Subcostal

Lumbar
Plexus

Sacral
Plexus

Saphenous

Common Peroneal

Tibial

Deep Peroneal

Superficial Peroneal

Autonomic Nervous System

The autonomic nervous system helps to regulate **homeostasis** by release of hormones, controlling heart rate, breathing rate, and other bodily functions. There are two divisions of the autonomic nervous system: the **Sympathetic Response**, and the **Parasympathetic Response**.

The Sympathetic Response is also known as "**fight-or-flight**". When the body is in a state of **stress**, the Sympathetic Response helps the body respond by releasing **norepinephrine** into the blood stream, which increases heart rate and blood sugar. The digestive organs will also shut down, and blood will be pulled from these organs and supplied to the muscles for use.

The Parasympathetic Response is also known as "**rest-and-digest**". When the body is in a state of **relaxation**, the Parasympathetic Response helps the body to calm itself. It decreases the body's heart rate, and increases blood flow to the digestive organs to increase **peristalsis**. The Parasympathetic Response, decreasing heart rate, and peristalsis are all controlled by Cranial Nerve X, the **Vagus Nerve**.

Sympathetic System

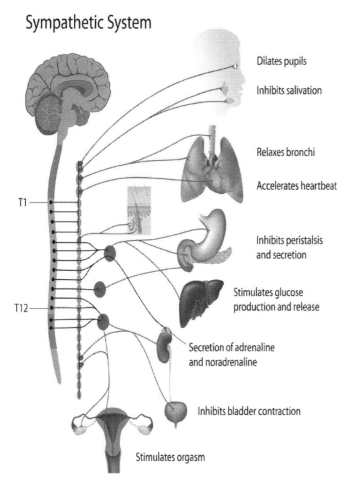

Parasympathetic System

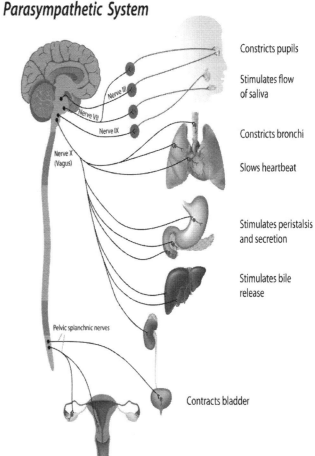

Respiratory System

- The Respiratory System has one essential function: to bring **oxygen** into the body, and eliminate wastes, such as **carbon dioxide**, from the body.

The main organs of the Respiratory System are the **lungs**. The left lung has two lobes and is smaller than the right lung, which has three lobes. This is due to the presence of the heart on the left side of the chest.

Conduction of air is controlled by the **nose**. Air enters the body through the nose, and is filtered by **hair** and **mucous**. The nose also warms the air as it enters the body.

The **larynx**, also known as the voice box, is a short tube located inferior to the pharynx. As air passes over the vocal cords in the larynx, the vocal cords vibrate, which produces **speech**.

Sitting atop the larynx is a flap of tissue known as the **epiglottis**. Upon swallowing, the epiglottis lies on top of the larynx, blocking any food or fluid from entering the larynx, which **prevents choking**.

Connecting to the larynx inferiorly is a tube of cartilage known as the **trachea**, or the wind pipe. The trachea is the primary passageway for air to enter into the lungs.

Once air enters the lungs, it goes into each lung through **bronchial tubes**, which branch off of the trachea. These tubes branch into smaller tubes called bronchioles. Bronchial tubes secrete **mucous**, which helps to trap any dirt or debris that have made it into the lungs.

At the end of the bronchioles are tiny **air sacs**, known as **alveoli**. The alveoli resemble a cluster of grapes. Capillaries attach to the alveoli and move blood across the surface of the alveoli. This allows carbon dioxide to detach from the erythrocytes and exit the blood stream, and also allows oxygen to enter the blood stream and attach to erythrocytes. Alveoli are where **gas exchange** occurs in the Respiratory System.

Respiration is accomplished by contraction of the **diaphragm**, a large muscle connected to the rib cage that separates the chest from the abdomen. The diaphragm creates a **vacuum** inside the chest. When it contracts, it descends, pulling the chest down. This allows air to enter into the lungs. When the diaphragm relaxes, it ascends up into the chest, which forces air out of the lungs.

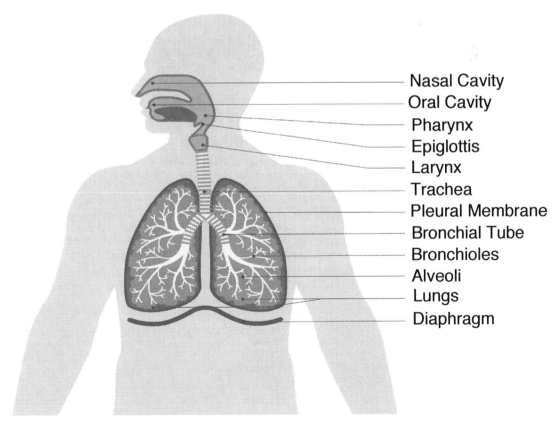

Nasal Cavity
Oral Cavity
Pharynx
Epiglottis
Larynx
Trachea
Pleural Membrane
Bronchial Tube
Bronchioles
Alveoli
Lungs
Diaphragm

Skeletal System

- The Skeletal System is a vital component of movement. We wouldn't be able to move if we didn't have bones! Muscles attach to bones, and when a muscle contracts, it pulls on a bone(or bones), which performs an action. Bones also produce blood cells, provide stability for the body, and protect structures and organs in the body. Needless to say, bones are extremely important!

There are **206** bones in the human body. Each bone can be classified as one of the following: **Long** bone, **Short** bone, **Irregular** bone, **Flat** bone, **Sesamoid** bone.

Long bones appear **longer** than they are **wide**. There are numerous long bones in the body, including, but not limited to, the clavicle, humerus, femur, metatarsals, and phalanges.

Short bones are **as long** as they are **wide**. Examples include the carpals and tarsals.

Irregular bones are bones that have generally **unusual shapes**. Examples include the mandible, vertebrae, and pubis.

Flat bones are named after how they look: **flat**. They are typically thin and flat. Examples include the scapula, ribs, and cranial bones.

Sesamoid bones are bones embedded **inside tendons**, and named after what they look like. They are rounded, and resemble **sesame seeds**. The primary examples are the patella and pisiform.

Joints

- Where bones come together is known as an **articulation**. Another name for articulation is "**joint**". Joints are where **movements** occur. We don't flex muscles, we flex joints!

All joints are classified as one of the following: **Synarthrotic**, **Amphiarthrotic**, or **Diarthrotic**. Synarthrotic joints are joints with little to **no movement** in them, such as the sutures in the skull. Amphiarthrotic joints are joints that are **slightly movable**, such as the intervertebral joints. Diarthrotic joints are **freely movable** joints, and have no real movement restrictions, such as in the shoulder or hip.

➤ *Easy to Remember: To remember the joint classifications, just think of "SAD". This tells you the order of joint classifications in order from least movable joint to most movable joint. Synarthrosis, Amphiarthrosis, Diarthrosis.*

Joints have several structures that help create and support them.

Between bones that articulate, on the **epiphyses**, there is **articular cartilage**. This type of cartilage is known as **hyaline** cartilage. It is a dense form of cartilage, very thick, and is a shock-absorber. Hyaline cartilage also **prevents friction** between the articulating bones, so bones don't rub against each other during movement.

Certain joints have a specific type of cartilage in them known as a **labrum**. The labrum, found in the glenohumeral joint and iliofemoral joint, is used to **deepen** the joint, providing a deeper socket for these ball-and-socket joints. This provides more **strength** and **stability** for the joint.

Bones are held together by **ligaments**. Ligaments are avascular, meaning they are not supplied with blood by blood vessels. Ligaments are strong, but do not stretch very far before injury can occur. Tearing of ligaments such as the Anterior Cruciate Ligament is common in activities such as sports, or in car accidents.

Four of the most important joints joined together by ligaments are located in the skull, between the cranial bones. These synarthrotic joints are called **sutures**. The **sagittal** suture runs along a sagittal plane on the top of the head, connecting the two **parietal bones**. The **coronal** suture runs on a coronal plane, connecting the **frontal** bone to the **parietal** bones. The **squamous** suture runs on a sagittal plane, but is located on the side of the skull, connecting the **parietal** and **temporal** bones together. Finally, the **lambdoid** suture, named for the Greek letter "lambda", connects the **occipital** bone to the **parietal** bones.

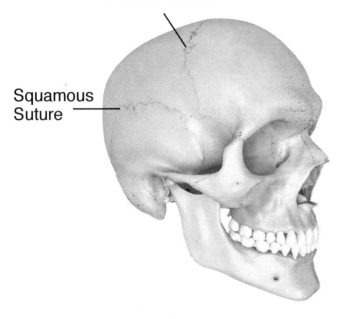

Coronal Suture

Squamous Suture

Muscles are held to bones via **tendons**. Tendons are similar to ligaments, but have a much more rich blood supply, and able to stretch further before injury occurs.

Inside the joint itself, a membrane is present, known as the **synovial membrane**. The synovial membrane produces a fluid that helps to **lubricate** the joint, known as the **synovial fluid**. Lubrication of the joint is key in keeping the joint functioning optimally. Surrounding the entire joint is thick, dense connective tissue known as the **joint capsule**. The joint capsule keeps everything inside the joint, such as the synovial fluid, and provides even more strength and support to the joint.

Synovial joint of the knee

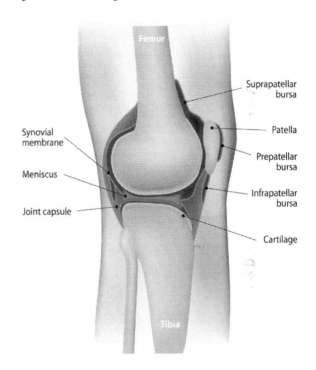

Femur

Suprapatellar bursa

Synovial membrane

Patella

Meniscus

Prepatellar bursa

Joint capsule

Infrapatellar bursa

Cartilage

Tibia

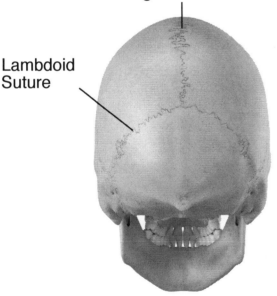

Sagittal Suture

Lambdoid Suture

Types of Diarthrotic Joints

- There are **six** different types of diarthrotic joints.

Ball-and-Socket joints feature one bone with a **ball** at the epiphysis, and another bone with a **socket**. The ball fits in the socket, creating a ball-and-socket joint. Examples include the shoulder and hip joints. Ball-and-socket joints have the most amount of movement, able to move the joint in really any direction.

Hinge joints act much like the hinge on a door, only opening and closing. Hinge joints only allow movement in **one plane**, allowing only **flexion** and **extension**. Examples include the elbow and knee joints.

Pivot joints allow only one type of movement: **rotation**. All they do is allow structures to turn. An example is the atlantoaxial joint, which lets us shake our head "no". This is rotation.

Plane/gliding joints are produced when the articulating bones have **flat** surfaces, and there is a **disc of cartilage** between the bones. This allows the joint to move, or glide, in any direction, although with slight movement. Examples include the joints between the carpals and tarsals.

Saddle joints are only located in one part of the body: the **metacarpophalangeal joint** of the **thumb**. Saddle joints are named after the appearance of the articulating bones. The articulating surfaces are both shaped like saddles. The two bones that create the saddle joint are the **first metacarpal** and the **trapezium**.

Ellipsoid/condyloid joints are extremely similar to ball-and-socket joints. On one bone, there is a **condyle**, which resembles a ball, but isn't as pronounced. This condyle fits into an **elliptical cavity** on another bone, which is similar to a socket, but not as deep. This allows movements such as flexion, extension, adduction, abduction, and circumduction. An example is the radiocarpal joint, created by the elliptical cavity of the radius meeting the condyle of the scaphoid.

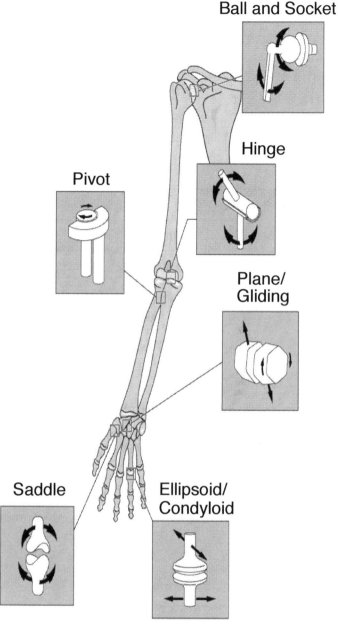

Skeleton Divisions

There are two divisions of the skeleton: the **Axial Skeleton** and the **Appendicular Skeleton**.

The Axial Skeleton contains all of the bones that do not correspond to any appendages: the **skull**, **vertebral column**, and **thoracic cage**. These bones make up the trunk.

The Appendicular Skeleton contains all of the bones that correspond to the appendages: the **humerus**, **radius**, **ulna**, **carpals**, **metacarpals**, **phalanges**, **femur**, **tibia**, **fibula**, **metatarsals**, **phalanges**, the **pectoral girdle**(clavicles and scapulae) and **pelvic girdle**(ilium, ischium, pubis, and sacrum).

Bones

Skull

The skull's primary function is to **protect** the **brain**. The bones that make up the skull are:

Parietal
Frontal
Temporal
Occipital
Zygomatic
Maxilla

Mandible
Vomer
Ethmoid
Sphenoid
Nasal
Lacrimal

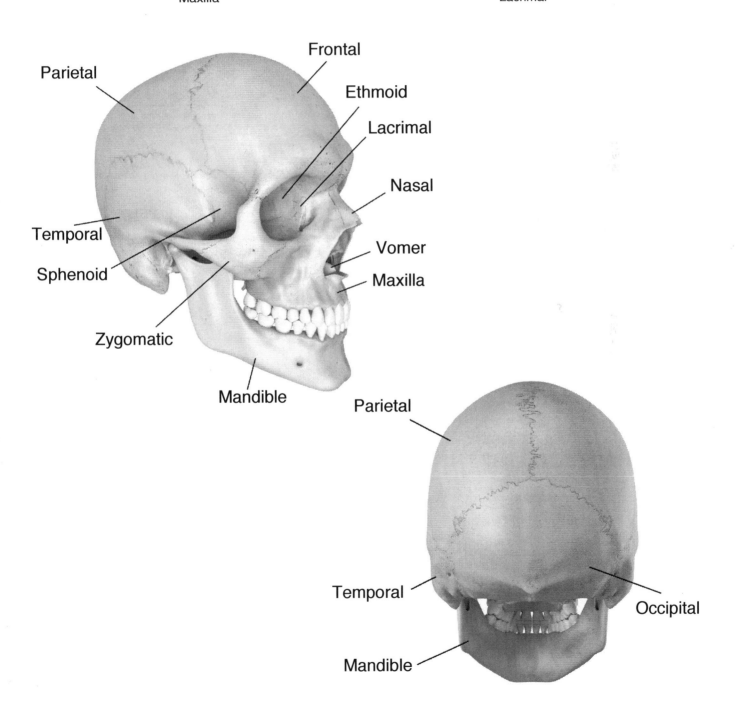

Vertebral Column

The vertebral column consists of **26** individual bones. Its primary function is to **protect** the **spinal cord**, which runs through it. There are **five** different regions of the vertebral column. They are:
Cervical(7 vertebrae)
Thoracic(12 vertebrae)
Lumbar(5 vertebrae)
Sacral(1 vertebrae)
Coccygeal(1 vertebrae)

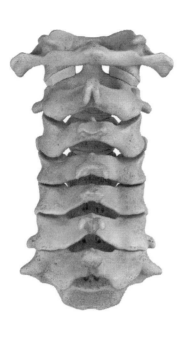

Cervical Vertebrae

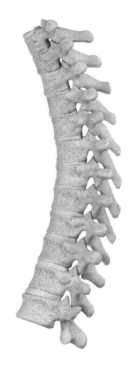

Thoracic Vertebrae

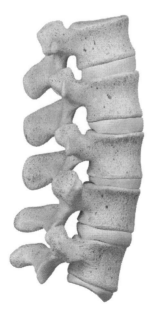

Lumbar Vertebrae

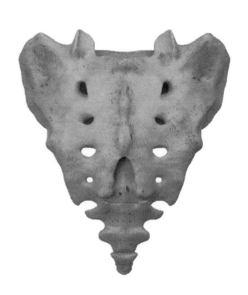

Sacrum and Coccyx

> ➤ *Easy to Remember: To remember how many vertebrae are in the cervical, thoracic, and lumbar regions, just think of breakfast, lunch, and dinner. You have breakfast(cervical) at 7, lunch(thoracic) at 12, and dinner(lumbar) at 5.*

Chest

The chest consists of the **rib cage**. The primary function of the rib cage is to **protect vital organs** inside the thorax, and **assist in breathing** by giving the **diaphragm** a place to attach. The rib cage consists of:
True ribs(superior seven ribs)
False ribs(inferior five ribs)
Floating ribs(ribs 11 and 12)

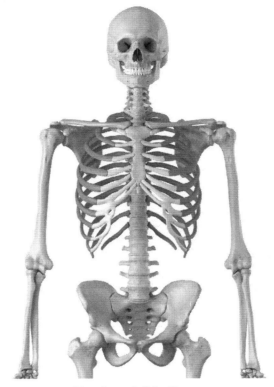

Pectoral Girdle

The pectoral girdle is responsible for holding the **upper limbs** to the **body**. The pectoral girdle consists of **four** bones:
Scapulae(two bones)
Clavicles(two bones)

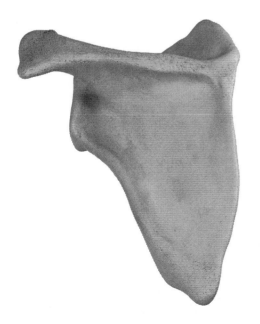

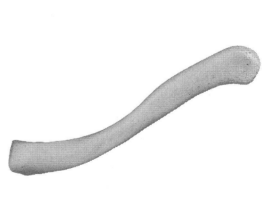

Scapula   Clavicle

Pelvic Girdle

The pelvic girdle is primarily responsible for holding the **lower limbs** to the **body**. The pelvic girdle contains:
Ilium(two bones)
Ischium(two bones)
Pubis(two bones)
Sacrum(one bone)

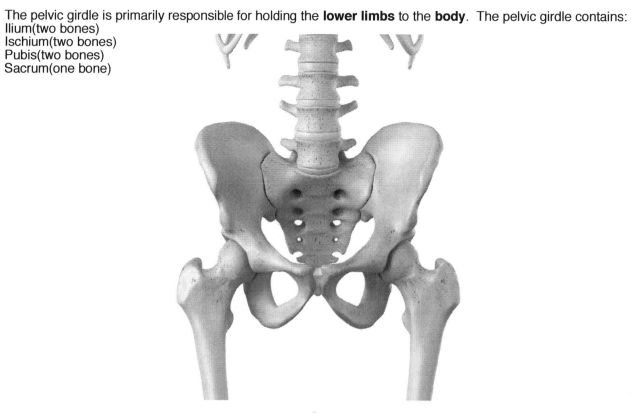

Arm

The arm contains **one** bone:
Humerus

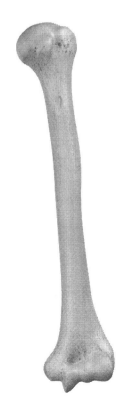

Forearm

The forearm contains **two** bones:
Radius
Ulna

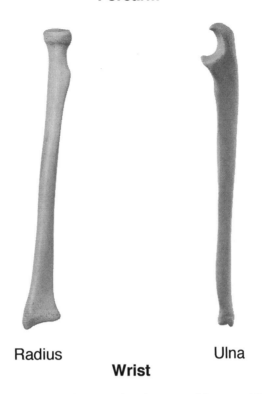

Radius   Ulna

Wrist

The wrist is located distally to the forearm, and it contains the **carpal** bones. The carpal bones are divided into two separate lines, each containing four bones. The proximal line is listed first, then the distal line:

Proximal Line: Distal Line:
Scaphoid   Trapezium
Lunate   Trapezoid
Triquetrum   Capitate
Pisiform   Hamate

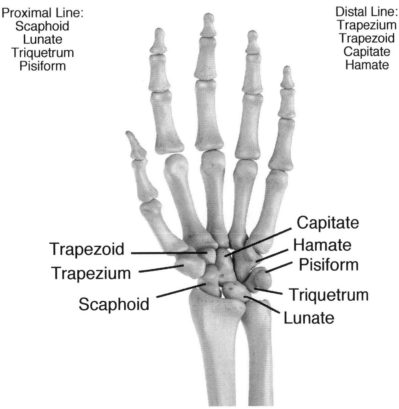

➢ *Easy to Remember: To remember the order of the carpals, think of this old saying: **S**ome **L**overs **T**ry **P**ositions **T**hat **T**hey **C**an't **H**andle(**S**caphoid, **L**unate, **T**riquetrum, **P**isiform, **T**rapezium, **T**rapezoid, **C**apitate, **H**amate)*

Hand

The hand contains **19** bones in each hand:
Metacarpals(5 bones)
Phalanges(14 bones)

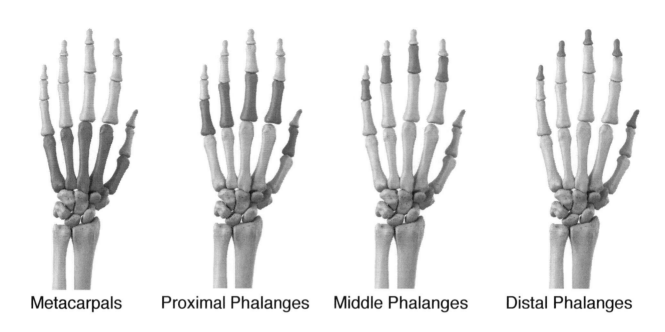

Metacarpals   Proximal Phalanges   Middle Phalanges   Distal Phalanges

Thigh

The thigh contains the **longest** and **strongest** bone in the body. This bone is:
Femur

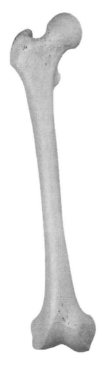

Leg

The leg contains **two** bones:
Tibia
Fibula

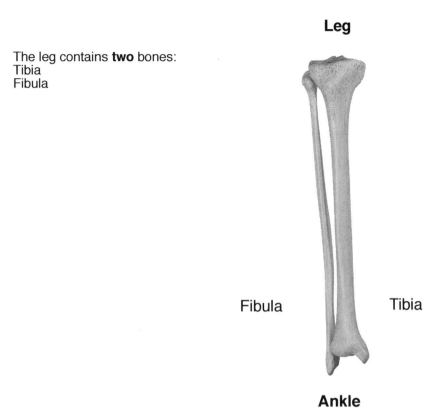

Fibula   Tibia

Ankle

The ankle is located distally to the leg, and it consists of the bones of the **tarsals**:

Calcaneus   Cuneiform I
Talus   Cuneiform II
Navicular   Cuneiform III
Cuboid

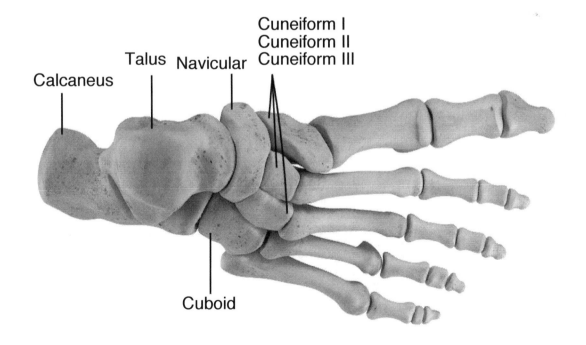

Cuneiform I
Cuneiform II
Talus Navicular Cuneiform III

Calcaneus

Cuboid

Foot

The foot contains **19** bones in each foot:
Metatarsals(5 bones)
Phalanges(14 bones)

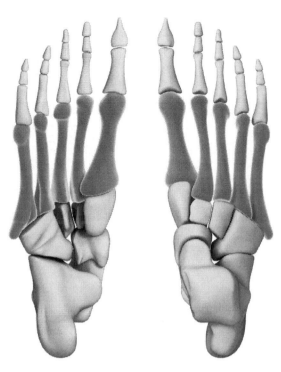

Metatarsals

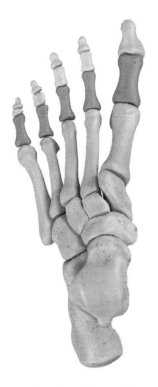

Proximal Phalanges

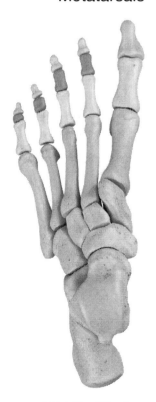

Middle Phalanges

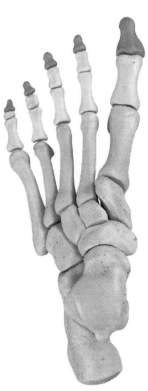

Distal Phalanges

Urinary System

The Urinary System is primarily responsible for **elimination** of **waste** from the body. It also assists in regulating the **pH level** of the body, and may also assist in reabsorption of substances back into the body.

The four main structures of the Urinary System are(in descending order) the **kidneys**, **ureters**, **urinary bladder**, and **urethra**.

Blood enters the kidneys through the renal arteries. Inside the kidneys, blood is **filtered** through the **nephrons**, which pulls waste products such as **urea** out of the blood. Inside each kidney, there are over one million nephrons. The waste products filtered out of the blood by the nephrons become **urine**. The nephrons also allow nutrients and water to be reabsorbed back into the blood stream.

Once urine has been created, it is sent from the kidneys to the urinary bladder through two small tubes known as ureters. The ureters only function as a **passageway** for urine.

Urine **collects** in the urinary bladder, until it is ready to be eliminated from the body. The urinary bladder expands as more urine is added to it. The urinary bladder can typically hold between 300-500 ml of fluid. Once urine is released from the urinary bladder, it passes through the urethra.

The urethra, much like the ureters, is a small tube that has one function: **transporting urine** from the urinary bladder **out of the body**.

The Urinary System

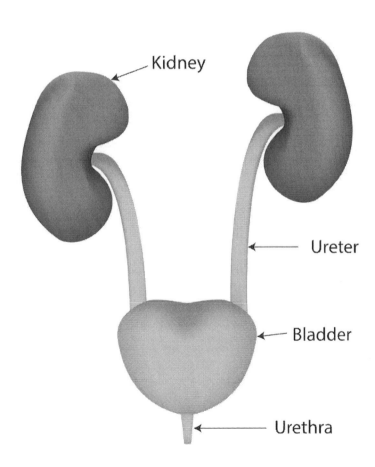

Kidney

Ureter

Bladder

Urethra

Anatomy and Physiology Matching

_____: Constant internal environment

_____: Suture connecting the two parietal bones

_____: Organ that creates bile and detoxifies blood

_____: Tissue responsible for separating structures

_____: Sensory receptor that detects pain

_____: Organ that filters blood and creates urine

_____: "Rest-and-digest" response

_____: Muscle contraction with constant tension and decreasing muscle length

_____: Gland responsible for the creation of T-Cells

_____: Muscle contraction with constant tension and increasing muscle length

_____: Region of the vertebral column with five bones

_____: Suture connecting the occipital bone and parietal bones

_____: Cell responsible for transporting oxygen and carbon dioxide

_____: Tissue responsible for protection, secretion, and absorption

_____: "Fight-or-flight" response

_____: Glands responsible for production of estrogen and progesterone

_____: Region of the vertebral column with seven bones

_____: Body plane that splits the body into superior and inferior

_____: Largest lymph vessel in the body

_____: Body plane that splits the body into anterior and posterior

A: Erythrocytes

B: Thymus

C: Homeostasis

D: Kidneys

E: Liver

F: Cervical Vertebrae

G: Transverse Plane

H: Epithelial Tissue

I: Thoracic Duct

J: Ovaries

K: Sagittal Suture

L: Concentric Contraction

M: Parasympathetic Response

N: Lambdoid Suture

O: Nociceptor

P: Lumbar Vertebrae

Q: Eccentric Contraction

R: Frontal Plane

S: Sympathetic Response

T: Connective Tissue

Anatomy and Physiology

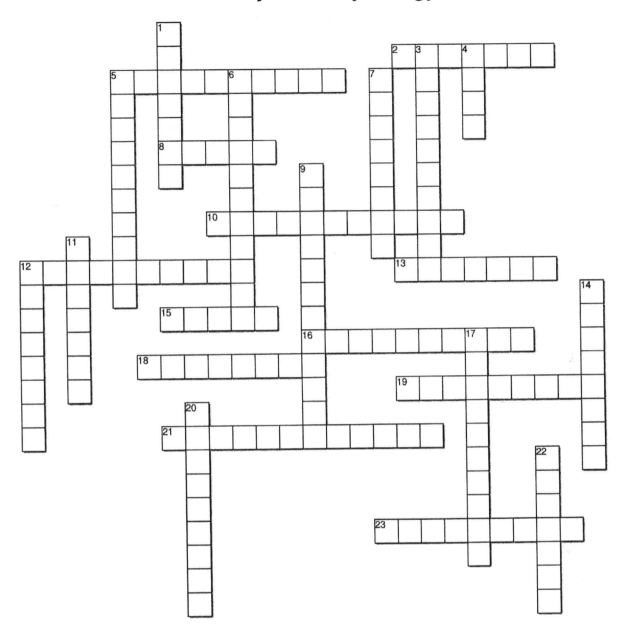

Across

2. Tissue that forms the brain, spinal cord, and nerves
5. Part of the brain regulating muscle tone and coordination
8. Largest artery in the body
10. Maintaining a constant internal environment
12. Study of the function of the human body
13. Air sacs where oxygen and carbon dioxide are exchanged
15. Organ that produces bile
16. Hormone produced by the thyroid
18. Carpal articulating with the radius
19. Valve located between the right atrium and right ventricle
21. Hormone produced by the ovaries
23. Cell that destroys pathogens

Down

1. Sphincter located between the esophagus and stomach
3. Tissue that forms glands and epidermis
4. Blood vessel that carries blood towards the heart
5. Contraction resulting in muscle tension increasing and muscle length decreasing
6. Cell that carries oxygen and carbon dioxide
7. Suture connecting the two parietal bones
9. Largest lymph vessel in the body
11. Most common form of cartilage in the body
12. Carpal bone that is a sesamoid bone
14. Suture connecting the occipital bone and parietal bones
17. Sensory receptor that detects pain
20. Carpal bone that helps create a saddle joint
22. Study of the structure of the human body

Anatomy and Physiology Fill-In-The-Blank

Anatomy is the study of the _____ of the human body.

Physiology is the study of the _____ of the human body.

Homeostasis

Homeostasis is the existence and maintenance of a constant _____, which is constantly changing due to stimuli such as hormones, temperature, and diet.

Regional Anatomy

Regional anatomy is the study of the body, broken down into different _____. To distinguish one structure from another, _____ are used.

- Superior: _____
- Inferior: _____
- Anterior: _____
- Posterior: _____
- Proximal: _____
- Distal: _____
- Medial: _____
- Lateral: _____
- Deep: _____
- Superficial: _____

Body Planes

A midsagittal plane splits the body into _____ left and right sides, running down the _____ of the body.

A sagittal plane splits the body into left and right, but not _____.

A transverse or horizontal plane splits the body into _____ and _____.

A frontal or coronal plane splits the body into _____ and _____.

Body Regions

The central body region contains all the structures located in the center of the body: the _____, _____, and _____.

The trunk can be divided into three regions: the _____, _____, and _____.

The upper limb can be broken down into four

regions: the _____, _____, _____, and _____.

The lower limb can be broken down into four regions: the _____, _____, _____, and _____.

Tissue

A tissue is made by a group of cells with similar _____ and _____. There are _____ types of tissue in the human body.

Epithelial tissue forms most _____, the _____ tract, the _____ tract, and the _____. It is responsible for _____, _____, and _____.

Muscular tissue creates _____. There are three types of muscles: _____, which connect to the skeleton, _____, which create the heart, and _____, which are found in places such as the digestive tract.

Nervous tissue forms the _____, _____, and _____. The primary cell of nervous tissue is known as a _____.

Neurons receive _____, brought into the cell by _____. The impulse is sent out of the neuron by way of the _____.

Connective tissue is the most _____ form of tissue in the body, creating structures such as bones, tendons, ligaments, cartilage, fascia, lymph, and blood. Connective tissue is responsible for _____ tissues, as well as _____ structures.

Blast cells are germ cells that _____ connective tissue.

Clast cells are cells that _____ connective tissue.

Blood is the most _____ form of connective tissue in the body, responsible for _____ of blood cells, hormones, nutrients, and waste products.

Erythrocytes, also known as _____ blood cells, are responsible for transporting _____ and _____ throughout the body. The cytoplasm is made of a protein called _____, which is what the elements attach to.

Leukocytes, also known as _____ blood cells, are the body's primary _____ against _____.

Thrombocytes, also known as _____, are responsible for _____ the blood.

Plasma is the _____ portion of blood, and allows the blood cells, hormones, nutrients, and waste products to be transported throughout the body.

Serous membranes are types of connective tissue that are used to _____ organs from one another. They accomplish this by _____ the organ.

The pericardium is located in the chest, and surrounds the _____.

The pleural membrane is located in the chest, and surrounds the _____.

The peritoneum is located in the _____ and _____.

The inner wall of a serous membrane, which comes into direct contact with the organ, is known as the _____ serous membrane.

The outer wall of a serous membrane, which comes into contact with other organs and bones, is known as the _____ serous membrane.

Cardiovascular System

The Cardiovascular System is responsible for _____ of nutrients and waste throughout the body.

The primary organ of the Cardiovascular System is the _____, which is responsible for _____ blood throughout the body.

Blood vessels are the main mode of _____ for blood. Arteries are blood vessels that carry blood _____ the heart. Veins are blood vessels that carry blood _____ the heart. Capillaries are microscopic _____, and are where gas exchange takes place between blood vessels and tissues.

Digestive System

The Digestive System is responsible for bringing food _____ the body, _____ of food, _____ of nutrients, and _____ of waste products.

The mouth, also known as the _____, is the first place digestion begins taking place. The _____ manually break down food by _____. The food mixes with _____, which breaks down carbohydrates. The _____ assists with mastication by pressing food against teeth.

Food moves from the mouth after swallowing through the _____, also called the throat.

Food moves into the _____, a long tube that runs from the pharynx inferiorly down to the _____. Smooth muscle in the esophagus contracts rhythmically, forcing food further down. This is known as _____.

Once food enters the stomach, both ends of the stomach close off, and the stomach begins _____ the food by churning it with powerful muscles. Once food is digested, it enters the _____.

The liver, an accessory organ, is responsible for _____ the blood. It also produces _____, which aids in the emulsification of fats.

The gallbladder is a small organ that is responsible for storing _____, and emptying it into the first part of the small intestine, known as the duodenum.

The pancreas produces _____, which increases glucose levels in the blood, and _____, which decreases glucose levels in the blood.

The small intestine consists of three parts: the _____, the _____, and the _____. Absorption of nutrients primarily takes place in the _____. Once nutrients have been absorbed by the small intestine, the food moves into the _____.

The large intestine is primarily responsible for absorption of _____ from feces, and elimination of _____ from the body.

Sphincters

A sphincter is a _____ band of muscle, which prevents food from moving backwards in the Digestive System.

The esophageal sphincter is located between the _____ and the _____.

The cardiac sphincter is located between the _____ and the _____.

The pyloric sphincter is located between the
_____ and the
_____.

The ileocecal sphincter is located between the
_____ and the
_____.

Endocrine System

The Endocrine System is responsible for
coordinating specific activities of cells and
tissues by releasing _____
into the body.

The adrenal glands secrete _____
and _____, which help
elevate blood pressure, heart rate, and blood
sugar.

The hypothalamus produces
_____, a hormone that increases
blood pressure and heart rate, and is
considered the reward center hormone.

The ovaries produce _____ and
_____, which are important to
female development and bone growth.

Pancreatic Islets are parts of the pancreas that
create _____ and
_____.

The pituitary gland, often considered the
"master gland", secretes _____
hormone, _____ to stimulate milk
production, and _____ hormone
to produce female egg cells and male sperm
cells.

The testes secrete _____, the
primary male hormone, responsible for
increasing bone and muscle mass.

The thyroid, located in the neck, produces
_____, which aids in decreasing
calcium levels in the blood stream.

Integumentary System

The Integumentary System is the body's first
line of _____ against
_____ and _____.
It's primary function is to
_____ the body.

The skin, the body's _____ organ,
helps to _____ the body.

The nails are responsible for _____
the fingers and toes from damage, and are
made of _____.

Glands

Inside the skin are glands. Sudoriferous glands
create and secrete _____. Sebaceous

glands create and secrete _____.

Sensory Receptors

Sensory receptors inside the skin help to detect
sensations and relay that information to the
_____.

Nociceptors are responsible for detection of
_____.

Meissner's Corpuscles are responsible for
detection of _____ pressure.

Pacinian Corpuscles are responsible for
detection of _____ pressure.

Lymphatic System

The Lymphatic System is vital in the body's
_____ against _____ and
_____.

Lymph is a fluid composed primarily of
_____, protein, leukocytes, urea, salts,
and glucose.

Lymph travels throughout the body through
_____, which are
similar to blood vessels, but only flow in one
direction: towards the _____. They
absorb foreign bodies and nutrients from
tissues. The largest _____ in
the body is located in the trunk, and is known as
the _____. It drains lymph
into the _____, where it
joins with blood.

Lymph nodes are large _____ of
lymphatic tissue, responsible for production of
_____.

The thymus is responsible for the production of
_____, also known as
_____, which are vital in regulation
of the body's immune system.

The spleen is responsible for _____
dead or dying _____.

Muscular System

Muscles are responsible for providing
movement, creating heat, and pumping blood
throughout the body.

Muscle Shapes

Muscles have many different shapes:

- Circular muscles are arranged in a
  _____ manner.
- Convergent muscles are _____ on
  one end and _____ together at another
  end.
- Parallel muscles have muscle fibers that all run
  in the _____ direction.

- Pennate muscles have an appearance resembling a _____.

Muscle Contractions

Muscle contractions result in _____ in a muscle.

Isometric contractions result in tension in a muscle _____ and the length of a muscle _____.

Isotonic contractions result in tension in a muscle _____ and the length of a muscle _____.

Concentric contractions result in tension in a muscle _____, then _____. The length of the muscle _____.

Eccentric contractions result in tension in a muscle _____, then _____. The length of the muscle _____.

Muscle Actions

Muscles perform numerous actions, including:

- Flexion: _____ the angle of a joint.
- Extension: _____ the angle of a joint.
- Adduction: Moving a structure _____ the midline.
- Abduction: Moving a structure _____ the midline.
- Protraction: Moving a structure _____.
- Retraction: Moving a structure _____.
- Inversion: Turning the _____ of the foot _____ towards the midline.
- Eversion: Turning the _____ of the foot _____ away from the midline.
- Elevation: Moving a structure _____.
- Depression: Moving a structure _____.
- Supination: Rotating the palm so it is facing _____.
- Pronation: Rotating the palm so it is facing _____.
- Rotation: _____ a structure around its long axis.
- Circumduction: _____ a structure around the _____ of a joint.
- Opposition: Moving structures in _____ directions.
- Lateral Deviation: Moving a structure from _____.
- Plantarflexion: Pointing toes _____.
- Dorsiflexion: Pointing toes _____.

A prime mover/agonist is the muscle that primarily performs a specific action, and is often the _____ muscle of a group of muscles that performs the action.

A synergist is a muscle that _____ the prime mover/agonist in performing the action.

An antagonist is a muscle that performs the _____ action of the prime mover/agonist.

A fixator is a muscle that _____ an area of joint while an action is being performed.

Nervous System

The Nervous System regulates vital functions, processes thought and mental input, and controls muscle.

There are two divisions of the Nervous System: the _____ Nervous System and the _____ Nervous System.

The Central Nervous System consists of the _____ and _____.

The brain consists of three parts: the _____, which is the largest portion of the brain, the _____, and the _____, which connects the brain to the spinal cord.

The Peripheral Nervous System consists of the body's _____. There are two divisions of the PNS: _____ Nerves, which emerge from the brain and contain _____ pairs, and _____ Nerves, which emerge from the spinal cord and contain _____ pairs.

Autonomic Nervous System

The Autonomic Nervous System helps to regulate _____ by release of hormones, controlling heart rate and breathing rate. There are two divisions of the Autonomic Nervous System: the _____ response, and the _____ response.

The Sympathetic Response is also known as "_____". When the body is in a state of _____, the Sympathetic Response helps the body respond by releasing _____ into the blood stream.

The Parasympathetic Response is also known as "_____". When the body is in a state of _____, the Parasympathetic Response helps the body to calm itself by decreasing heart rate and increasing blood flow to the digestive organs to increase _____. The Parasympathetic Response is controlled by the _____ Nerve.

Respiratory System

The Respiratory System functions to bring _____ into the body and eliminate wastes, such as _____ from the body.

The main organs of the Respiratory System are the _____. The left lung has _____ lobes and is smaller than the right lung, which has _____ lobes.

Conduction of air is controlled by the _____, which also filters air via _____ and _____.

The larynx, also known as the _____, is responsible for producing _____.

The epiglottis is a flap of tissue that prevents food or fluid from entering the larynx upon swallowing, which prevents _____.

The trachea is a tube of cartilage, also known as the _____. The trachea transports air into the lungs.

The trachea branches off into bronchial tubes. The bronchial tubes branch into smaller tubes called bronchioles. These tubes contain _____ to help trap any dirt or debris which have entered the lungs.

At the end of the bronchioles are tiny air sacs known as _____, which resemble a cluster of grapes. This is where oxygen and carbon dioxide are exchanged in the blood stream.

Respiration is accomplished by contraction of the _____, a large muscle connected to the rib cage that separates the chest from the abdomen. This muscle creates a vacuum inside the chest.

Skeletal System

The Skeletal System is a vital component of movement. It also helps to produce _____ cells, provide _____ for the body, and _____ structures and organs in the body.

There are _____ bones in the human body.

Long bones appear _____ than they are _____.

Short bones are _____ as they are _____.

Irregular bones are bones that have generally _____ shapes.

Flat bones are named after how they look: _____.

Sesamoid bones are bones embedded inside _____, and named after what they look like: _____.

Joints

Where bones come together is known as an _____.

Synarthrotic joints are joints with little to _____ movement.

Amphiarthrotic joints are joints that are _____ moveable.

Diarthrotic joints are joints that are _____ moveable.

Between bones that articulate, on the epiphyses, there is _____ cartilage. This type of cartilage is known as _____ cartilage, which prevents _____ between the articulating bones.

Certain joints, such as the glenohumeral and iliofemoral joints, have a specific type of cartilage in them known as a _____, which is used to _____ the joint, providing more strength and stability for the joint.

Bones are held together by _____.

Four of the most important joints are located in the skull, between the cranial bones. These synarthrotic joints are called _____.

The sagittal suture is located between the _____ bones.

The coronal suture is located between the _____ and _____ bones.

The squamous suture is located between the _____ and _____ bones.

The lambdoid suture is located between the _____ and _____ bones.

Muscles are held to bones via _____.

Inside of a joint itself, a membrane is present, known as the _____ membrane, which produces _____ fluid. This fluid helps lubricate the joint. Surrounding the entire joint is thick, dense connective tissue known as the _____, which keeps everything inside the joint, providing strength and support for the joint.

Types of Diarthrotic Joints

There are _____ different types of diarthrotic joints.

- Ball-and-socket joints feature one bone with a _____ at the epiphysis, and another bone with a _____.
- Hinge joints allow movement in _____ plane, allowing only _____ and _____.
- Pivot joints only allow _____ to take place.
- Plane/gliding joints are produced when the articulating bones have _____ surfaces, and there is a _____ of cartilage between the bones.
- Saddle joints are only located in one part of the body: the _____ joint of the _____.
- Ellipsoid/condyloid joints are extremely similar to ball-and-socket joints. On one bone, there is a _____, which resembles a ball, but isn't as pronounced. This fits into an _____ cavity on another bone, which is similar to a socket, but not as deep.

Skeletal Divisions

There are two divisions of the skeleton: the _____ Skeleton, and the _____ Skeleton.

The Axial Skeleton contains the _____, _____, and _____.

The Appendicular Skeleton contains all the bones that correspond to the _____.

The skull's primary function is to _____ the brain. The bones that make up the skull are: Parietal, Frontal, Temporal, Occipital, Zygomatic, Maxilla, Mandible, Vomer, Ethmoid, Sphenoid, Nasal, Lacrimal.

The vertebral column consists of 26 individual bones. Its primary function is to _____ the spinal cord. There are five different regions of the vertebral column: Cervical(____ vertebrae), Thoracic(____ vertebrae), Lumbar(____ vertebrae), Sacral(____ vertebrae), Coccygeal(____ vertebrae).

The chest consists of the rib cage. The primary function of the rib cage is to _____ vital organs inside the thorax, and assist in breathing by giving the diaphragm a place to attach. The rib cage consists of: True ribs(superior _____ ribs), False ribs(inferior ____ ribs), Floating ribs(ribs ___ and ___).

The pectoral girdle is responsible for holding the upper limbs to the body. The pectoral girdle consists of ____ bones: Scapulae(___ bones), Clavicles(___ bones).

The pelvic girdle is primarily responsible for holding the lower limbs to the body. The pelvic girdle contains: Ilium(___ bones), Ischium(___ bones), Pubis(___ bones), Sacrum(___ bone).

The arm contains one bone: _____.

The forearm contains two bones: _____ and _____.

The wrist contains the _____ bones: Scaphoid, Lunate, Triquetrum, Pisiform, Trapezium, Trapezoid, Capitate, Hamate.

The hand contains ___ bones: Metacarpals(___ bones), Phalanges(___ bones).

The thigh contains the _____ and _____ bone in the body, the _____.

The leg contains two bones: _____ and _____.

The ankle consists of the _____: Calcaneus, Talus, Navicular, Cuboid, Cuneiform I, Cuneiform II, Cuneiform III.

The foot contains ___ bones: Metatarsals(___ bones), Phalanges(___ bones).

Urinary System

The Urinary System is primarily responsible for _____ of waste from the body, and assisting in regulating the _____ level of the body.

There are four main structures of the Urinary System: the _____, _____, _____, and _____.

The kidneys are responsible for _____ the blood, pulling waste products such as _____ out of the blood. The waste products filtered out of the blood by the nephrons inside the kidneys become _____.

Urine exits the kidneys and into the ureters, small tubes that provide a _____ for urine to travel from the kidneys to the bladder.

The urinary bladder _____ urine and stores it until it is ready to be eliminated from the body.

Once urine is ready to leave the body, it leaves the urinary bladder and enters the urethra. The urethra _____ urine _____ the body.

Anatomy and Physiology Matching

C   P
K   N
E   A
T   H
O   S
D   J
M   F
L   G
B   I
Q   R

Anatomy and Physiology Answers

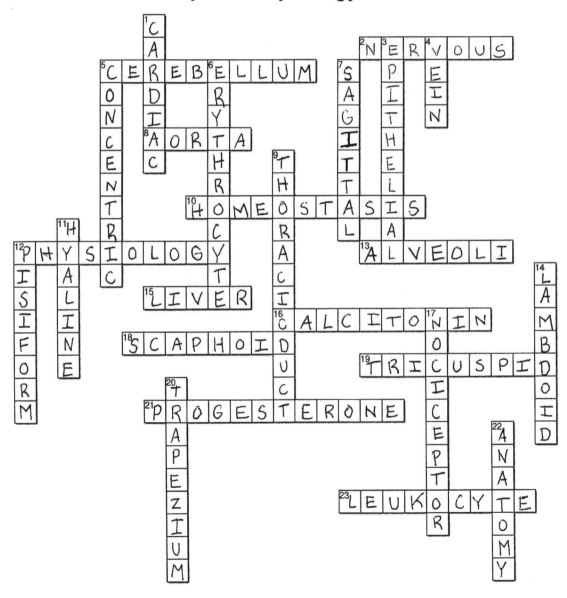

Anatomy and Physiology Practice Exam

1. The sympathetic nervous response is also referred to as
A. Housekeeping
B. Rest and digest
C. Fight or flight
D. Central

2. A sudoriferous gland is a type of exocrine gland that produces what substance
A. Oil
B. Sweat
C. Testosterone
D. Milk

3. The longest vein in the body, located on the medial aspect of the leg and thigh
A. Great saphenous
B. Femoral
C. External iliac
D. Brachial

4. The pituitary gland produces all of the following hormones except
A. Growth hormone
B. Testosterone
C. Follicle-stimulating hormone
D. Prolactin

5. Perirenal fat surrounds the
A. Rectum
B. Bladder
C. Liver
D. Kidneys

6. Primary function of a gland
A. Secretion
B. Protection
C. Absorption
D. Contraction

7. Branching muscle tissue is also called
A. Smooth
B. Skeletal
C. Cardiac
D. Striated

8. What aspect of the body is being studied in anatomy
A. Structure
B. Function
C. Diseases
D. Movement

9. Mastication is more commonly known as
A. Chewing
B. Swallowing
C. Sneezing
D. Defecating

10. The pulmonary arteries carry blood from the right ventricle to
A. Left atrium
B. Rest of the body
C. Aorta
D. Lungs

11. Beta cells produce
A. Bile
B. Glucagon
C. Somatostatin
D. Insulin

12. Where two bones come together
A. Fracture
B. Articulation
C. Contracture
D. Ellipsoid

13. T-lymphocytes are produced by which gland
A. Thymus
B. Thalamus
C. Pituitary
D. Pineal

14. Light pressure is detected by
A. Nociceptors
B. Pacinian corpuscles
C. Merkel discs
D. Meissner's corpuscles

15. The phrenic nerve emerges from the
A. Neck
B. Chest
C. Lumbar
D. Brain

16. Another name for a leukocyte is
A. Thrombocyte
B. Red blood cell
C. Platelet
D. White blood cell

17. The cervical plexus emerges from which sets of vertebrae
A. C1-C7
B. C1-C4
C. T1-T6
D. L1-S4

18. There are seven vertebrae in which region of the vertebral column
A. Thoracic
B. Cervical
C. Lumbar
D. Coccygeal

19. Erythrocytes
A. Carry oxygen and carbon dioxide throughout the body
B. Are also called neutrophils and perform phagocytosis
C. Produce thrombi at an area of trauma
D. Allow transport of blood cells throughout the body

20. Storage of bile is controlled by the
A. Gallbladder
B. Liver
C. Small intestine
D. Stomach

21. Absorption of nutrients primarily takes place in what part of the small intestine
A. Jejunum
B. Ileum
C. Duodenum
D. Cecum

22. The superior seven pairs of ribs are also called
A. Inferior ribs
B. False ribs
C. Superior ribs
D. True ribs

23. Waste moves through the large intestine in the following order
A. Transverse colon, ascending colon, sigmoid colon, descending colon
B. Sigmoid colon, descending colon, transverse colon, ascending colon
C. Ascending colon, transverse colon, descending colon, sigmoid colon
D. Descending colon, ascending colon, transverse colon, sigmoid colon

24. Peristalsis is controlled by which of the following types of muscle
A. Cardiac
B. Skeletal
C. Smooth
D. Striated

25. Vitamin D is produced in the following organ
A. Liver
B. Skin
C. Pancreas
D. Spleen

26. Glucagon is produced by
A. Delta cells
B. Beta cells
C. Alpha cells
D. Theta cells

27. Part of the respiratory passage that divides into the left and right bronchus
A. Larynx
B. Pharynx
C. Trachea
D. Epiglottis

28. Which of the following is not one of the four types of tissue
A. Nervous
B. Connective
C. Epithelial
D. Skeletal

29. The largest internal organ in the body
A. Liver
B. Stomach
C. Brain
D. Spleen

30. Enzyme located in the saliva which aids in digestion of carbohydrates
A. Epinephrine
B. Prolactin
C. Amylase
D. Parotid

31. The esophagus passes through the following structure on its way to the stomach
A. Peritoneum
B. Liver
C. Pericardium
D. Diaphragm

32. Heat creation is produced by which type of muscle tissue
A. Smooth
B. Cardiac
C. Skeletal
D. Adipose

33. The functional unit of tissue is called
A. Cell
B. Nerve
C. Blood
D. Muscle

34. Most superior portion of the sternum
A. Costal cartilage
B. Body
C. Xiphoid process
D. Manubrium

35. Which of the following molecules attaches to hemoglobin
A. Nitrogen
B. Oxygen
C. Helium
D. Argon

36. Breaking down food, absorption of nutrients, and elimination of waste is the function of which body system
A. Urinary
B. Digestive
C. Cardiovascular
D. Lymphatic

37. Non-striated muscle is
A. Involuntary
B. Voluntary
C. Controlled easily
D. Controlled by concentration

38. Connective tissue connecting bone to bone
A. Fascia
B. Tendon
C. Ligament
D. Dermis

39. There are how many pairs of spinal nerves in the peripheral nervous system
A. 24
B. 12
C. 18
D. 31

40. All of the following carry blood away from the heart except
A. Capillaries
B. Arteries
C. Arterioles
D. Veins

41. The ovaries and testes are examples of
A. Exocrine glands
B. Digestive organs
C. Endocrine glands
D. Cardiovascular vessels

42. Chyme moves from the stomach into the small intestine through which sphincter
A. Ileocecal
B. Cardiac
C. Pyloric
D. Esophageal

43. Epithelial tissue
A. Holds tissue together and separates tissues
B. Provides protection, secretes substances, and absorbs substances
C. Is found inside joints and helps to lubricate joints
D. Allows nerve impulses to be transmitted from the brain to muscles

44. The adrenal glands are located atop which organs
A. Large intestine
B. Small intestine
C. Kidneys
D. Ureters

45. Dopamine is an example of a
A. Hormone
B. Synapse
C. Neuron
D. Dendrite

46. The largest veins in the body, responsible for returning deoxygenated blood to the heart
A. Aorta
B. Vena Cava
C. Pulmonary arteries
D. Pulmonary veins

47. Function of serous membranes
A. Secreting sebum
B. Connect organs
C. Creating blood
D. Separate organs

48. Which of the following is not a structure in the digestive system
A. Gallbladder
B. Spleen
C. Liver
D. Pancreas

49. The first cervical vertebrae is also called the
A. Occiput
B. Axis
C. Atlas
D. Dens

50. Pepsin is located in the
A. Stomach
B. Small intestine
C. Pancreas
D. Gallbladder

Anatomy and Physiology Practice Exam Answer Key

01. C	26. C
02. B	27. C
03. A	28. D
04. B	29. A
05. D	30. C
06. A	31. D
07. C	32. C
08. A	33. A
09. A	34. D
10. D	35. B
11. D	36. B
12. B	37. A
13. A	38. C
14. D	39. D
15. A	40. D
16. D	41. C
17. B	42. C
18. B	43. B
19. A	44. C
20. A	45. A
21. A	46. B
22. D	47. D
23. C	48. B
24. C	49. C
25. B	50. A

For detailed answer explanations, watch the
video at mblextestprep.com/resources.html

Pathology

On the MBLEx, you will be asked several questions about pathology. These questions are meant to ensure you, the student, understand diseases and the disease process, and can properly assess a client and determine any potential contraindications.

In this section, we will discuss many subjects, covering a wide range of information.

Information covered in this section includes:

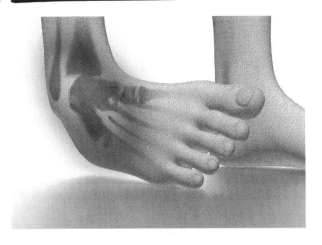

Pathology of the Cardiovascular System
Pathology of the Digestive System
Pathology of the Endocrine System
Pathology of the Integumentary System
Pathology of the Lymphatic System
Pathology of the Muscular System
Pathology of the Nervous System
Pathology of the Respiratory System
Pathology of the Skeletal System
Pathology of the Urinary System
Cancers
Medications
CPR
First Aid

This information is followed by four assignments:

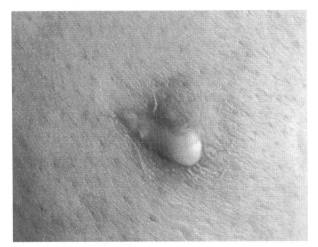

Pathology Matching
Pathology Crossword
Medications Word Search
Pathology Fill-In-The-Blank

The end of the section has a 50 question practice exam on Pathology. These questions ARE NOT the exact same questions will you see on the MBLEx. They are meant to test information that MAY be seen on the MBLEx.

While taking the practice exam, make sure to utilize your test-taking strategies(page 3) to optimize your test scores.

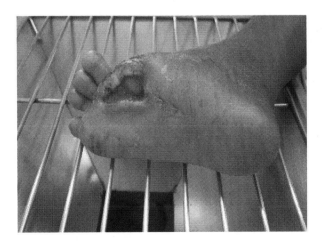

Pathology of the Cardiovascular System

Anemia
(an-: without; -emia: blood)

Anemia is a disease of the blood, resulting in a lack of **oxygen** and an over-abundance of carbon dioxide in the blood. There are many different types of anemia, ranging from iron-deficient anemia, to sickle cell anemia. Anemia is the most common blood condition in the United States, with an estimated 3.5-4 million people afflicted with it.

Iron-Deficient Anemia, again, is the most common form of anemia. The cells in the blood that are responsible for carrying oxygen and carbon dioxide throughout the body are the erythrocytes, or red blood cells. In the cytoplasm of erythrocytes, there is a protein present known as hemoglobin, which is made of iron. The hemoglobin attracts oxygen and carbon dioxide, allowing these molecules to attach to the erythrocytes.

In Iron-Deficient Anemia, the primary cause is a lack of iron being consumed. Less iron being consumed results in less **hemoglobin** in the erythrocytes, which in turn causes a lack of oxygen and carbon dioxide attaching to the red blood cells.

People with anemia may feel sluggish, tired, have an increased heart rate, may show paleness in the skin, shortness of breath, and experience dizziness, all due to a lack of sufficient oxygen reaching tissues.

Treatments for anemia vary depending on the type, but may include increasing iron intake, bone marrow transplants, or blood transfusions.

Aneurysm
(Greek "aneurysma": a widening)

An aneurysm is a condition of the arteries, resulting in a **bulge** in the wall of an artery. There are several different forms and causes of aneurysms.

Aneurysms are the result of a part of an arterial wall becoming weakened. When the wall of the artery becomes weakened, it forces the wall out, creating a pouch or bubble. Most commonly, aneurysms are the result of hypertension putting too much pressure or strain on the artery.

When the arterial wall stretches due to weakness, it makes it much easier for the artery to rupture. Because the artery carries oxygen-rich blood, this makes aneurysms very dangerous, as any rupture will severely cut off blood flow to the structure supplied with blood by the artery.

Common locations for aneurysms include the abdominal aorta and the brain. Aneurysms may be treated surgically before rupture to prevent major medical emergencies in the future. Beta blockers are commonly used as medications before surgery is required.

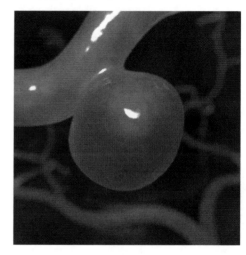

Aneurysm

Arrhythmia
(a-: without; rhythm: rhythm)

Arrhythmia is a condition of the heart, which results in the heart's natural **rhythm** being altered. There are several different forms of arrhythmia. Some of the most common forms of arrhythmia are Atrial Fibrillation, Bradycardia, and Tachycardia.

Atrial Fibrillation, the most common form of arrhythmia, results when the atria, the heart's upper chambers, contract irregularly, which sends blood into the ventricles at uncoordinated times. This is caused by an electrical signal from the SA Node not firing correctly, which disrupts the timing of the atria contracting. This can affect the ability of the heart to consistently deliver oxygenated blood to the body.

Bradycardia(brady-: slow; -cardia: heart) results in the heart rate being reduced to a rate of contraction that is considered too slow to deliver substantial oxygen to the body.

Tachycardia(tachy-: rapid; -cardia: heart) results in the heart rate being increased to a rate of contraction that is considered too rapid. In Tachycardia, the ventricles of the heart are contracting too rapidly, which may cause a lack of oxygen-rich blood from reaching the body, as the quick contractions do not allow the ventricles to properly fill with blood before being pumped out to the rest of the body.

Treatments vary, depending on the type of arrhythmia a person suffers from. Medical devices, such as pacemakers, may be implanted into the body to help regulate and control heart rhythm(IE, if a person's heart rate drops too low, the pacemaker will stimulate the heart muscle and cause it to contract, increasing heart rate back to safe levels). Alternative methods to controlling arrhythmia, such as massage therapy and yoga, may be applied in some cases.

Heart Murmur

A heart murmur is a condition of the heart, which results in blood flowing **backwards** in the heart. A "murmur" refers to the sound of blood flowing through the heart.

Heart murmurs may not require any medical attention, depending on the cause. Other times, medical attention may be needed. Most commonly, heart murmurs are the result of a **bicuspid/mitral valve** prolapse, where the valve is pulled backwards into the left atrium. This allows blood to flow backwards in the heart, which may reduce the ability of the heart to pump enough oxygen-rich blood to the body.

Heart murmurs may require the person to take anticoagulants to prevent the formation of blood clots, may be treated for hypertension if it is resulting in heart murmurs, or may need surgery to repair the malfunctioning valve.

Hypertension
(hyper-: above; -tension: tension)

Hypertension is a condition of the cardiovascular system, resulting in **elevated blood pressure**. There are numerous factors that may contribute to the development of hypertension. For an average healthy adult, systolic blood pressure(pressure felt in arteries when the heart beats) is around 120 mmHg, and diastolic pressure(pressure felt in arteries when the heart is at rest) is around 80 mmHg. To be diagnosed with hypertension, a person's systolic pressure would be 140 mmHg and diastolic pressure would be 90 mmHg.

Hypertension may have no underlying cause, or may be the result of factors such as dysfunction of the adrenal glands or thyroid, dietary issues such as obesity or high sodium intake, kidney disease, and alcohol consumption.

Untreated, hypertension may lead to numerous serious medical conditions, such as myocardial infarction, stroke, atherosclerosis, and aneurysm. Luckily, hypertension is very easy to detect, and very treatable. Often times, treatment is as simple as making lifestyle or dietary changes, such as consuming less sodium and increasing exercise. Other times, hypertension may require the use of medications such as beta blockers, statins, and diuretics.

Main complications of hypertension

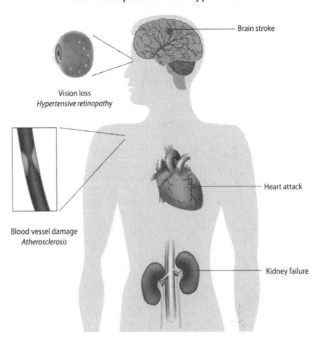

Side effects of hypertension

Migraine Headaches

Migraine Headaches are a type of headache that affect the brain, which results in most side effects experienced. Symptoms include nausea, fatigue, extreme pain, loss of sight, and many more.

Migraines have been referred to as "**vascular** headaches", due to the involvement of blood vessels. In migraines, when the brain is stimulated by a trigger, neurons rapidly send impulses which affects the blood vessels surrounding the meninges, three layers of connective tissue that surround and protect the brain. At first, the blood vessels constrict, which does not result in pain. A short time after constricting, the blood vessels will dilate, which places immense pressure on the meninges, which results in severe pain.

Migraines have numerous causes, which may be from exposure to substances like tyramine(a naturally occurring chemical found in foods such as aged cheese, alcoholic beverages, and cured meats), caffeine, stress, or even hormonal imbalance during stages such as menstruation. Migraines may even be considered hereditary.

Myocardial Infarction
(myo-: muscle; -cardia: heart; infarct: obstruction of blood flow)

A Myocardial Infarction, or heart attack, is a condition that affects the heart muscle, reducing blood flow throughout the body.

An Infarction is an obstruction of blood flow to a specific part of the body. In this case, blood flow to the heart is obstructed. The two arteries that supply blood to the heart muscle are known as the coronary arteries. When an abundance of substances such as plaque build up inside these arteries, it restricts blood flow to the heart muscle. When blood flow is restricted, the tissue does not receive adequate oxygen, which results in **necrosis** of the affected tissue. When too much cardiac muscle dies, the body experiences a myocardial infarction, or heart attack.

Myocardial Infarctions may be the result of atherosclerosis(athero-: fatty plaque), a condition which causes the artery walls to harden and thicken, due to a build-up of plaque in the arteries. Hypertension, smoking, and obesity may also contribute to the development of atherosclerosis.

A person who has suffered from a myocardial infarction may have a coronary bypass surgery performed, an angioplasty or stent placed in the affected artery, or may not need any surgery and only requires medications such as aspirin, beta blockers, and statins.

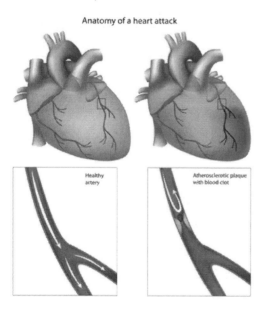

Anatomy of a heart attack

Healthy artery

Atherosclerotic plaque with blood clot

Plaque buildup in the arteries, resulting in ischemia and necrosis of cardiac tissue

Phlebitis
(phleb-: vein; -itis: inflammation)

Phlebitis is a condition of the cardiovascular system, affecting the **veins**, causing them to become **inflamed**. Blood clots may form in these veins.

Phlebitis may have numerous causes, including trauma to a vein, and immobility. Trauma to a

vein results in what is known as superficial phlebitis, usually the result of IV catheters being placed into a vein via needles.

Deep vein thrombosis is another type of phlebitis, taking place deeper in the body. Deep vein thrombosis(DVT) is most commonly caused by immobility of a limb. The body's veins move and stretch with the rest of the body during movement. If the veins are immobilized, they will become irritated, due to blood pooling in the veins. The blood pooling may result in blood clot formation. If a blood clot dislodges from its location and flows freely in the blood stream, it is known as an embolus, which could become lodged in other blood vessels throughout the body, cutting off blood flow and resulting in ischemia. Depending on the part of the body this takes place, it could even lead to possible death.

Treatments of phlebitis include anticoagulants for deep vein thrombosis such as heparin, ibuprofen, and antibiotics for superficial phlebitis.

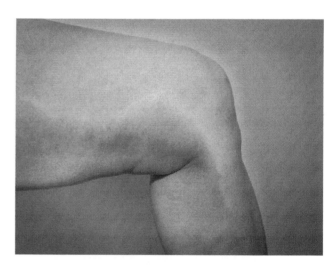

Deep vein thrombosis

Raynaud's Syndrome

Raynaud's Syndrome is a condition that results in **constriction** of the blood vessels in the **fingers** and **toes**, reducing **circulation** to these areas. This constriction is known as "vasospasm". Primary Raynaud's Syndrome occurs independently, while Secondary Raynaud's Syndrome is typically associated with other conditions.

The primary contributors to Raynaud's Syndrome are cold temperatures, stress, and cigarette smoking. Raynaud's Syndrome is typically not a debilitating disease. During a flare-up, the skin typically turns white, the person may experience numbness or pain, and the affected areas become very cold.

Secondary Raynaud's Syndrome may be associated with conditions such as lupus or scleroderma, and develops later in life than Primary Raynaud's Syndrome.

Treatments for Raynaud's Syndrome include exercise, reducing stress, not smoking, and avoiding cold temperatures whenever possible. Secondary Raynaud's Syndrome may require medications such as statins to help regulate blood pressure and cholesterol.

Varicose Veins
(varicose: abnormally swollen)

Varicose veins are the abnormal swelling of veins in the body, most commonly seen in the **legs**, but may be present in any vein. There are many different types, ranging from regular varicose veins, to spider veins, and even hemorrhoids.

Inside the veins, there are valves that push deoxygenated blood back up to the heart. Typically, as a person ages, the valves stop working as efficiently, which allows blood to pool **backwards** in the veins. This added pressure causes irritation and swelling of the veins. Blood pooling in the veins may also lead to complications such as the development of blood clots.

Because veins are much more superficial than arteries, when a vein becomes swollen, it is often visible. Varicose veins often present with a purple color, may look cord-like, and may even cause pain and discomfort. Causes of varicose veins include sitting or standing for prolonged periods, age, and even pregnancy.

Treatment is often unnecessary, outside of self-care. Self-care may include wearing compression socks, exercise, diet, and elevating the legs to help circulation. If treatment is required, there are a number of different things that can be done, all the way up to removing the varicose vein from the body
.

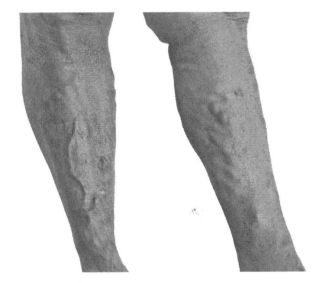

Varicose Veins

Pathology of the Digestive System

Diverticulitis
(diverticula: tubular sac branching off a cavity;
-itis: inflammation)

Diverticulitis is a condition affecting the large intestine, but may also affect other structures such as the abdomen, or the entire cardiovascular system. If a person is affected by diverticulosis, they have small pouches that develop in the large intestine. In certain cases, these pouches may become **inflamed** and/or **infected**, which then becomes diverticulitis.

Diverticulitis, because it puts strain on sections of the large intestine that are already weakened, may result in ulcerations, or open sores. These open sores may lead to infection, and leaking of feces into the abdomen, which results in peritonitis(inflammation of the peritoneum, a very serious condition that requires medical attention).

Diverticulitis may be treated in several different ways, depending on the severity. Pain medication may help with discomfort in less severe cases. In recurring diverticulitis, scarring may be present, which could lead to backing up of fecal content in the large intestine. Infections will require antibiotics.

Diverticulosis
(diverticula: tubular sac branching off a cavity;
-osis: condition)

Diverticulosis is a condition affecting the large intestine, which presents with **pouches** forming in the walls of the large intestine, typically in the descending and/or sigmoid colons. It is a common condition seen in roughly half of people over the age of 65.

During peristalsis, the smooth muscle located in the walls of the large intestine contract, forcing food to move further through the organ and eventually out of the body. If the large intestine does not contain enough fecal matter, as in the case of a low-fiber diet, the contractions may result in weakening of the wall of the large intestine. As a result, small pouches may develop.

If a person develops diverticulosis, small pieces of feces, nuts, seeds, etc, may become stuck inside the pouches. If feces becomes trapped in a pouch, the large intestine will absorb all of the water from it, and it will become very solid and extremely hard to remove. This may result in pain in the abdomen.

Treatment primarily includes increasing intake of fiber via fruits and vegetables, and increasing fluid intake to make passing of stool easier to manage.

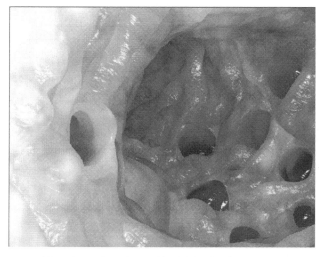

Pouches developed inside a large intestine

Hepatitis
(hepat-: liver; -itis: inflammation)

Hepatitis is a condition that results in **inflammation** of the **liver**. There are numerous causes of hepatitis, which affect numerous different organ systems. Most commonly, hepatitis is the result of a **viral** infection, but may also result from toxic substances entering into the body, such as alcohol. Short-term symptoms of hepatitis include jaundice(yellowing of the skin due to increased bilirubin in the blood stream), fever, and nausea. Long-term symptoms include cirrhosis(destruction of healthy liver cells), scarring of the liver, liver cancer, and liver failure.

There are five known hepatitis viruses: Hepatitis A, B, C, D, and E. Each varies in mode of contraction, and severity in symptoms.

Hepatitis A is the most common form, and is typically transmitted through ingestion of fecal matter(most commonly seen in parts of the world with low sanitation standards). People infected with Hepatitis A most frequently make a full recovery, and develop an immunity to the virus.

Hepatitis B is typically transmitted through exposure to body fluids such as blood. The virus produces symptoms for a period greater than Hepatitis A, but most people will develop an immunity to it after about four weeks. A small percentage of people who contract Hepatitis B will become chronically affected by it. Vaccines for Hepatitis B are available.

Hepatitis C, much like Hepatitis B, is contracted through exposure to body fluids such as blood. Hepatitis C is a chronic condition which damages the liver even further each time the person's symptoms are in the acute stage. Hepatitis C is one of the leading causes of liver failure.

Hepatitis D is an infection that only results in symptoms if the person is also infected with the Hepatitis B virus. When this occurs, major complications may arise. Because Hepatitis D is only activated by the Hepatitis B virus, the Hepatitis B vaccine may contribute to the prevention of Hepatitis D.

Hepatitis E, like Hepatitis A, is contracted through exposure to fecal matter. It is most commonly seen in developing countries, where sanitation standards may not be high. Hepatitis E, if severe, may lead to liver failure, despite being an acute infection.

Treatments vary, depending on severity. Immunizations are available for Hepatitis B, and medications may help reduce the symptoms.

A hiatal hernia results from part of the stomach protruding upwards through the diaphragm, into the chest. Gastroesophageal Reflux Disease may result from this type of hernia, where stomach acids leak from the stomach backwards into the esophagus.

An umbilical hernia, most commonly seen in infants, is caused by the small intestine protruding through the abdominal wall and into the umbilicus. This condition usually resolves on its own.

An inguinal hernia, most commonly seen in men, is caused by the small intestine protruding through the wall of the abdomen, which typically descends into the scrotum. This may cause trauma to the testes. Sometimes, the small intestine may even drop farther down the body, into the thigh.

Treatments may include dietary changes in cases such as a hiatal hernia, weight loss, medication such as antacids, or even surgery to repair the hernia.

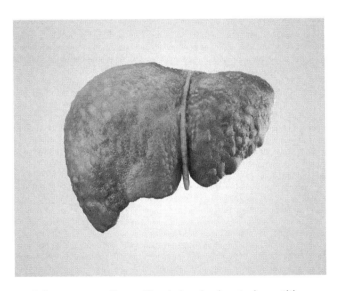

A liver presenting with cirrhosis due to hepatitis

Hernia
(hernia: a rupture)

A hernia is a rupture in a muscle or connective tissue, allowing an organ or other tissue to **protrude** through its normal location. There are many different types of herniae in the digestive system, including hiatal, umbilical, and inguinal.

A hernia is caused by a weakness in the affected tissue, and/or straining of the tissue. When the tissue tears, the organ, usually the small intestine, protrudes through it. This can lead to many complications, such as organ strangulation, constipation, pain, or even trauma to other structures, such as the testes.

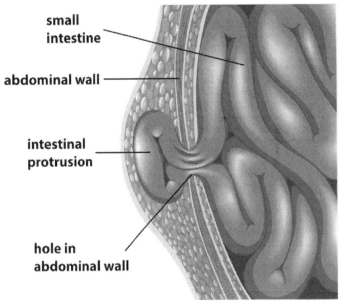

Strangulated Hernia

small intestine

abdominal wall

intestinal protrusion

hole in abdominal wall

Pathology of the Endocrine System

Addison's Disease

Addison's Disease is an autoimmune disorder affecting the adrenal glands, which results in a lack of cortisol and/or aldosterone production.

Addison's Disease is caused by damage to the **adrenal cortex** by the body's immune system. Damage to these glands results in an inability to produce cortisol, which regulates stress levels in the body by helping control blood sugar, blood pressure, and metabolism, and aldosterone, which aids in reabsorption of water and sodium back into the blood stream.

Addison's Disease may result in fatigue, weight loss, low blood pressure, hair loss, and nausea. It may become life-threatening if not treated.

Treatment primarily consists of hormone replacements, which may be taken orally or injected.

Addison's disease

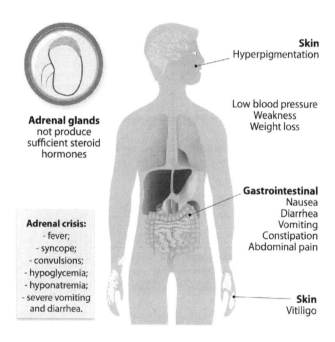

Adrenal glands
not produce
sufficient steroid
hormones

Skin
Hyperpigmentation

Low blood pressure
Weakness
Weight loss

Gastrointestinal
Nausea
Diarrhea
Vomiting
Constipation
Abdominal pain

Adrenal crisis:
- fever;
- syncope;
- convulsions;
- hypoglycemia;
- hyponatremia;
- severe vomiting
and diarrhea.

Skin
Vitiligo

Cushing's Disease

Cushing's Disease is a disease of the pituitary gland, which results in hyper-production of adrenocorticotropic hormone(ACTH).

Cushing's Disease is the result of hyperplasia(excessive growth) of the pituitary gland, or development of a tumor. This causes too much ACTH to be released in the body, which stimulates hyper-production of **cortisol**.

Cushing's Disease may result in weight gain around the face and torso, weakening of bone, thinning of skin, and fatigue, amongst other complications.

Treatments for Cushing's Disease include surgery to remove a tumor, and hormone therapy to reduce the production of cortisol.

SYMPTOMS
of Cushing's syndrome

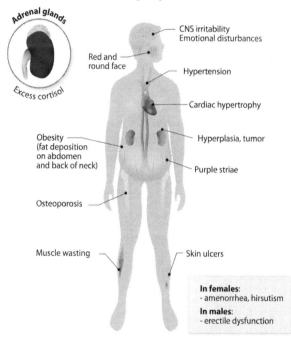

Adrenal glands

Excess cortisol

CNS irritability
Emotional disturbances

Red and
round face

Hypertension

Cardiac hypertrophy

Obesity
(fat deposition
on abdomen
and back of neck)

Hyperplasia, tumor

Purple striae

Osteoporosis

Muscle wasting

Skin ulcers

In females:
- amenorrhea, hirsutism
In males:
- erectile dysfunction

Diabetes Mellitus

Diabetes Mellitus is a condition of the endocrine system that affects **insulin** function in the body.

There are three types of diabetes: Diabetes Type I, Diabetes Type II, and Gestational Diabetes.

Diabetes Type I is often known as juvenile diabetes, as it begins in childhood. In Type I, the body's immune system attacks the pancreas, the organ that produces insulin. This results in the body not producing enough insulin, which the body needs in order to convert glucose to energy.

Diabetes Type II, the most common form of diabetes, is caused by the body having an insulin resistance. The insulin in the body is unable to break down glucose, which causes high levels of sugar in the blood stream. Obesity is a common cause of Diabetes Type II.

Gestational Diabetes is only present during pregnancy. Gestational Diabetes typically affects less than 10% of all pregnant women, and typically resolves after pregnancy ends.

Treatment for Diabetes Type I is primarily insulin injections. Treatment for Diabetes Type II includes medications, but exercise and dietary changes are most common. Treatment for Gestational Diabetes includes exercise, regulating weight gain during pregnancy, and possibly insulin medication depending on the severity.

Grave's Disease

Grave's Disease is an autoimmune disorder, in which the body's immune system attacks the thyroid gland, causing an increase in thyroid hormone production(**hyperthyroidism**).

Grave's Disease can affect numerous parts of the body, resulting in sensitivity to heat, weight loss, the development of a goiter(enlargement of the thyroid), bulging of the eyes, and irregular heart rhythm. Women are more likely to develop Grave's Disease, as well as people under the age of 40.

Treatment for Grave's Disease include medications such as beta blockers and anti-thyroid medications. If medication isn't helpful, surgical removal of the thyroid may be an option.

Hypothyroidism

Hypothyroidism is a primarily autoimmune disorder affecting the thyroid gland, resulting in a lack of **thyroid hormone** being produced.

When the body's immune system attacks the thyroid, it destroys healthy thyroid cells. When too many of these cells have been destroyed, the thyroid may not produce sufficient amounts of thyroid hormone. Hypothyroidism may also be the result of a previously inflamed thyroid, which can also damage thyroid cells.

Lack of thyroid hormone may result in weight gain, fatigue, hair loss, sensitivity to cold, and pain throughout the body.

Synthetic thyroid hormones may be prescribed to increase thyroid hormone levels in the body.

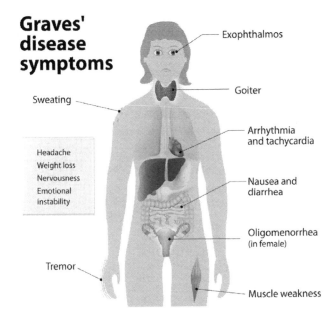

Graves' disease symptoms

- Exophthalmos
- Goiter
- Sweating
- Arrhythmia and tachycardia
- Headache
- Weight loss
- Nervousness
- Emotional instability
- Nausea and diarrhea
- Oligomenorrhea (in female)
- Tremor
- Muscle weakness

Pathology of the Integumentary System

Acne

Acne is an infection of the skin, resulting from numerous factors. Acne may result in whiteheads, blackheads, or even cysts if left untreated.

Acne is caused by an increased production of sebum on the skin, which results in blocked pores. These blocked pores may become **infected**, which may develop into pustules. There are several contributing factors that lead to the development of acne, including **testosterone** production, stress, hormonal imbalances, and poor personal hygiene.

Treatment includes over the counter skin care products for mild acne, or in the case of severe acne, medications such as birth control pills to regulate hormone levels in women, and antibiotics to eliminate bacterial growth. Other treatments include light therapy and chemical peels.

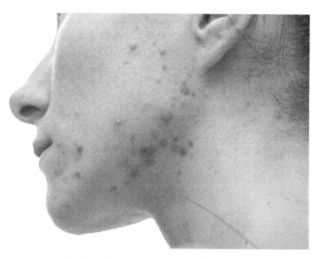

Localized skin infection commonly seen with acne

Athlete's Foot
(tinea: fungus; pedis: foot)

Athlete's Foot(also known as Tinea Pedis) is a **fungal** infection of the foot. Despite the name, anyone may develop Athlete's Foot, not just athletes. Athlete's Foot, like other fungal infections such as ringworm and jock itch, is highly contagious.

Athlete's Foot is caused by exposure to fungus on the foot. When a person wears tight-fitting shoes, it provides an environment for the fungus to thrive: a warm, humid, dark space. The fungus spreads, growing between the toes, then expanding across the foot. The infection causes the skin to become dry and scaly, which may result in breaking of the skin and bacterial infection.

Treatment of Athlete's Foot primarily consists of over the counter medications, in addition to self-care, such as ensuring the foot and footwear are dry as much as possible, wearing shower shoes in public bathing areas, etc.

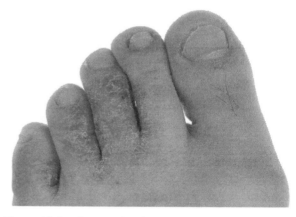

Fungal infection on the feet, known as Tinea Pedis

Boil

A boil is a **bacterial** infection of a hair follicle, also known as a **furuncle**. A group of these infections together in one localized area is known as a carbuncle.

A boil typically results from small cuts in the skin(caused by things like shaving), allowing staphylococci bacterium to enter the body and reproduce. Boils can be red, inflamed, and painful to the touch. The lump initially produced by the infection begins to soften over a few days, and becomes much more painful. Pus develops on the affected area.

Boils are treated by lancing(draining) the area with application of antibacterial soap and water, or in more severe cases, prescription of antibiotics to combat the bacterial infection.

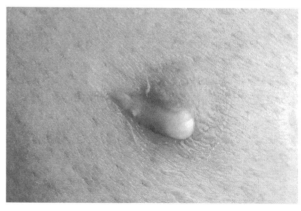

Boil

Burns

Burns are a skin condition in which the skin is damaged due to exposure to **heat** or **chemicals**. This may result in inflammation, blister formation, or necrosis, depending on the severity of the burn.

Burns of the skin can be categorized as first, second, third, or fourth degree, with first being the least severe.

A first degree burn only affects the epidermis. It may lead to pain and inflammation of the skin, but nothing more. A common first degree burn is a sun burn. The pain and inflammation subsides in a day or two, and the skin returns to normal.

A second degree burn is more severe. In a second degree burn, the burn moves through the epidermis and into the dermis. Because the burn goes deeper into the skin, it causes more damage, which can be seen by blistering. Blisters form to help repair the damage done by the burn. Second degree burns may result in scarring if they are too severe.

Third degree burns move even deeper into the skin, reaching the subcutaneous layer of the skin. Third degree burns often cause severe tissue damage and necrosis. Skin grafts may be needed to help repair an area affected by a third degree burn.

While first, second, and third degree burns are most common, a fourth degree burn moves completely through all layers of the skin, and goes deeper into tissues beneath the skin, such as tendons, ligaments, muscles, and bones.

Treatment for burns often depends on the severity of the burn. Application of aloe vera may help reduce the pain in first degree burns. Second degree burns may require bandages with topical antibiotic cream to prevent infection. Third degree burns, again, may require surgery and skin grafts to repair the affected areas.

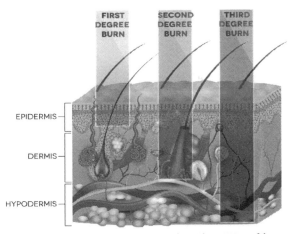

Depth of skin affected by varying degrees of burns

Cellulitis
(cell: cell; -itis: inflammation)

Cellulitis is a bacterial infection of the skin, causing symptoms such as inflammation of the infected area, fever, pain, and blisters.

Cellulitis is caused by **staphylococci** bacterium entering the body through exposure to **wounds**, most commonly on the legs. The infection typically stays localized, but continues to spread to surrounding tissues as the bacteria grows. The infection can present with well-defined borders of infection. If the infection enters the blood stream, it may result in septicemia, a potentially life-threatening condition.

Spider or insect bites may also introduce the bacterium into the body. Any insect bite should be cleaned thoroughly to prevent infection.

Treatment for cellulitis includes antibiotic medication, taken orally. Cellulitis is not typically contagious.

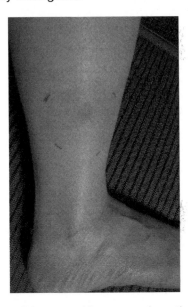

Cellulitis caused by a scorpion sting

Decubitus Ulcer
(decubitus: the act of lying down; ulcer: open sore)

A decubitus ulcer is a condition affecting the skin, resulting in the development of open sores.

Decubitus ulcers are also known as **bed sores** or **pressure ulcers**. When the body is in a static position for an extended period of time, such as when lying down, the parts of the body coming in contact with the bed, floor, or chair experience **ischemia**, a reduction of blood flow to the tissues due to pressure. When ischemia is present for too long, the tissue experiences **necrosis** due to a lack of oxygen. The dead tissue becomes ulcerated, and bacterial infection may occur.

People who are prone to decubitus ulcers are the elderly, disabled people, and people confined to a bed or wheelchair.

Treatments for decubitus ulcers vary, depending on the severity of the ulceration. If an infection is present, antibiotics may be prescribed. If there is an abundance of necrotic tissue, cleaning of the area(debridement) may be performed. If there is ischemia, but no ulcer, massage and application of heat may help bring blood back into the area.

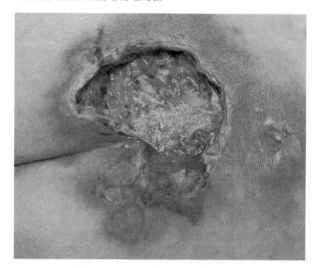

Open sore resulting from sustained ischemia and necrosis

Herpes Simplex
(herpein: to creep; simplex: simple)

Herpes Simplex is a **viral** infection of the skin. There are two types of Herpes Simplex: Herpes Simplex I, which causes sores around the mouth, and Herpes Simplex II, which causes sores around the genitals.

Herpes Simplex is highly contagious, passing between people via direct contact. During an acute outbreak, a sore may appear on the skin, most commonly the mouth, face, or genitals. This sore disappears after a short time. Despite not having any sores present, a person may still be able to transmit the virus to another asymptomatically.

While there is no cure for Herpes Simplex, medications may be prescribed to reduce the chance of spreading the infection to others.

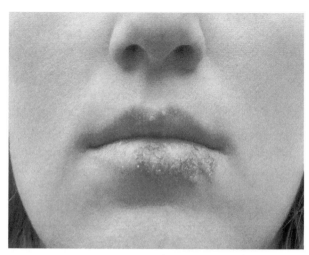

Sore development on the face and lips, typically seen with Herpes Simplex

Impetigo
(impetere: to attack)

Impetigo is a **bacterial** infection of the skin, most commonly seen in children. Impetigo is often confused with Hand, Foot, and Mouth Disease, which is a viral infection.

Impetigo is a highly contagious infection, caused by staphylococci or streptococci, which most commonly enter the body through already damaged skin, but may affect healthy skin as well. When the bacteria enters the skin, it produces sores that blister and leak a yellow, crust-like fluid. These sores typically develop around the mouth, nose, and ears.

Depending on the severity of the infection, impetigo may be treated with topical antibiotic cream for less severe cases, or with oral antibiotics for more severe cases. Recovery time is typically around one week with the use of medication.

Psoriasis
(psora-: to itch; -iasis: condition)

Psoriasis is an **autoimmune** disorder of the skin, resulting in the production of thick, dry, scaly patches. Psoriasis has periods of exacerbation and remission, where the patches appear and then resolve themselves.

The exact cause of psoriasis is unknown. Certain triggers, such as stress, may cause the body's immune system to attack the skin. Normally, skin cells have a life span of 3-4 weeks, and ultimately flake off the body. When the immune system attacks the skin, the body responds by increasing production of epithelial cells at an extremely rapid pace, which is much faster than the cells are being destroyed. This rapid pace of cell production is what produces the patches on the skin.

There is no cure for psoriasis, but treatments

are available to help manage the condition. Treatments include topical creams(which may contain steroids), exposure to sunlight, and application of aloe vera.

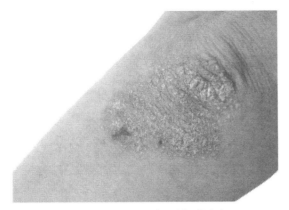

Increased buildup of epithelial tissue

Ringworm
(dermato-: skin; phyt-: plant; -osis: condition)

Ringworm(also known as dermatophytosis) is a **fungal** infection of the skin, similar to Athlete's Foot. Despite the name, it is not a parasitic infection. It results in a ring-like area of infection.

Fungus, like the kind found in ringworm, live on the dead cells of the body, such as the epidermis. When ringworm is contracted, it forms red blisters and a ring of infection begins to show, which then spreads as the infection grows through the skin.

Ringworm is contagious, and may be spread from person to person. It is especially common in athletes, whose bodies come in close contact with one another, such as wrestlers.

Treatment includes good personal hygiene, and most commonly application of antifungal ointment to the affected area. More severe cases may require oral antifungal medication.

Sebaceous Cyst

A sebaceous cyst is a condition affecting the skin, but may affect other tissues as well.

A **sebaceous** gland produces oil, and secretes oil onto the surface of the skin. If a blockage of a sebaceous gland occurs, oil cannot escape the gland, and bacteria may infect the area. If too much bacteria is present, the body may develop connective tissue that surrounds the infected sebaceous gland, trapping it inside. This is a sebaceous cyst.

Sebaceous cysts may be large or small. They may be painful to the touch, or may lead to localized infections known as abscesses. Cysts may need to be removed surgically. If the entire cyst membrane is not removed, there may be a chance of the cyst returning in the future.

Treatment, if necessary, includes moist compresses on the area to help drain the cyst, or possible surgery if there is a risk of infection.

Wart

Warts(also known as verrucae), are small benign growths on the skin, caused by the **human papilloma virus(HPV)**.

Warts are contagious, and may be spread by direct skin contact. The human papilloma virus stimulates the skin to produce more keratin, which causes a hard, thick overgrowth on a small localized area. This is a wart.

Warts may be located in numerous locations on the body, including the hands, feet(plantar warts), and genitals(genital warts).

Warts often go into remission on their own, and treatment is not necessary. Treatment options include cryotherapy to freeze the wart, excising (cutting out) the wart, or electrosurgery to burn the wart.

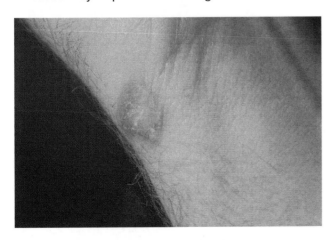

Circular rash seen with ringworm

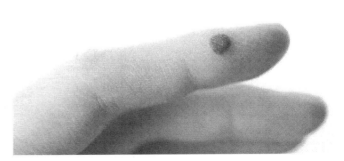

Wart

Pathology of the Lymphatic System

Allergy

An allergy is a reaction of the body's immune system in response to substances that normally **do not affect people**. Common substances people may be allergic to include dust, pollen, mold, certain foods, pet dander, and medication.

Allergies may be mild, or may be severe and result in serious conditions such as anaphylactic shock. Anaphylactic shock requires the use of an epinephrine shot to reverse the effects of the allergen. Less severe allergies may result in a runny nose, itchy eyes or skin, and hives.

Typical treatments of allergens include the use of antihistamines, decongestants, and steroid nasal sprays. Avoiding the allergen is advised.

Lupus Erythematosus
(lupus: wolf; erythemat-: red skin; -osus: pertaining to)

Lupus Erythematosus is an autoimmune disorder affecting the **connective tissues** of the entire body, but can be physically seen in the skin by the formation of a **butterfly rash** that appears on the face during flare-ups. This rash is similar in shape to the markings found on the face of a wolf, which is where lupus gets its name.

Symptoms of Lupus Erythematosus include fever, the formation of a butterfly rash, joint pain, discomfort, fatigue, and sensitivity to sunlight. It may also contribute to the development of other medical conditions, such as Raynaud's Syndrome.

There is no cure for Lupus Erythematosus, but treatment is available to help manage the condition. Non-steroidal anti-inflammatory drugs may help with systemic inflammation in non-severe cases. Topical corticosteroid creams may help alleviate rashes. Blood thinners may also be used in more severe cases.

Lymphedema
(lymph: lymph; -edema: swelling)

Lymphedema is a condition of the lymphatic system that results in increased **interstitial fluid** in a limb, which causes **swelling**.

Causes of lymphedema vary. Most commonly, it results from damage to the lymph nodes and vessels during treatment for cancer(such as a mastectomy, where breast tissue and lymph channels may be completely removed). This results in lymph not draining properly. Other causes include obesity and advanced age.

While there is no cure for lymphedema, treatments may help reduce the amount of fluid in the area by stimulating lymph circulation. Massage therapy is highly effective at increasing lymph circulation. Compression clothing may help move lymph. Exercise is also extremely helpful in increasing lymph flow.

Pitting Edema
(edema: swelling)

Pitting edema is a form of lymphedema that produces **pits** in the skin after pressure is applied and released. Lymphedema does not leave pits, and the skin rebounds immediately due to the amount of fluid in the area.

Pitting edema may be non-serious, or may have severe underlying causes. A common cause of pitting edema is pregnancy, due to the body creating much more fluid than it normally has. This increases fluid retention. Other, more serious causes, include heart failure, liver failure, or most commonly amongst these, **renal** failure. If these organs are not functioning properly, fluid is not properly drained from the body, which increases swelling.

For serious cases of pitting edema, it is recommended to visit a doctor to find the underlying cause. Once the cause is determined, a proper treatment plan may be developed. Typically, if a person is suffering from organ failure, diuretics may be prescribed to help drain excess fluid from the body. Keeping limbs such as the legs elevated may also help reduce swelling.

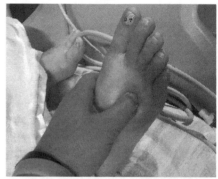
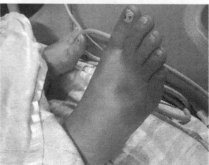

Pitting edema resulting from pregnancy

Pathology of the Muscular System

Adhesive Capsulitis
(capsul-: capsule; -itis: inflammation)

Adhesive capsulitis is a condition of the muscular system, which results in restricted range-of-motion at the shoulder joint. Another name for adhesive capsulitis is "Frozen Shoulder".

Surrounding the glenohumeral joint is connective tissue known as the joint capsule. This joint capsule holds everything in the joint in place, such as the bones themselves, synovial membrane, synovial fluid, etc. If there is irritation or over-use of the shoulder joint, **adhesions** may form between the joint capsule and the head of the humerus. These adhesions can decrease range-of-motion in the joint, and make movement in the joint uncomfortable.

The **subscapularis** muscle is often called the "Frozen Shoulder Muscle", due to its possible role in adhesive capsulitis. If the subscapularis is hypertonic, it may pull back on the humerus, which can restrict range-of-motion.

Treatments include stretching exercises and massage therapy to help break up the adhesions restricting range-of-motion, or to relax the subscapularis.

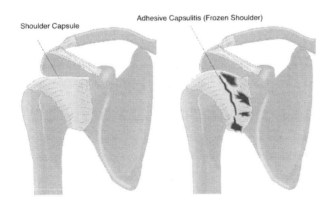

De Quervain's Tenosynovitis
(teno-: tendon; synov-: synovial; -itis: inflammation)

De Quervain's Tenosynovitis is a form of tenosynovitis that specifically affects the **thumb**.

De Quervain's Tenosynovitis is caused by **over-use** of the thumb, which contributes to straining of the tendons around the thumb, and their protective sheaths. This may cause pain around the thumb, inflammation, and difficulty in moving the area.

Treatments primarily consist of rest and ice to reduce pain and inflammation in the area. Any repetitive actions that are causing the inflammation should be stopped to allow irritation to subside.

Golfer's Elbow

Golfer's Elbow is a form of tendonitis that affects and weakens the **flexors** of the wrist. Golfer's Elbow is also known as Medial Epicondylitis, inflammation of the **medial epicondyle**.

Golfer's Elbow is caused by repetitive motions such as elbow flexion, which put strain on the tendons connecting the flexors of the wrist to the humerus, at the medial epicondyle.

Treatment typically involved rest and ice on the medial epicondyle to reduce inflammation. Any repetitive actions that are causing the inflammation should be stopped to allow irritation to subside.

Strain

A strain is an injury to a **tendon** or **muscle**, usually caused by over-exertion or over-use.

Activities such as exercise are a common cause of strains. Much like burns, there are three grades of strains: grade 1, grade 2, and grade 3. The less severe the strain, the lower the grade.

A grade 1 strain results in slight tearing of a tendon or muscle. An example could be a person's muscles being sore after exercise. The muscles have experienced slight tears during exercise, but will heal after a day or two.

A grade 2 strain results in more tearing of a muscle or tendon. Grade 2 strains may require surgery to repair, or may heal on their own with rest. There may be accompanying bruising and inflammation around the strain.

A grade 3 strain results in complete tearing of a muscle, or more commonly, a tendon. Surgery is required to repair a grade 3 strain. The quadriceps and biceps brachii are two muscles prone to grade 3 strains more than others. Grade 3 strains will inhibit movement involved with the muscle involved, due to its inability to pull on the bone.

Treatment varies depending on the severity of the strain. Grade 1 strains should be able to receive massage and heat therapy after 24-48 hours to increase circulation and promote healing. Grade 2 strains may need to rest longer before receiving treatment. Grade 3 strains would require surgery to repair.

➤ *Easy to Remember: To remember the difference between a strain and sprain, look for the "t" in "strain"! "T" for "tendon"!*

Tendonitis
(tendon-: tendon; -itis: inflammation)

Tendonitis is an injury that results in **inflammation** of a **tendon**.

Tendonitis is a mostly repetitive strain injury, caused by repeated use of one specific muscle, which can over-exert the tendon. When the tendon is over-exerted, it may tear slightly, which causes pain and inflammation.

There are several different types of tendonitis, including Golfer's Elbow(inflammation of the tendon at the medial epicondyle of the humerus), Tennis Elbow(inflammation of the tendon at the lateral epicondyle of the humerus), and Jumper's Knee(inflammation of the patellar tendon). All these conditions are caused by repetitive movements.

Treatment for tendonitis is primarily rest and application of ice to reduce any inflammation. Repetitive actions causing the inflammation should be stopped until the irritation subsides.

Tennis Elbow

Tennis Elbow is a form of tendonitis that affects and weakens the **extensors** of the wrist. Tennis Elbow is also known as Lateral Epicondylitis, inflammation of the **lateral epicondyle**.

Tennis Elbow is caused by repetitive motions such as elbow extension, which put strain on the tendons connecting the extensors of the wrist to the humerus, at the lateral epicondyle.

Treatment typically involved rest and ice on the lateral epicondyle to reduce inflammation. Any repetitive actions that are causing the inflammation should be stopped to allow irritation to subside.

Tenosynovitis
(teno-: tendon; synov-: synovial; -itis: inflammation)

Tenosynovitis is a repetitive strain injury that results in **inflammation** of a **tendon** and its **protective sheath**.

Tenosynovitis primarily affects the hands, wrists, and feet due to the length of the tendons in these areas. The longer the tendon is, the easier it becomes to strain. Because there may be inflammation, pain may be present, and it may be difficult to move the affected area.

A common type of tenosynovitis is known as De Quervain's Tenosynovitis, which causes inflammation around the thumb due to overuse.

Tenosynovitis is typically treated the same as any strain, with rest and ice to reduce pain. Less commonly, tenosynovitis may be the result of bacterial infection, which may produce a fever. If a fever is present, medications such as antibiotics and antipyretics may be prescribed to combat bacterial growth and fever.

Tennis Elbow
Right arm, lateral (outside) side

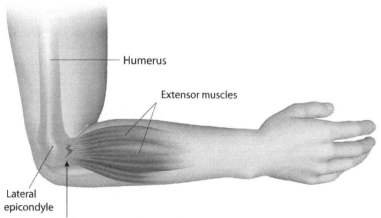

Humerus

Extensor muscles

Lateral epicondyle

Injured common extensor tendon

Pathology of the Nervous System

Bell's Palsy

Bell's Palsy is a condition affecting the **facial nerve**, causing **paralysis** on one side of the **face**.

The exact cause of Bell's Palsy is unknown, but is likely the result of an attack to the facial nerve(cranial nerve VII) by the Herpes Simplex virus. The inflammation damages the nerve, causing the muscles of the side of the face controlled by the facial nerve to become paralyzed or severely weakened. The side of the face affected may also become numb.

Bell's Palsy is mostly a temporary condition, and should resolve over the course of a month or two. In some cases, it can become permanent.

A person with Bell's Palsy may take corticosteroids to help treat the muscle weakness. Self care, including facial exercises, are recommended.

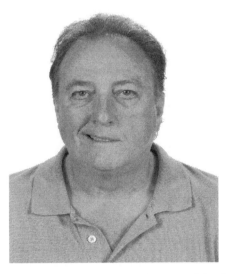

Patient with paralysis of the left side of the face

Carpal Tunnel Syndrome

Carpal Tunnel Syndrome is a condition caused by compression of the **median nerve** between the carpals and the **transverse carpal ligament**.

Several factors may contribute to the development of carpal tunnel syndrome, although the most common cause is repetitive movements. These repetitive movements can cause straining of the tendons that run through the carpal canal, which can place pressure on the median nerve. If the transverse carpal ligament tightens, it can also place pressure on the median nerve. When pressure is placed on the median nerve, numbness, pain, or tingling sensations may be experienced in the thumb, index, ring, and lateral side of the ring finger.

Several treatments are available for carpal tunnel syndrome. Self-care is recommended, including stretching the forearm and wrist flexors, massaging the transverse carpal ligament and hand muscles, and icing the area. Because carpal tunnel syndrome is often caused by repetitive actions, ceasing these actions is recommended. Non-steroidal anti-inflammatory medications may be prescribed. Surgery to remove the transverse carpal ligament may also be an option if the condition is severe.

Carpal Tunnel Syndrome

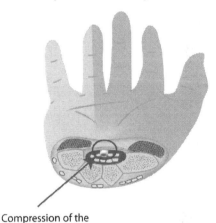

Compression of the
median nerve

Encephalitis
(encephal-: brain; -itis: inflammation)

Encephalitis is primarily a **viral** infection that results in **inflammation** of the **brain**.

Causes of encephalitis vary, but may include mosquito-borne viruses, such as West Nile, the Herpes Simplex virus, and the Rabies virus. Symptoms of encephalitis are usually mild, with the infected person suffering no more than flu-like symptoms, but severe cases may result in brain damage or death.

Because most cases of encephalitis are mild, treatment often consists of bed rest, and letting the virus work through its course. Antiviral medications may also be administered via an IV if the infection is more severe.

Multiple Sclerosis
(scler-: hard; -osis: condition)

Multiple Sclerosis is an **autoimmune** disorder, affecting the **myelin sheaths** that protect the axons of the nervous system.

The cause of Multiple Sclerosis is unknown, but may be hereditary, and even environmental factors have been linked to the development of the disease. The disease begins with the body's immune system attacking the myelin sheaths, the protective fatty layers surrounding axons. These sheaths help to insulate the axons and prevent damage to the axons. When the myelin sheath is attacked and destroyed, it exposes the axons, which can have many different effects. Impulses traveling along an axon may terminate at the site of myelin degeneration, which may cause loss of functions. Scar tissue may form over the axons, which leads to extreme pain.

There is no cure for Multiple Sclerosis. People may be prescribed disease-altering drugs, that may suppress the functions of the immune system. People may seek other means of managing Multiple Sclerosis and the accompanying pain and fatigue, including massage therapy, yoga, and meditation.

➤ *Easy to Remember: Match up MS with MS, "Multiple Sclerosis" and "Myelin Sheaths"!*

MULTIPLE SCLEROSIS

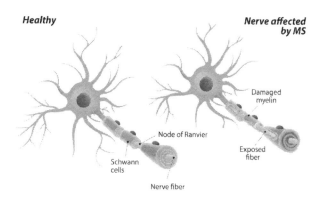

Healthy   Nerve affected by MS

Damaged myelin

Node of Ranvier

Exposed fiber

Schwann cells

Nerve fiber

Paralysis
(paraleyin: disable)

Paralysis is a loss of **function** of a part of the body. This condition can affect a small area, or a large portion of the body.

Paralysis is caused by **damage** to a nerve that innervates a muscle or muscles. When a nerve is damaged, it can cause weakness(partial paralysis) in a muscle, making it extremely difficult to use, or even result in complete loss of function. The three main types of paralysis that result in complete loss of function are

paraplegia, quadriplegia, and hemiplegia.

Paraplegia is paralysis affecting the lower limbs. This is typically caused by an injury to the spinal cord, but may also be caused by conditions such as spina bifida.

Quadriplegia is paralysis affecting all four limbs. This is typically caused by an injury to the spinal cord around the C4 vertebrae , which eliminates nerve supply to the limbs.

Hemiplegia is paralysis that affects one side (hemisphere) of the body . This is typically caused by a stroke, transient ischemic attack, or even multiple sclerosis.

Treatment for paralysis may be helpful in cases of partial paralysis, where there is still some function. Physical and occupational therapy may also help the nervous tissue regenerate.

Parkinson's Disease

Parkinson's Disease is a motor disease that results in **trembling** due to a loss of the neurotransmitter **dopamine**.

There is no known cause of Parkinson's Disease . Neurons in the brain that produce dopamine are gradually destroyed. Dopamine is the neurotransmitter that stabilizes the body during motor movements, especially fine movements like writing. When dopamine levels in the body drop, trembling and shaking increases. Over time, as dopamine levels drop, the trembling increases. As dopamine continues to drop, larger movements become affected, like walking and talking.

While there is no cure for Parkinson's Disease, treatments are available to help manage the condition, including dopamine replacement medications.

Sciatica

Sciatica is a condition causing pain radiating down the buttocks, posterior thigh, and leg.

Sciatica is most commonly caused by a **herniated disc** in the lumbar vertebrae, which puts compression on the nerves that comprise the **sciatic nerve**. Bone spurs may also place pressure on the nerves.

Piriformis Syndrome is often confused with sciatica. Piriformis Syndrome is caused by tightness in the piriformis muscle, which may place substantial pressure on the sciatic nerve.

Treatment for sciatica may include physical therapy, anti-inflammatory medications, or surgery if the condition is severe enough.

Thoracic Outlet Syndrome

Thoracic Outlet Syndrome is a condition caused by **compression** of **nerves** and **blood vessels** passing through the **thoracic outlet**.

Thoracic Outlet Syndrome may be caused by tight muscles, including **pectoralis minor** and **scalenes**, obesity, and tumors in the neck, such as those seen in Non-Hodgkin's Lymphoma.

Pressure placed on the nerves and blood vessels may cause pain, numbness, and weakness in the upper limb.

Treatments primarily consist of stretching of the tight muscles to release pressure on the nerves and blood vessels. In the case of a tumor, surgery to remove the tumor may be required.

Thoracic Outlet Syndrome

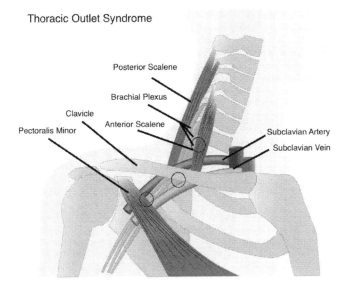

Trigeminal Neuralgia
(neur-: nerve; -algia: pain)

Trigeminal Neuralgia is a chronic condition causing extreme **pain** in the **face**.

The **trigeminal nerve** (cranial nerve V) sends sensory information from the face to the brain. When a blood vessel comes into contact with the trigeminal nerve at the brain stem, it results in dysfunction of the trigeminal nerve. This dysfunction results in hyper-sensitivity of the face, making even light touch extremely painful.

Treatments for trigeminal neuralgia include medications to reduce pain, botox injections, or possible surgery.

Pathology of the Respiratory System

Asthma

Asthma is a chronic respiratory disease that causes **constriction** of the **airways**, restricting oxygen intake.

Asthma affects the **smooth** muscle in the walls of the bronchial tubes. Typically, when a person inhales an irritant(such as dust or smoke), the smooth muscle spasms and constricts in an effort to reduce the irritant moving further into the lungs. The bronchi will also produce an excessive amount of **mucous**, which further restricts the flow of oxygen into the lungs.

Symptoms include wheezing, chest tightness, and shortness of breath. Treatment varies depending on the severity in acute stages. If it is mild, medication may not be required. If symptoms are more severe, bronchodilators may be required to calm and open the airways. In extreme cases, where regular bronchodilators do not work, medical attention should be sought. A nebulizer, with inhalable steroids, should be used with asthma attacks.

Asthma usually begins in childhood, but may disappear with age. Other times, it remains a chronic condition. Other factors such as smoking or obesity may lead to the development of asthma.

Bronchitis
(bronch-: bronchi; -itis: inflammation)

Bronchitis is an inflammatory disease of the respiratory system, restricting oxygen intake.

There are two different types of bronchitis: acute bronchitis and chronic bronchitis. Acute bronchitis is the result of a **primary** infection of the respiratory system, such as influenza or pneumonia. These diseases affect the bronchial tubes, causing them to become irritated and inflamed. When these diseases resolve, the bronchitis will also resolve. Chronic bronchitis is the result of **constant irritation** to the bronchial tubes, caused by things such as **cigarette smoking** or exposure to things like dust. When exposure to the irritant ceases, the bronchitis will also cease.

With both forms of bronchitis, there is an increased amount of mucous produced in the lungs, which makes breathing difficult. Increased coughing may be a side effect of the increase in mucous.

Treatments vary depending on which type of bronchitis is involved. Acute bronchitis may require nothing more than a bronchodilator or cough suppressant. Because acute bronchitis is usually caused by a viral infection, antivirals may be prescribed to stop the advancement of the virus. Chronic bronchitis often requires the use of a bronchodilator, but not much else.

Pathology of Asthma

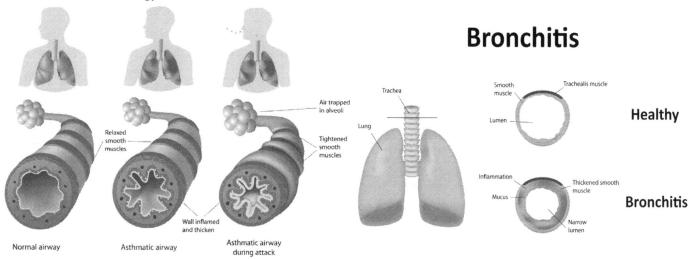

95

Emphysema
(emphyso: inflate)

Emphysema is a chronic condition of the lungs, resulting in difficulty bringing oxygen into the body and eliminating carbon dioxide from the body.

Emphysema is caused by over-exposure to substances such as **cigarette smoke**. Constant irritation of the lungs by smoke can lead to degeneration of the **alveoli**, air sacs at the end of bronchial tubes where gas exchange takes place. When the alveoli degenerate, they lose surface area, which is what capillaries move across to eliminate carbon dioxide from the body and bring oxygen into the body. Lack of enough alveoli surface area makes gas exchange extremely difficult.

Emphysema causes shortness of breath. A person with emphysema may be much more likely to develop a collapsed lung due to damage to the lungs.

Breathing exercises and oxygen supplementation may help control emphysema. If needed, bronchodilators can help relax the airways. If infections such as pneumonia occur, antibiotics may help.

Influenza
(Italian "influenza": influence)

Influenza is a highly contagious **viral** infection that primarily affects the lungs.

There are many different strains of the flu virus. It is constantly mutating, so treatment can be difficult. **Vaccinations** are the primary form of prevention for influenza.

Influenza, during acute stages, results in fever, general malaise, body aches, runny nose, and cough. Symptoms generally last no more than a week. Depending on the person involved, it can be a moderate infection, or can be life-threatening. Children and the elderly are much more likely to have serious cases of influenza than the general population.

Pneumonia
(pneumo: lung)

Pneumonia is a highly contagious infection of the lungs, resulting in a buildup of **fluid** in the **alveoli**.

The primary cause of pneumonia is **bacterial** infection(staphylococci), but may also be caused by a virus or fungi. When the lungs are infected with pneumonia, the person may experience fever, nausea, shortness of breath, coughing, and chest pain. Pneumonia can be life-threatening for young children and the elderly, but is mostly a moderate condition in the general population.

Pneumonia is typically treated with antibiotics. Cough medicine and antipyretics may be prescribed to aid with coughing and to lower fever.

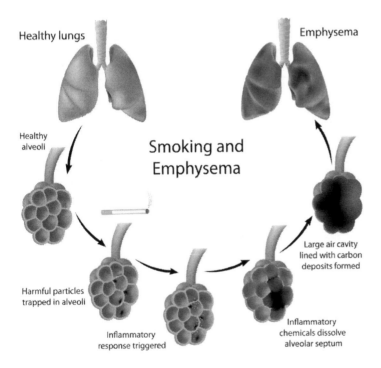

Healthy lungs

Emphysema

Healthy alveoli

Smoking and Emphysema

Harmful particles trapped in alveoli

Inflammatory response triggered

Inflammatory chemicals dissolve alveolar septum

Large air cavity lined with carbon deposits formed

PNEUMONIA

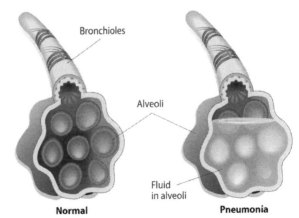

Bronchioles

Alveoli

Fluid in alveoli

Normal

Pneumonia

Pathology of the Skeletal System

Bursitis
(burs-: bursa; -itis: inflammation)

Bursitis is a condition that results in **inflammation** of a **bursa**, a small sac filled with synovial fluid.

Bursae are located all over the body, typically between a tendon and bone to prevent friction and irritation. When there is repeated stress placed on the bursa, it can become inflamed. Bursitis may affect many different joints, including the knee, shoulder, elbow, hip, and ankle.

Bursitis is most often caused by repetitive motions in the affected joint, which may irritate the bursa. Trauma may also result in bursitis, such as fractures or tendonitis.

Bursitis is easily treatable, primarily with rest and ice. Depending on the severity, the bursa may also need to be surgically drained or removed, or injected with corticosteroids to reduce the inflammation.

Dislocation

A dislocation is when a bone at an articulation becomes **displaced** from its normal location. A dislocation, in the acute stage, results in immobilization of the joint and temporary deformation. It may also be painful and result in inflammation around the joint.

Dislocations are most commonly the result of trauma to the joint, which pushes a bone out of place. The most common areas for dislocations are the fingers and shoulder, but dislocations may occur in many other joints as well, such as the knee or hip.

Dislocations may result in tearing of tendons, ligaments, muscles, or in the case of the shoulder or hip, the labrum(circular cartilage surrounding the joint). The dislocated joint, while most commonly returns to normal strength and function after being relocated, may become prone to dislocations in the future. This may cause arthritis to develop.

Shoulder Dislocation

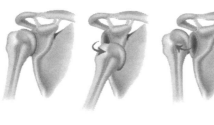

| Normal anatomy | Anterior dislocation | Posterior dislocation |

Treatments for dislocations in the acute stage include relocation of the bone back to its normal location, keeping the joint immobilized to allow the joint and surrounding structures to properly heal, and depending on the severity, surgery may be required.

Fracture

A fracture is a **break** in a bone. There are several different types of fractures, including transverse, greenstick, oblique, and spiral.

Types of Bone Fractures

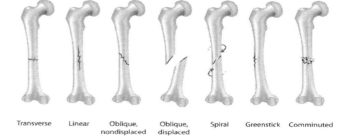

Transverse   Linear   Oblique, nondisplaced   Oblique, displaced   Spiral   Greenstick   Comminuted

Fractures are the result of trauma to a bone. Despite many different types of fractures, every fracture is categorized as one of the following: Simple or Compound. A **simple** fracture is a fracture that **does not break through** the skin, and does not damage any surrounding tissue. A **compound** fracture, which is much more severe, **breaks through** the skin and damages surrounding tissues. Compound fractures are much more prone to infection due to exposure to the outside environment.

Fractures result in deformity of the affected bone, pain, immobilization of the area, and inflammation. In the case of compound fractures, external bleeding may also occur.

Despite most fractures being the result of blunt trauma, certain diseases that weaken the bones may also cause fractures, such as osteoporosis.

Fractures should be treated immediately. A cast or splint may be applied, depending on which bone is fractured. Other fractures, such as vertebrae fractures, may need more extensive treatment, including metal plates or bone grafts.

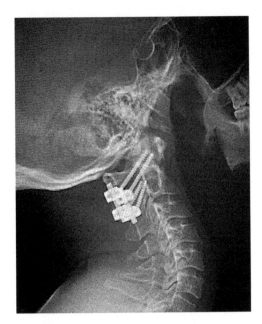

Spinal fusion post-surgery due to
fractured cervical vertebrae

Gout

Gout is a form of arthritis, mostly seen around the base of the **big toe**, but may also affect other joints in the body, such as the hands and fingers.

Gout is the result of an over-abundance of **uric acid** crystals in the body. Gravity pulls the uric acid crystals down the body, where they collect in the most distal points in the limbs, the big toes, hands and fingers. Gout is typically the result of the kidneys not excreting enough uric acid, or the body producing too much uric acid.

Gout may be extremely painful in the acute stage as the crystals collect in the joints. Inflammation may set in, which can increase the pressure and pain in the joint. Loss of range-of-motion may also occur. Untreated, gout may result in kidney stones.

Treatments for gout include non-steroidal anti-inflammatory drugs and/or corticosteroids to reduce pain and inflammation. Gout may also require the use of certain medications that prevent the creation of uric acid in the body.

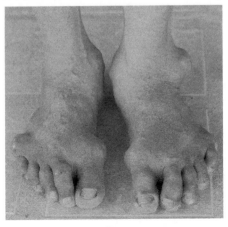

Gout

Herniated Disc

A herniated disc is a condition affecting the vertebral column, which may cause intense pain and numbness.

An intervertebral disc, located between two vertebrae, is made of two parts: the nucleus pulposus, and the annulus fibrosus. The nucleus pulposus is a gelatinous substance located in the center of the disc. The annulus fibrosus is the part of the disc made of thick cartilage. If a tear occurs in the **annulus fibrosus**, the **nucleus pulposus** may **protrude** through the torn section, which may place pressure on spinal nerves emerging from the spinal cord. This is a herniated disc.

A herniated disc is primarily caused by degeneration of a disc, which takes place gradually. This makes injury of the disc much easier in actions such as lifting and twisting. Other times, trauma may cause a herniated disc, such as in car accidents.

Herniated discs may result in pain and/or numbness due to the disc placing pressure on the spinal nerves. Because numbness may occur, weakness in the muscles innervated by the nerves may also set in due to impaired function.

Treatment for a herniated disc varies depending on the severity. Pain medication may help control pain. Muscle relaxers may help take pressure off the area of the herniation. Physical therapy may also contribute to lessening the effects of the herniated disc. Very rarely, surgery may be required.

Spinal disc herniation

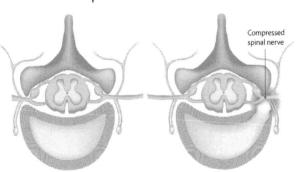

Normal disc   Herniated disc

Kyphosis
(kyph-: hill; -osis: condition)

Kyphosis is a condition affecting the **thoracic** vertebrae, resulting in **hyper-curvature**. Another name for kyphosis is "Dowager's Hump".

A kyphotic curvature in the vertebrae is a curvature that moves posteriorly. If the curvature is exaggerated, it is known as kyphosis. Kyphosis has many different causes. Kyphosis may be caused by extremely tight muscles(such as **pectoralis minor** and **serratus anterior**) pulling the scapulae anteriorly, which rounds the back. It may also be the result of bone degeneration(osteoporosis), disc degeneration(ankylosing spondylitis), or even birth defects.

Kyphosis may cause pain in the back, and difficulty in movement and breathing as a result. It may also result in the lumbar vertebrae losing its curvature, a condition known as **flat back**.

Kyphosis may vary from mild to severe, depending on the cause. Treatments include exercises that strengthen the muscles of the back, stretching of tight muscles that may contribute to kyphosis, braces to keep the vertebrae properly aligned, and possibly even surgery if it's warranted.

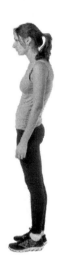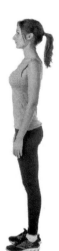

Hyper-curvature of the thoracic vertebrae, resulting in a hunched appearance

Lordosis
(lord-: curve; -osis: condition)

Lordosis is a condition affecting the **lumbar** vertebrae, resulting in **hyper-curvature**. Another name for lordosis is "Swayback".

A lordotic curvature in the vertebrae is a curvature that moves anteriorly. If the curvature is exaggerated, it is known as lordosis. Lordosis has many different causes. Lordosis may be caused by tight muscles(such as **psoas major**, **iliacus**, **quadratus lumborum**, and **rectus femoris**), weak muscles(such as **rectus abdominis** and the **hamstrings**), obesity, or bone diseases(such as osteoporosis). Pregnancy is also a common cause of lordosis, but the condition typically subsides post-pregnancy.

Lordosis may place excessive pressure on the vertebrae, and alter a person's stance and gait.

Treatment primarily includes strengthening weak muscles, stretching tight muscles, and lifestyle changes, such as adjusting posture, diet, and exercise.

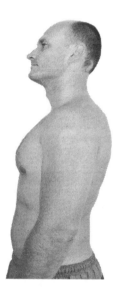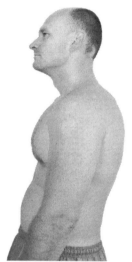

Hyper-curvature of the lumbar vertebrae

Osgood-Schlatter Disease

Osgood-Schlatter Disease is a repetitive strain injury, caused by over-use of the **patellar** tendon.

Osgood-Schlatter Disease primarily affects adolescents, particularly those involved in sports. Over-use of the **quadriceps** during activities such as running and jumping can cause tightness in the patellar tendon. When the patellar tendon tightens, it pulls proximally on the tibial tuberosity. Because the bone is still growing, the force of the patellar tendon on the tibial tuberosity can cause an **over-growth of bone**, resulting in a bony lump. Males are more likely to develop this condition than females, but instances in females are increasing as participation in sports by females increases.

Osgood-Schlatter Disease may cause pain, but it varies from person to person. The pain may be mild, or it may be more intense, making movement of the knee difficult.

Despite complications from Osgood-Schlatter Disease being rare, inflammation of the area may persist over time. The bony lump produced by increased bone production may also remain.

Treatment is mild, usually nothing more than pain relievers, rest, and ice. Exercises that stretch the quadriceps are recommended.

Osteoarthritis
(osteo-: bone; arthr-: joint; -itis: inflammation)

Osteoarthritis is the most common form of arthritis, which is **inflammation** of a **joint**.

Osteoarthritis, also known as "wear-and-tear arthritis", is caused by damage to the **hyaline cartilage** separating one bone from another. The cartilage between bones reduces friction between the bones, and absorbs shock in the joint. Over time, the articular cartilage may begin to break down and wear away. This causes irritation in the joint and increases friction between the bones, which causes inflammation. As this persists, damage to the bone may take place. The most common location of osteoarthritis is the knee, but in massage therapists, it may also affect the metacarpophalangeal joint of the thumb(saddle joint).

Osteoarthritis may cause pain, difficulty moving the affected joint, and bone spurs in the joint due to increased friction between the bones. When the condition advances to the point of the joint being mostly unusable, joint replacement surgery may be recommended.

Treatment includes non-steroidal anti-inflammatory drugs, lifestyle and dietary changes if caused by obesity, and alternative methods such as yoga.

OSTEOARTHRITIS

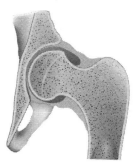

NORMAL JOINT   DESTRUCTION OF CARTILAGE

BONE

CARTILAGE   THINNING CARTILAGE   BONE ENDS RUB TOGETHER   BONE SPUR   THINNED CARTILAGE

Osteoporosis
(osteo-: bone; por-: porous; -osis: condition)

Osteoporosis is a condition that causes weakness and **degeneration** in the **bones**.

Osteoporosis mainly affects post-menopausal women. After menopause, a woman's body produces less **estrogen**. Estrogen, during growth stages of a person's life, help the bones grow and mature. When estrogen levels drop post-menopause, osteoclast levels increase, and more bone is destroyed than is created. When this occurs, the bones become brittle, weak, and prone to fracture.

Osteoporosis, in addition to making bones brittle, may also contribute to the development of kyphosis and back pain. One of the most common places for fracture to occur is in the neck of the femur. The femur, which is normally the strongest bone in the body, should be able to support roughly 2,000 pounds of pressure per square inch. When the femur becomes weakened, it makes it incredibly easy to break. If a fracture takes place around the hip joint, joint replacement surgery is often required.

Treatments for osteoporosis include estrogen replacement therapy, and weight-bearing exercise earlier in life before any symptoms of osteoporosis surface. Weight-bearing exercise, such as squats and dead-lifts, helps to strengthen the bones, which substantially reduces the risk of developing osteoporosis in older age.

OSTEOPOROSIS

NORMAL BONE   OSTEOPOROSIS

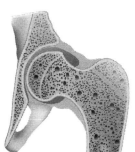

Rheumatoid Arthritis

Rheumatoid Arthritis is an **autoimmune** disorder, resulting in inflammation, pain, and deformity of the joints around the hands and wrists.

Around synovial joints, there is a membrane called the synovial membrane, which supplies joints with synovial fluid. In rheumatoid arthritis, the body's immune systems attacks the **synovial membranes**, destroying them. This is especially common in the metacarpophalangeal joints. After the synovial membranes have been destroyed, extremely thick, fibrous material replaces them, which not only makes movement painful and difficult, but can also cause deformity, turning the fingers into an adducted position.

There is no cure for rheumatoid arthritis, but treatments include non-steroidal anti-inflammatory drugs, corticosteroids, and physical therapy.

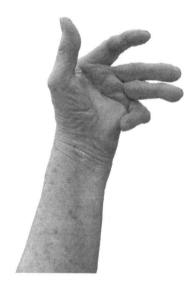

Deformity of the hand resulting
from rheumatoid arthritis

Scoliosis
(scoli-: crooked; -osis: condition)

Scoliosis is a condition causing the vertebral column, usually in the thoracic region, to be pulled into a **lateral** position.

The causes of scoliosis are unknown, but there may be a hereditary link. Scoliosis typically develops around the beginning stages of puberty. Scoliosis is mostly mild in severity, but can become much more prominent, which can put incredible strain on the ribs, vertebrae, and hips. With scoliosis, one hip may be higher than the other, which causes a discrepancy in gait. Tight muscles may also contribute to the development of scoliosis, as seen in cases such as a hypertonic rhomboid major and minor unilaterally, which pulls the vertebrae to one side.

If scoliosis is severe, damage to the heart or lungs may occur, due to the deformity of the rib cage. Back pain may also persist.

Treatment, while commonly unnecessary, may include the use of braces to correct posture, the use of chiropractic therapy, massage therapy, or in severe cases, surgery with metal rod implantation.

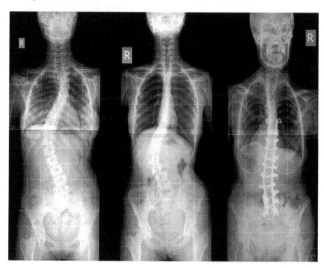

Before and after x-rays of a scoliosis
patient with rod implantation

Sprain

A sprain is an injury to a **ligament**.

Sprains are much less likely to be caused by repetitive motions, unlike strains. Sprains typically occur quickly, causing tears in a ligament. Like strains, sprains may be broken down in severity by using grades: grade 1, grade 2, and grade 3.

A grade 1 sprain is caused by stretching of a ligament, but does not cause major tearing. Common grade 1 sprains may be caused by activities such as running. After 24/48 hours, the ligament should return to normal, and any pain and/or inflammation should subside.

A grade 2 sprain, such as a high ankle sprain, causes tearing of a ligament and presents with bruising and inflammation. Grade 2 sprains may require surgery to repair, or they may heal on their own, depending on the severity of the tear.

A grade 3 sprain is a complete rupture of a ligament, and much like a grade 3 strain, does

101

require surgery to repair. The most common form of grade 3 sprain is a torn anterior cruciate ligament(ACL, the ligament holding the femur and tibia together), most commonly caused by sports, or automobile accidents.

Sprains take much longer to heal than strains, due to ligaments being avascular, compared to muscles and tendons, which have a rich blood supply. Treatment for sprains vary depending on the severity of the sprain. The less severe, the more likely it is that rest, ice, and elevation will suffice. Surgery is only required when there is no chance of the ligament repairing itself.

Temporomandibular Joint Dysfunction

Temporomandibular Joint Dysfunction(TMJD) is a condition affecting the mandible, causing simple tasks such as **chewing** to become **painful** and **difficult**.

The temporomandibular joint is the joint that connects the mandible to the temporal bone. Between the bones, there is a small disc of cartilage, used to prevent friction between the bones and to make movement smooth. If there is arthritis in the joint, or the disc is damaged, it can result in Temporomandibular Joint Dysfunction. This can cause pain, difficulty in moving the jaw, and produce a clicking sensation when the jaw opens. Often times, the muscles that connect to the mandible(temporalis, lateral pterygoid) may tighten and pull the mandible out of place.

Treatments vary depending on the primary cause, ranging from prescription muscle relaxants and pain relievers, to physical and massage therapy.

Pathology of the Urinary System

Cystitis
(cyst-: bladder; -itis: inflammation)

Cystitis is a **bacterial** infection, resulting in **inflammation** of the **bladder**. Often, it can involve the entire urinary system, and is then known as a Urinary Tract Infection(UTI). Cystitis is most common in women, as the female urethra is shorter than the male urethra, giving bacteria a shorter passage to the bladder.

Cystitis is caused most commonly by E. Coli entering the urethra, then reproducing. The increased amount of bacterium in the urethra causes the infection to spread upwards, into the bladder. Cystitis can cause numerous symptoms, including blood in the urine, burning sensations while urinating, and a frequent urge to urinate. If untreated, the infection may spread to the kidneys. When this happens, it is known as pyelonephritis.

Cystitis, because it is a bacterial infection, is treated with antibiotics.

Cystitis

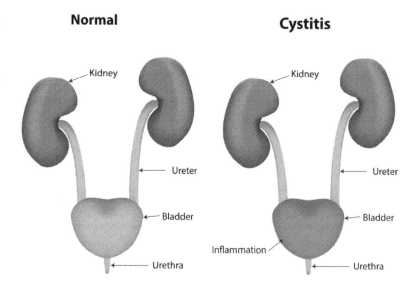

Normal	Cystitis

Cancers

Basal Cell Carcinoma
(carcin-: cancer; -oma: tumor)

Basal Cell Carcinoma is a type of **skin** cancer typically seen around the face, head, neck, and arms.

Basal Cell Carcinoma is the **most common** form of skin cancer, caused by exposure to ultraviolet light. The tumor grows extremely slowly, which makes Basal Cell Carcinoma much more treatable than other types of skin cancer. Because it is much more treatable, it is considered the **least serious** form of skin cancer.

Basal Cell Carcinoma is considered a malignant form of cancer, due to its ability to spread to the tissues immediately surrounding it. It will very rarely spread to other organs, however.

Treatment for Basal Cell Carcinoma includes surgical excision of the tumor, freezing the tumor, or in more serious cases, medications that prevent the cancerous cells from spreading to other tissues.

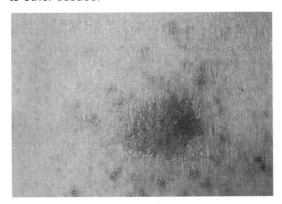

Tumor seen in basal cell carcinoma

Malignant Melanoma
(melan-: black; -oma: tumor)

Malignant Melanoma is a type of **skin** cancer that may affect any part of the skin, and can also affect other tissues such as the eyes and internal organs.

Malignant Melanoma is the **least common** form of skin cancer, but it is the **most serious**. It is caused by exposure to ultraviolet light. The cells in your body that produce skin pigment, **melanocytes**, become stimulated by exposure to ultraviolet light, and reproduce, causing darker skin. In Malignant Melanoma, the melanocytes reproduce uncontrolled. This uncontrolled reproduction results in a tumor, and these cancerous cells can easily spread throughout the body and damage other organs and tissues.

Dermatologists use the ABCDE method to diagnose Malignant Melanoma:

- A: Asymmetrical; moles are typically symmetrical, but melanoma tumors have an unusual shape, and the sides don't match.
- B: Borders; the borders of the growth change over time. This is a sign of significantly increased melanin production.
- C: Color; moles are typically some shade of brown. If there are multiple shades or colors, or if the tumor is black, this may be a sign of increased melanin production.
- D: Diameter; if a growth is 6mm or greater in diameter(the distance through it), this may be a sign of melanoma.
- E: Evolving; moles typically look the same over time. If a mole or growth begins to evolve or change in any way, this may be a sign of melanoma.

Malignant Melanoma most commonly begins to appear on a part of the body that doesn't have any prior lesions, like moles. If a new growth appears where there was nothing prior, this may be a sign of melanoma. Less commonly, moles may become cancerous.

Malignant Melanoma, if caught early enough, is easily treatable. Later stages, where it has grown beyond the skin, need more advanced treatments, including surgery to remove any tumors or cancerous lymph nodes, chemotherapy, and radiation therapy.

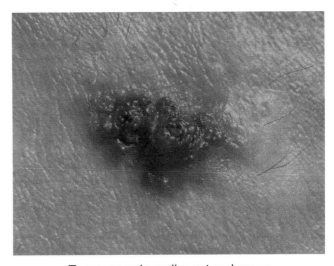

Tumor seen in malignant melanoma

Non-Hodgkin's Lymphoma
(lymph-: lymph; -oma: tumor)

Non-Hodgkin's Lymphoma is a type of cancer of the **lymphatic** system, caused by the development of tumors by lymphocytes.

In the body, lymphocytes, like every cell, go through their normal life cycle, and die when they are supposed to. In Non-Hodgkin's Lymphoma, the lymphocytes don't die, but continue reproducing. This causes an **excessive amount** of **lymphocytes** to build up in the lymph nodes.

People with Non-Hodgkin's Lymphoma may experience swollen lymph nodes around the neck, groin, and axilla, fatigue, weight loss, and fever.

Often times, Non-Hodgkin's Lymphoma isn't serious, and treatment is only required when it becomes advanced. Advanced Non-Hodgkin's Lymphoma is treated with chemotherapy and radiation therapy to destroy the cancerous cells.

Squamous Cell Carcinoma

Squamous Cell Carcinoma is a form of **skin** cancer that in many cases is not serious, but has the ability to spread to other parts of the body. Squamous Cell Carcinoma is **more serious** and **less common** than **Basal Cell Carcinoma**, but **not as serious** and **more common** than **Malignant Melanoma**.

Squamous Cell Carcinoma, much like Basal Cell Carcinoma and Malignant Melanoma, is most often caused by exposure to ultraviolet light. Tumors most commonly develop on areas of the body commonly exposed to sunlight, such as the head, neck, arms, and hands. Tumors may be flat, scaly, and firm, and appear around the mouth, in the mouth, and on the lips.

Much like Basal Cell Carcinoma, treatment for Squamous Cell Carcinoma is relatively easy, with several different methods, from surgical excision and freezing of the tumor, to radiation therapy for more advanced tumors.

Medications

There are many different types of medications used to treat many types of illnesses, diseases, and infections. Among the most common are:

- **Analgesics**, which help to **relieve pain**. Examples include acetaminophen and non-steroidal anti-inflammatory drugs.

- **Antacids**, which reduce the activity of **acids** in the stomach.

- **Antibiotics**, which are used to combat **bacterial** growth. Examples include penicillin, amoxicillin, and erythromycin.

- **Anticoagulants**, which are used to reduce the formation of **blood clots**. Examples include aspirin, heparin, and warfarin.

- **Antifungals**, which aid in destroying **fungus**. Examples include terbinafine and fluconazole.

- **Antihistamines**, which reduce the effects of **histamines** on the body, including runny nose and itching.

- **Anti-inflammatory agents**, which help to reduce **inflammation**. Examples include non-steroidal anti-inflammatory drugs such as ibuprofen.

- **Antipyretics**, which help to reduce **fever**. Examples include ibuprofen and aspirin.

- **Antivirals**, which aid in preventing **virus** reproduction. Examples include amantadine and rimantadine.

- **Beta blockers**, which help to reduce **blood pressure**. Examples include acebutolol. nadolol, and nebivolol.

- **Bronchodilators**, which aid in **dilation** of the **bronchial tubes**. Examples include albuterol and salmeterol.

- **Decongestants**, which reduce **inflammation** in the **nasal cavity**. Examples include pseudoephedrine and phenylephrine.

- **Diuretics**, which increase the production of **urine**. Examples include bumetanide, amiloride, and mannitol.

- **Insulin**, which **lowers** the amount of **sugar** in the blood stream.

- **Local anesthetics**, which are used to **numb** an area. They are most commonly administered via **needle injection**. Examples include lidocaine and nitracaine.

- **Sedatives**, which are used to **calm** and **relax** the body. Examples include diazepam and clonazepam.

- **Statins**, which aid in lowering **cholesterol** levels in the blood stream. Examples include atorvastatin, rosuvastatin, and lovastatin.

CPR and First Aid

CPR

CPR, which stands for **Cardiopulmonary Resuscitation**, is extremely important to know and understand how to perform. Refer to REMSA guidelines for appropriate instruction. CPR consists of alternating **chest** compressions and **breathing** support in cases where cardiac arrest has occurred.

First Aid

There are many different ways to care for a person with a medical emergency, depending on the type of injury and the severity. When using first aid, **universal precautions** should be administered. Universal precautions are treating every person and fluid as if they were **contaminated** or **infectious**. Universal precautions are extremely important in containing blood-borne pathogens. Any time there is exposure to any type of bodily fluid, **gloves** and other **personal protective equipment** should be worn, and contact with blood should be avoided at all costs.

Heat Injuries

There are three main types of heat injuries, that don't involve burns: heat exhaustion, heat cramps, and heat stroke. **Heat exhaustion** is caused by a person having a **high body temperature** with **excessive sweating**. Sweating is a product of homeostasis, which is trying to cool the body. If the person continues to sweat, it means the body isn't properly cooling down. This can lead to **heat cramps**, which cause tightening and involuntary **spasms** of the **muscles** due to dehydration and loss of electrolytes, such as sodium and potassium. **Heat stroke** is when a person has an **extremely high body temperature**, with a **lack of sweating**. This occurs when a person is severely dehydrated, and has no more fluid to use as sweat to try cooling the body down. This can be potentially fatal.

Cold Injuries

There are two main types of cold injuries: hypothermia and frostbite. **Hypothermia** is caused by the body temperature dropping **below 90 degrees**. This can be potentially fatal. **Frostbite** is caused by a formation of **ice crystals** in **soft tissues**, typically the fingers, toes, and parts of the face such as the nose and ears. If the tissues are frozen for too long, they experience **necrosis**.

The Rule of 9's

The **Rule of 9's** is used to determine the extent of **burns** by the total body area involved. Each percentage represents the percentage of the body damaged by burns:

Head and Neck: 9%
Right Arm : 9%
Left Arm: 9%
Right Leg: 18%
Left Leg: 18%
Thorax: 18%
Abdomen: 9%
Lower Back: 9%
Groin: 1%

Wounds

Wounds are the result of a **breakage** in the skin, which exposes underlying tissues. There are several different types of open wounds.

- An **incision**, such as produced during surgery, is a **clean cut** through tissue.

- A **laceration** is a cut that produces **jagged edges**.

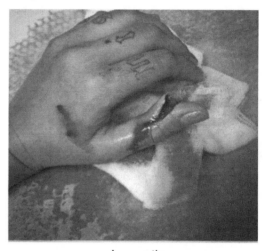

Laceration

- An **abrasion** is produced by **scraped skin**.

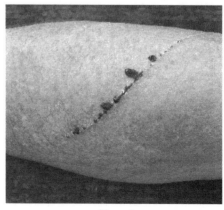

Abrasion

- A **puncture** is caused by an object **piercing** the skin, producing a **hole**.

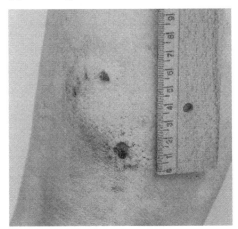

Puncture

Wounds should be cleansed with soap and water, and a sterile bandage should be applied to stop bleeding.

Bites and Stings

Bites and stings are similar to wounds. If an **animal bite** produces a puncture in the skin, a sterile bandage should be applied after **forcing bleeding** to flush out bacteria from the area and cleansing with soap and water.

Insect stings, such as bee stings, should be **scraped** with a hard, flat, sharp object such as a knife in order to remove any stinger left in the skin. The area should be cleansed with soap and water. If anaphylactic shock is suspected, EMS should be contacted.

Snake bites require EMS contact, and the bitten area should be immobilized **below the heart**. The area should be cleansed with soap and water.

Spider bites and **scorpion stings** should be cleansed with soap and water, and the area should also be immobilized **below the heart**.

Orthopedic Injuries

As previously discussed, strains, sprains, and fractures are all forms of **orthopedic injuries**. Strains and sprains are primarily treated with the use of **PRICE**: **Protect**, **Rest**, **Ice**, **Compression**, **Elevation**. The damaged area should be protected from further injury, rested to allow proper healing, iced to reduce inflammation, compression to help further reduce inflammation, and elevated to assist in proper circulation and reduce inflammation.

Poisoning

Poisoning may occur in several different ways. Poisoning via **inhalation**, such as carbon monoxide poisoning, may require the person be given an **antidote**, or require breathing support by way of an **oxygen mask**.

Injection poisoning introduces harmful substances into the body via **needles**, **insect stings**, **sharp objects**, or **bites**. The poison usually requires the use of an **antidote** to treat.

Absorption of poison typically includes exposure to substances such as **pesticides**. The area affected should be cleansed thoroughly with water.

Ingestion is introducing harmful substances through **swallowing**. Depending on the substance ingested, the person may be required to induce **vomiting**, or need to drink milk or water.

Patholog Matching

_____: Hyper-curvature of the thoracic vertebrae caused by tight pectoralis minor and serratus anterior

_____: Protrusion of the nucleus pulposus through the annulus fibrosus

_____: Inflammation of the liver

_____: Erosion of the articular cartilage, causing inflammation in a joint

_____: Swelling of veins due to malfunctioning valves

_____: Injury to a ligament caused by over-stretching

_____: Lack of cortisol production caused by damage to the adrenal cortex

_____: Epidermal growth caused by the human papilloma virus

_____: Fungal infection of the skin causing a circular rash

_____: Autoimmune disorder causing dry, scaly patches to form on the skin

_____: Swelling of a limb due to excessive interstitial fluid in an area

_____: Degeneration of alveoli, reducing gas exchange

_____: Constriction of blood vessels in the hands and feet, reducing blood flow

_____: Bacterial infection causing inflammation of the bladder

_____: Paralysis of one side of the face due to damage to the facial nerve

_____: Necrosis of heart tissue

_____: Compression of the brachial plexus and blood vessels caused by tight scalenes and pectoralis minor

_____: Bacterial infection of a hair follicle, also known as a furuncle

_____: Form of tendonitis causing inflammation at the lateral epicondyle of the humerus

_____: Highly contagious viral infection of the respiratory tract

A: Varicose Veins

B: Emphysema

C: Thoracic Outlet Syndrome

D: Kyphosis

E: Psoriasis

F: Boil

G: Hepatitis

H: Myocardial Infarction

I: Raynaud's Syndrome

J: Wart

K: Tennis Elbow

L: Bell's Palsy

M: Cystitis

N: Sprain

O: Osteoarthritis

P: Herniated Disc

Q: Influenza

R: Lymphedema

S: Ringworm

T: Addison's Disease

Pathology

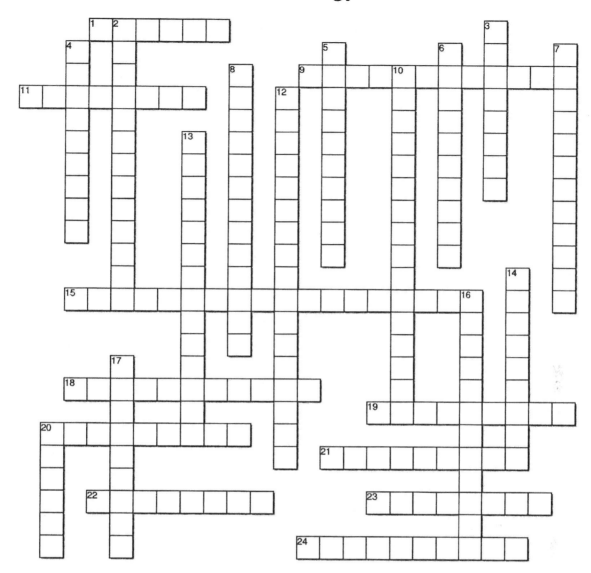

Across

1. Injury to a muscle or tendon
9. Blood pressure of 140/90 or above
11. Hyper-curvature of the thoracic vertebrae
15. Least serious, most common, slowest growing skin cancer
18. Tendonitis affecting the lateral epicondyle of the humerus
19. Inflammation of the liver most commonly due to viral infection
20. Lateral curvature of the vertebrae
21. Autoimmune disorder attacking epithelial cells in the skin
22. Bulging of an artery due to weakness in the wall
23. Hyper-curvature of the lumbar vertebrae
24. Inflammation of bronchial tubes

Down

2. Inflammation of a tendon and its sheath
3. Bladder infection
4. Destruction of lung alveoli
5. Increased amounts of interstitial fluid in a limb
6. Paralysis of one side of the face
7. Inflammation of the brain
8. Viral infection resulting in cold sores
10. Constriction of arteries in the hands and feet
12. Autoimmune disorder which attacks myelin sheaths in the CNS
13. Development of pouches in the wall of the large intestine
14. Inflammation of a vein
16. Fungal infection of the foot
17. Viral infection of the respiratory tract
20. Injury to a ligament

Medications

Find the medications based on what they're used for!

```
W  J  A  P  K  D  H  D  W  E  A  N  T  I  F  U  N  G  A  L
V  S  M  C  I  Q  T  N  J  Q  W  W  B  Y  E  Y  X  F  J  X
C  B  L  X  A  E  N  I  M  A  T  S  I  H  I  T  N  A  U  N
M  I  A  Z  N  A  N  T  I  B  I  O  T  I  C  L  H  S  B  Q
N  A  Q  W  T  K  T  F  U  K  C  D  L  O  L  B  V  R  R  G
A  N  T  I  I  N  F  L  A  M  M  A  T  O  R  Y  O  P  X  Z
T  D  R  U  V  Z  U  J  Z  S  L  H  C  G  O  N  A  B  V  J
H  B  Q  E  I  I  N  M  X  J  R  A  H  X  C  N  E  L  W  O
P  Y  R  F  R  U  N  Z  I  C  L  F  O  H  T  K  V  V  X  E
B  R  M  B  A  I  N  B  V  A  U  G  O  I  N  I  I  O  D  X
P  Y  A  I  L  S  D  X  N  I  T  D  P  P  A  M  T  N  W  C
K  A  Z  U  G  Y  S  E  A  F  I  Y  Z  S  T  X  A  Z  R  X
B  G  S  X  Z  F  S  N  D  L  R  J  R  G  S  V  D  S  Z  N
S  N  J  X  U  T  T  N  A  E  B  T  P  G  E  D  E  G  I  W
I  Z  Y  B  H  A  N  T  T  A  N  A  L  G  E  S  I  C  P
O  S  Q  E  C  A  O  I  F  T  K  P  I  P  N  U  E  N  J  O
G  T  T  I  R  R  C  I  S  V  Z  I  Z  L  O  M  M  B  H  S
E  I  D  J  S  N  G  K  W  S  L  K  W  U  C  C  B  Y  A  Y
C  T  N  A  L  U  G  A  O  C  I  T  N  A  E  H  G  S  M  J
C  I  T  E  R  U  I  D  E  F  L  B  Y  R  D  V  I  K  O  M
```

Numbs a localized area	Pain reliever	Reduces activity of acid in stomach
Combats growth of bacteria	Prevents blood clots	Destroys fungus
Reduces effects of histamines on the body	Reduces inflammation	Reduces fever
Combats virus reproduction	Dilates bronchial tubes	Reduces inflammation in the nasal cavity
Increases production of urine	Helps control diabetes	Calms and relaxes the body

111

Pathology Fill-In-The-Blank

Pathology of the Cardiovascular System

Anemia is a lack of _____ and an over-abundance of carbon dioxide in the blood. The most common cause is a lack of _____ in the body, which causes a decrease in the amount of _____ produced in erythrocytes.

An aneurysm is a _____ in the wall of an artery, caused by a weakened arterial wall. Aneurysms are most commonly caused by _____ putting too much pressure or strain on the artery. Aneurysms may burst open, causing severe internal hemorrhaging.

Arrhythmia is a condition of the heart, resulting in the heart's natural _____ being altered. Three common types of arrhythmia include Atrial Fibrillation, in which the atria contract irregularly, Bradycardia, which causes the heart to beat too _____, and Tachycardia, which causes the heart to beat too _____.

A heart murmur results in blood flowing _____ in the heart due to malfunctioning _____, typically the bicuspid/mitral valve. Formation of blood clots may result, in addition to fatigue due to lack of sufficient oxygen reaching tissues.

Hypertension is also known as _____, and may be caused by poor diet, adrenal dysfunction, and kidney disease. Hypertension may lead to serious medical conditions, such as myocardial infarction. Hypertension may be treated with medications such as _____, beta blockers, and diuretics.

Migraine headaches are also known as _____ headaches. Migraines are typically caused by dilation of extracranial blood vessels, which places pressure on the meninges, resulting in severe pain. Migraines may be produced by exposure to caffeine and other chemicals, stress, and hormonal imbalances, such as during menstruation.

Myocardial Infarctions, also known as _____, are caused by obstruction of blood flow to the heart muscle. This lack of blood flow can result in _____ of the heart muscle, which can lead to a myocardial infarction.

Phlebitis is _____ of a _____, which may develop blood clots. Trauma and immobility are likely causes of phlebitis, along with pregnancy. Deep vein thrombosis may result, in which blood clots form in the blood vessels involved. _____ are typically prescribed for deep vein thrombosis.

Raynaud's Syndrome is a disease that results in _____ of the blood vessels in the fingers and toes, which restricts _____ supply to these areas. Primary Raynaud's Syndrome occurs independently of other conditions, while Secondary Raynaud's Syndrome is associated with other conditions. Exposure to cold temperatures, stress, and cigarette smoking are all contributing factors to the development of Primary Raynaud's Syndrome. Treatments can include exercise, not smoking, and possibly exposing the affected areas to warmth.

Varicose veins are a form of phlebitis that results in swollen veins. Varicose veins are caused by dysfunction of the _____ inside the veins, which are responsible for helping push blood back up the body towards the heart. This causes blood to pool backwards, putting pressure on the veins, causing them to become swollen and much more visible.

Pathology of the Digestive System

Diverticulitis, which only occurs if someone has diverticulosis, is an _____ of diverticular pouches, which can result in abscesses and ulceration of the large intestine. Can result in peritonitis, which requires medical attention.

Diverticulosis, a condition affecting the large intestine, results in the development of small _____ forming in the walls of the large intestine. These occur when the large intestine contracts without substances to press against, which causes the walls of the large intestine to become weakened.

Hepatitis is a _____ infection that causes _____ of the _____. Symptoms include yellowing of the skin(jaundice), fever, and nausea. Hepatitis may be acute or chronic, depending on which infection the person contracts.

A hernia is a _____ of an organ through its surrounding connective tissue membrane. A hernia may cause pain, discomfort, or possible impairment of organ function depending on the organ and severity of the hernia.

Pathology of the Endocrine System

Addison's Disease is an _____ disorder affecting the _____ glands, which results in a lack of cortisol and/or aldosterone production. Addison's Disease is caused by damage to the _____ cortex, which limits the body's ability to produce stress hormones.

Cushing's Disease is a condition caused by excessive growth of the _____ gland, or the development of a tumor on the gland. This causes an increased production of ACTH, which stimulates hyper-production of _____.

Diabetes Mellitus affects _____ function in the body. Diabetes Type I is caused by a decrease in _____ levels in the body, which reduces the breakdown of glucose. Diabetes Type II is caused by the body having an _____ resistance. Gestational Diabetes is only present when a person is _____.

Grave's Disease is an _____ disorder, which affects the _____ gland, causing an increase in production of _____ hormone. Grave's Disease can cause sensitivity to heat, weight loss, development of a goiter, bulging of the eyes, and irregular heart rhythm.

Hypothyroidism is an _____ disorder affecting the _____ gland, resulting in a lack of _____ hormone being produced. This can result in weight gain, fatigue, hair loss, sensitivity to cold, and body pain.

Pathology of the Integumentary System

Acne is an infection of the skin, typically caused by blockage of a pore due to excessive oil on the skin. The pore may become _____. Increased oil on the skin may be caused by increased _____ production, stress, hormonal imbalances, and poor personal hygiene.

Athlete's Foot, also known as Tinea Pedis, is a highly contagious _____ infection found on the feet. As the infection spreads, it can cause drying and cracking of the feet, and may itch. Bacterial infection may result from breaking of the skin.

A boil is a _____ infection of a hair follicle, also known as a _____. Boils usually result from small cuts in the skin, which allow _____ to enter the body and reproduce. Pus may develop in the affected area.

Burns are the result of damage to the skin caused by _____ or _____. First degree burns affect the _____. Second degree burns move deeper into the skin, and may result in the formation of _____. Third degree burns move into the _____ layer of the skin, and cause necrosis. Fourth degree burns move beyond the skin, and can damage tissues such as muscles, tendons, ligaments, and bones.

Cellulitis is a _____ infection of the skin, caused by _____ entering the body through exposure to _____, most commonly on the legs. The infection presents with well-defined borders of inflammation.

A decubitus ulcer is also known as a _____ ulcer or _____ sore. Decubitus ulcers are caused by prolonged _____ being placed on a part of the body, resulting in lack of blood flow to the area. If ischemia is excessive, _____ of the affected tissue may result, which could become infected.

Herpes Simplex is a highly contagious _____ infection of the skin. In the acute stage of infection, a person may develop a _____ around the mouth, often the result of stress.

Impetigo is an acute _____ infection, resulting in the formation of sores that form around the mouth, nose, and hands. These sores may develop blisters that leak a yellow, crust-like fluid. Impetigo is highly contagious, and most commonly seen in _____.

Psoriasis is an _____ disorder, in which the body's epithelial tissues are attacked. The epithelial cells quickly regenerate, which produces an excessive amount of epithelial cells. This causes thick, dry, possibly itchy patches of skin.

Ringworm is a _____ infection of the skin, similar to Athlete's Foot. Ringworm presents with a _____-like area of infection. Ringworm is contagious and common in athletes who play contact sports.

A sebaceous cyst is caused by blockage of a _____ gland. Bacteria may infect the gland as a result of the blockage. The body may develop connective tissue around the gland to prevent the infection from spreading.

A wart is a _____ infection, caused by the _____. A wart stimulates the excessive growth of keratin, which causes a hard, thick overgrowth on a small localized area. Warts are contagious.

Pathology of the Lymphatic System

An allergy is a reaction of the body's immune system in response to substances that normally _____ affect people. Common substances people may be allergic to include dust, pollen, mold, certain foods, pet dander, and medication.

Lupus Erythematosus is an _____

disorder affecting the _____ tissues of the entire body, and may present with a _____ rash that appears on the face during flare-ups. Symptoms include fever, joint pain, discomfort, fatigue, and sensitivity to sunlight.

Lymphedema is a condition that results in increased amounts of _____ fluid in a limb, which causes _____. Causes vary, from damage to a lymph node or vessel, obesity, and advanced age.

Pitting edema is a form of edema that produces _____ in the skin after pressure is applied and released. Pitting edema may have serious under-lying causes, including _____ failure.

Pathology of the Muscular System

Adhesive capsulitis results in restricted range-of-motion at the shoulder joint, caused by _____ forming between the joint capsule and the head of the humerus. It may also be caused by a hypertonic _____ muscle. Another name for adhesive capsulitis is "_____ Shoulder".

De Quervain's Tenosynovitis is a form of tenosynovitis(inflammation of a tendon and its sheath) that specifically affects the _____, caused by _____.

Golfer's Elbow is a form of tendonitis that results in pain and inflammation at the _____ epicondyle of the humerus. The _____ of the wrist are affected.

A strain is an injury to a _____ or _____, usually caused by over-exertion or over-use.

Tendonitis is an injury that results in _____ of a _____. Tendonitis is most commonly a repetitive strain injury.

Tennis Elbow is a form of tendonitis that results in pain and inflammation at the _____ epicondyle of the humerus. The _____ of the wrist are affected.

Tenosynovitis is a repetitive strain injury that results in _____ of a _____ and its protective _____. Tenosynovitis primarily affects the hands, wrists, and feet due to the _____ of _____ in these areas.

Pathology of the Nervous System

Bell's Palsy results in paralysis of one side of the face as a result of damage to the _____ nerve.

Carpal Tunnel Syndrome is caused by compression of the _____ nerve between the carpals and the transverse carpal ligament. This can result in loss of function and pain in the hand.

Encephalitis results in _____ of the _____, most commonly caused by a _____ infection, examples of which include mosquito-borne diseases, Herpes Simplex, and Rabies.

Multiple Sclerosis is an _____ disorder, in which the body's immune system attacks the _____ surrounding the axons in the central nervous system. This causes degeneration of the myelin, and can cause extreme pain, discomfort, and loss of function.

Paralysis is a loss of _____ of a part of the body. Paralysis is typically caused by _____ to a nerve that innervates a muscle. Paraplegia is when a person's _____ are paralyzed. Quadriplegia is when all _____ limbs are paralyzed. Hemiplegia is when one _____ of the body is paralyzed.

Parkinson's Disease is a motor disease that results in _____ due to a loss of the neurotransmitter _____. This can lead to debilitation of movements such as walking and talking over longer periods.

Sciatica, most commonly caused by a _____ in the lumbar vertebrae, results in pain radiating down the buttocks, posterior thigh, and leg, due to compression of the _____ nerve.

Thoracic Outlet Syndrome is caused by _____ of nerves and blood vessels passing through the _____ outlet. It is commonly caused by tight muscles, including the _____ minor and _____. Obesity and tumors in the neck may also contribute.

Trigeminal Neuralgia is a chronic condition affecting the _____, caused by compression of the _____ nerve. This makes any pressure on the face extremely painful.

Pathology of the Respiratory System

Asthma is a chronic respiratory disease in which the _____ muscles in the respiratory tract spasm, causing a constriction of the airways. Commonly caused as a result of inhaling an irritant such as dust or smoke.

Bronchitis is _____ of the bronchial tubes, which restricts the airways and makes breathing difficult. Acute bronchitis is the result of a _____ infection of the respiratory system such as influenza. Chronic bronchitis is the result of irritants constantly entering the lungs, such as _____ and dust.

Emphysema results in the degeneration of the _____ in the lungs due to exposure to irritants such as _____. This decreases the intake of oxygen and elimination of waste, such as carbon dioxide.

Influenza is a highly contagious _____ infection, which results in fever, general malaise, body aches, runny nose, and cough.

Pneumonia is a highly contagious _____ infection of the lungs, which results in a buildup of _____ in the _____.

Pathology of the Skeletal System

Bursitis is _____ of a _____, a small sac filled with synovial fluid. Common causes for bursitis include repetitive motions, and trauma.

A dislocation is when a bone becomes _____ from its normal location. This results in immobilization of the joint and temporary deformation. Most commonly caused by trauma to a joint.

A fracture is a _____ in a bone. A simple fracture is a fracture that does not _____ the skin. A compound fracture is a fracture that _____ the skin.

Gout is a form of arthritis, most commonly seen around the base of the _____, caused by an over-abundance of _____ acid crystals in the body.

A herniated disc is caused by protrusions of the _____ through the _____ of an intervertebral disc, which may place pressure on spinal nerves emerging from the spinal cord.

Kyphosis, also known as Dowager's Hump, is a condition causing _____ of the _____ vertebrae. Common causes include tight muscles, such as _____ and _____, osteoporosis, and ankylosing spondylitis. Can result in _____ in the lumbar region.

Lordosis, also known as Swayback, is a condition causing _____ of the _____ vertebrae. Common causes include tight muscles, such as psoas major, iliacus, quadratus lumborum, and rectus femoris, weak muscles such as rectus abdominis and the hamstrings, obesity, and

osteoporosis.

Osgood-Schlatter Disease is a type of repetitive strain injury, caused by over-use of the _____ tendon and the _____ muscle group. This can cause an over-growth of bone at the _____ tuberosity.

Osteoarthritis is the most common form of arthritis, also known as "wear-and-tear" arthritis. It is caused by progressive damage to the _____ separating one bone from another. Erosion of the cartilage takes place, which irritates the joint, causing inflammation and pain. The most common location for massage therapists to develop osteoarthritis is in the _____ joint.

Osteoporosis is a condition that causes weakness and _____ in the _____. Commonly caused by a decrease in the hormone _____.

Rheumatoid Arthritis is an _____ disorder, which results in inflammation, pain, and deformity of the joints around the hands and wrists. Caused by destruction of the _____ membrane, which is then replaced by thick, fibrous material.

Scoliosis is caused by a _____ curvature of the thoracic vertebrae, which can be caused by hyper-tonic muscles unilaterally, such as the _____, congenital deformities, and poor posture.

A sprain is an injury to a _____. A grade 1 sprain is stretching of a ligament without _____. A grade 2 sprain is _____ of a ligament, but may heal on its own without surgery. A grade 3 sprain is a complete _____ of a ligament, and does require surgery to repair.

Temporomandibular Joint Dysfunction is a condition of the mandible, causing simple tasks such as _____ to become painful and difficult. Can be caused by arthritis in the joint, or damage to the disc between the articulating bones.

Pathology of the Urinary System

Cystitis is a _____ infection, which results in _____ of the _____. Often, it can involve the entire urinary system, which is known as a Urinary Tract Infection.

Cancers

Basal Cell Carcinoma is a malignant form of _____ cancer. It is the _____ common, _____ growing,

_____ serious type of skin cancer. Typically affects parts of the body exposed to sunlight, such as the face, neck, and arms.

Malignant Melanoma is a malignant form of _____ cancer. It is the _____ common, _____ growing, _____ serious type of skin cancer. Caused by over-exposure to sunlight, which can cause the _____ to reproduce uncontrolled.

Non-Hodgkin's Lymphoma is a type of cancer of the _____ system, caused by the development of tumors by _____.

Squamous Cell Carcinoma is a malignant form of _____ cancer. It is _____ serious and _____ common than Basal Cell Carcinoma. Tumors appear in areas exposed to sunlight, such as the face, head, and arms.

Medications

- Analgesics help to relieve _____.

- Antacids reduce the activity of _____ in the stomach.

- Antibiotics are used to combat _____ growth.

- Anticoagulants reduce the formation of _____.

- Antifungals aid in destroying _____.

- Antihistamines reduce the effects of _____ on the body.

- Anti-inflammatory agents reduce _____.

- Antipyretics are used to help reduce _____.

- Antivirals aid in preventing _____ reproduction.

- Beta blockers help reduce _____.

- Bronchodilators aid in _____ of the _____.

- Decongestants reduce _____ in the _____ cavity.

- Diuretics increase the production of _____.

- Insulin is responsible for _____ the amount of _____ in the blood stream.

- Local anesthetics are used to _____ an area, most commonly administered via _____.

- Sedatives are used to _____ and _____ the body.

- Statins aid in lowering _____ levels in the blood stream.

117

CPR and First Aid

CPR

CPR stands for

_____, and consists
of alternating _____ compressions and
_____ support.

First Aid

Universal precautions are treating every person
and fluid as if they were
_____ or
_____. This helps contain
blood-borne pathogens. Gloves and other
_____ should
be worn any time there is exposure to any type
of bodily fluid.

Heat Injuries

Heat exhaustion is caused by a person having a
_____ body temperature with excessive
_____.

Heat cramps cause involuntary _____
of the _____ due to dehydration
and loss of electrolytes.

Heat stroke is when a person as an extremely
_____ body temperature, with a lack of
_____, and can potentially be
fatal.

Cold Injuries

Hypothermia is caused by the body temperature
dropping below _____ degrees, and can be
potentially fatal.

Frostbite is caused by a formation of _____
crystals in _____ tissues, which may
result in necrosis of the affected tissues.

The Rule of 9's

The Rule of 9's is used to determine the extent
of _____ by the total body area
involved. Each percentage represents the
percentage of the body damaged by burns.

Wounds

Wounds are the result of a _____ in
the skin, which exposes underlying tissues.

An incision is a _____
through tissue.

A laceration is a cut that produces
_____ edges.

An abrasion is produced by _____
skin.

A puncture is caused by an object
_____ the skin, producing a
_____.

Bites and Stings

An animal bite requires application of a sterile
bandage after forcing _____ to
flush out bacteria from the area and cleansing
with soap and water.

Insect stings should be _____ with a
hard, flat, sharp object to remove any stinger
left in the skin.

Snake bites require EMS contact, and the bitten
area should be immobilized below the
_____.

Spider bites and scorpion stings should be
cleansed with soap and water, and the area
should be immobilized below the
_____.

Orthopedic Injuries

Orthopedic injuries, such as strains and sprains,
are primarily treated with the use of PRICE:
_____, _____,
_____, _____,
_____.

Poisoning

Inhaled poisons, such as carbon monoxide,
may require the use of an
_____, or breathing support by
way of an _____ mask.

Injection poisoning introduces harmful
substances into the body via
_____, insect stings, sharp
objects, or bites.

Absorption of poison typically includes
exposure to substances such as
_____.

Ingestion is introducing harmful substances
through _____. Induced
_____ may be required.

Matching Answers

D   R
P   B
G   I
O   M
A   L
N   H
T   C
J   F
S   K
E   Q

Pathology Answers

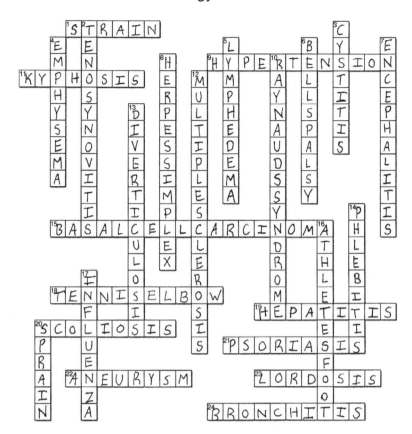

Medications

Find the medications based on what they're used for!

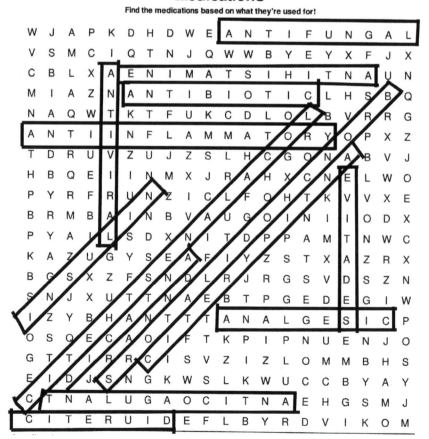

Pathology Practice Exam

1. Most common form of arthritis
A. Rheumatoid arthritis
B. Gouty arthritis
C. Osteoarthritis
D. Periostitis

2. Loss of density in bone, caused by a decrease in the hormone estrogen in the body
A. Osteomyelitis
B. Menopause
C. Osteoporosis
D. Scoliosis

3. Cellulitis
A. Bacterial infection resulting in yellow scabs around the nose
B. Viral infection resulting in yellow scabs around the mouth
C. Bacterial infection involving the skin and surrounding tissues
D. Viral infection causing cold sores to appear around the mouth

4. Aneurysm
A. Bulge in an artery wall, usually caused by a weakened artery due to a condition such as hypertension
B. Inflammation of a vein due to trauma, resulting in blood clot formation
C. Blood clot in the blood stream becoming lodged in the heart, lungs, or brain, resulting in death of tissue
D. Ischemia in the myocardium due to a blockage in the coronary arteries, resulting in myocardial infarction

5. Pain felt at the medial epicondyle of the humerus is associated with
A. Tennis elbow
B. Golfer's elbow
C. Carpal tunnel syndrome
D. Synovitis

6. Bradycardia is a form of
A. Aneurysm
B. Heart murmur
C. Infarction
D. Arrhythmia

7. Bacterial infection resulting in honeycomb sores around the mouth and nose
A. Boil
B. Impetigo
C. Psoriasis
D. Meningitis

8. Lordosis is also known as
A. Swayback
B. Dowager's hump
C. Scoliosis
D. Bamboo spine

9. Decrease in oxygen traveling throughout the body
A. Hypoplasia
B. Hypoglycemia
C. Hypoxia
D. Hyperplasia

10. Achilles tendonitis can be caused by a strain to the
A. Pes anserinus
B. Patellar tendon
C. Calcaneal tendon
D. Ischial tuberosity tendon

11. While at work, Chris falls and lands on his back, injuring it. The next day, he calls to make a massage appointment, hoping the massage will help with his pain. The appropriate response would be
A. Reschedule the massage and refer the client to a physician
B. Perform the massage and do compression onto the back
C. Perform the massage and apply heat to the affected area
D. Perform the massage and do passive joint mobilization on the vertebrae

12. The most common site of sprain
A. Shoulder
B. Knee
C. Elbow
D. Ankle

13. Nausea, vomiting, and fatigue with yellowing of the skin may be the result of
A. Hepatitis
B. Food poisoning
C. Diarrhea
D. Meningitis

14. Spasm of capillaries in the fingers and toes, restricting circulation
A. Cyanosis
B. Raynaud's syndrome
C. Emphysema
D. Diabetes mellitus

15. Signs of inflammation include
A. Heat, pain, redness, coldness
B. Pain, edema, swelling, redness
C. Swelling, heat, redness, pain
D. Redness, pain, heat, dehydration

16. Squamous cell carcinoma is what type of tumor
A. Benign
B. Malignant
C. Idiopathic
D. Lymphatic

17. A client who suffers from pitting edema would be referred to which doctor
A. Dermatologist
B. Nephrologist
C. Cardiologist
D. Gastroenterologist

18. Ischemia may ultimately result in
A. Phlebitis
B. Arteriosclerosis
C. Necrosis
D. Varicose veins

19. Anticoagulants are medications that prevent
A. Blood vessel dilation
B. Inflammation
C. Mucous production
D. Blood clotting

20. All of the following are contagious conditions except
A. Mononucleosis
B. Herpes Simplex
C. Psoriasis
D. Tinea Pedis

21. Encephalitis
A. Inflammation of the brain caused by a viral infection
B. Aneurysm in the cerebrum causing brain damage
C. Blockage of a coronary artery, resulting in necrosis of myocardium
D. Inflammation of the meninges, leading to migraine headaches

22. Inflammation of a bursa sac, usually present due to trauma
A. Synovitis
B. Bursitis
C. Osteoarthritis
D. Bruxism

23. Medication prescribed to fight off bacterial infections
A. Anti-inflammatory Agents
B. Antivenoms
C. Antipyretics
D. Antibiotics

24. Pacemakers are commonly implanted in patients who suffer from
A. Arrhythmia
B. Emphysema
C. Angina pectoris
D. Heart murmur

25. Virus resulting in the development of warts
A. Herpes simplex
B. Human papilloma virus
C. Epstein-Barr virus
D. Urticaria

26. Excessive death of myocardium results in
A. Arrhythmia
B. Stroke
C. Myocardial infarction
D. Heart murmur

27. Grade 3 sprain
A. Complete rupture of a ligament
B. Partial tearing of a tendon
C. Complete rupture of a tendon
D. Partial tearing of a ligament

28. A lack of hemoglobin in erythrocytes may result in
A. Decreased immune response
B. Raynaud's syndrome
C. Myocardial infarction
D. Anemia

29. Due to having a shorter urethra, women are more prone to developing the following condition than men
A. Prostatitis
B. Nephritis
C. Cystitis
D. Cholecystitis

30. In a client with lordosis, the following muscle might be weakened, resulting in an exaggerated anterior tilt of the pelvis
A. Psoas major
B. Latissimus dorsi
C. Quadratus lumborum
D. Rectus abdominis

31. Viral or bacterial infection resulting in severe increases of fluids in the lungs
A. Pneumonia
B. Asthma
C. Bronchitis
D. Emphysema

32. Dopamine is a neurotransmitter which helps to stabilize the body in specific movements. A lack of dopamine in the body would result in
A. Anemia
B. Alzheimer's disease
C. Parkinson's disease
D. Sleep apnea

33. A cardiologist is a doctor who specializes in the
A. Lungs
B. Heart
C. Liver
D. Bladder

34. A blood pressure reading of 140/90 results in a person being diagnosed with
A. Hypertension
B. Hypotension
C. Hyperemia
D. Myocardial infarction

35. The most common type of diabetes
A. Insulin-dependent diabetes
B. Diabetes type I
C. Juvenile diabetes
D. Diabetes type II

36. Emphysema
A. Spasm of smooth muscle surrounding bronchial tubes, reducing inhalation
B. Inflammation of bronchial tubes due to inhalation of smoke from cigarette smoking
C. Destruction of alveoli, resulting in decreased oxygen intake
D. Bacterial infection of the lungs, reducing carbon dioxide output

37. Paralysis of one half of the face, caused by stimulation of the Herpes Simplex virus, which affects the Facial nerve
A. Graves disease
B. Cerebral palsy
C. Trigeminal neuralgia
D. Bell's palsy

38. Chronic inflammation located at the tibial tuberosity, caused by overuse of the quadriceps
A. Osgood-Schlatter disease
B. Grave's disease
C. Raynaud's disease
D. Knock-knee

39. Viral infection resulting in inflammation of the liver
A. Nephritis
B. Hepatitis
C. Mononucleosis
D. Encephalitis

40. Varicose veins most often occur in
A. Legs
B. Arms
C. Thighs
D. Ankles

41. Portion of an intervertebral disc that protrudes through the annulus fibrosus during a disc herniation
A. Spinal cord
B. Annulus pulposus
C. Facet cartilage
D. Nucleus pulposus

42. Autoimmune disorder affecting myelin sheaths in the central nervous system
A. Multiple sclerosis
B. Myasthenia gravis
C. Parkinson's disease
D. Alzheimer's disease

43. Paralysis of the lower limbs
A. Quadriplegia
B. Hemiplegia
C. Paraplegia
D. Triplegia

44. Fungal infection affecting the epidermis, resulting in a circular rash
A. Cordyceps
B. Athlete's foot
C. Ringworm
D. Whitlow

45. A common treatment for bursitis
A. Lymphatic drainage
B. Heat and compression
C. Rest and ice
D. Cold compress and friction

46. Chris has recently recovered from a severe pneumonia infection. A massage technique that may aid in lung decongestion would be
A. Vibration
B. Effleurage
C. Tapotement
D. Friction

47. Analgesics are used to combat
A. Pain
B. Obesity
C. Inflammation
D. Gout

48. Benign tumors
A. Spread to other parts of the body through lymph
B. Do not spread to other locations in the body
C. Spread to other parts of the body through blood
D. Spread to other parts of the body through interstitial fluid

49. Overproduction in melanocytes results in a tumor known as
A. Sarcoma
B. Carcinoma
C. Melanoma
D. Lymphoma

50. Lice, scabies, and ticks are all types of
A. Parasites
B. Bacterium
C. Fungi
D. Viruses

Pathology Practice Exam Answer Key

01. C	26. C
02. C	27. A
03. C	28. D
04. A	29. C
05. B	30. D
06. D	31. A
07. B	32. C
08. A	33. B
09. C	34. A
10. C	35. D
11. A	36. C
12. D	37. D
13. A	38. A
14. B	39. B
15. C	40. A
16. B	41. D
17. B	42. A
18. C	43. C
19. D	44. C
20. C	45. C
21. A	46. C
22. B	47. A
23. D	48. B
24. A	49. C
25. B	50. A

For detailed answer explanations, watch the
video at mblextestprep.com/resources.html

Kinesiology

A large portion of a massage therapist's knowledge should be about muscles, bones, attachment sites, and actions. All of this information may be seen on the MBLEx.

In this section, we will discuss many subjects, covering a wide range of information.

Information covered in this section includes:

Muscle Actions
Bony Landmarks
Muscles of the Head
Muscles of the Neck
Muscles of the Back
Muscles of the Chest
Muscles of the Abdomen
Muscles of the Arm
Muscles of the Forearm
Muscles of the Pelvis
Muscles of the Thigh
Muscles of the Leg

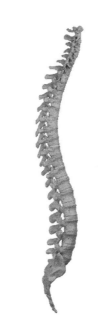

This information is followed by seven assignments:

Kinesiology Matching
Kinesiology Crossword
Muscle Action Fill-In-The-Blank
Bony Landmark Fill-In-The-Blank
Muscle Fill-In-The-Blank
Muscle Labeling
Bone Labeling

The end of the section has a 50 question practice exam on Kinesiology. These questions ARE NOT the exact same questions will you see on the MBLEx. They are meant to test information that MAY be seen on the MBLEx.

While taking the practice exam, make sure to utilize your test-taking strategies(page 3) to optimize your test scores.

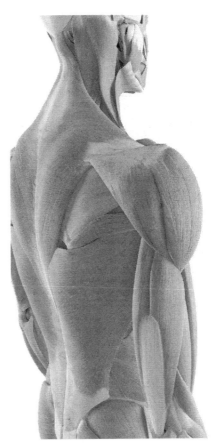

Muscle Actions

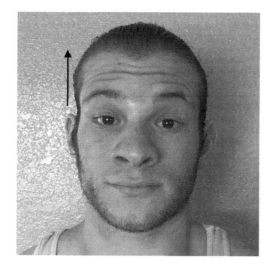

Eyebrow Elevation

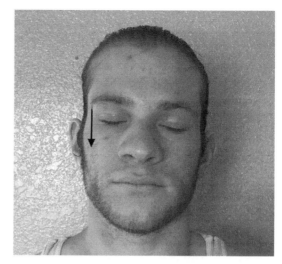

Eyelid Depression

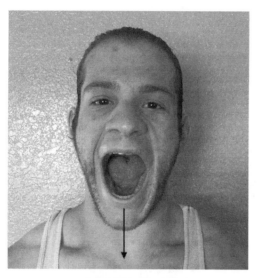

Jaw Depression

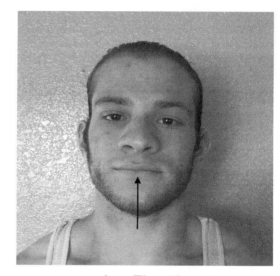

Jaw Elevation

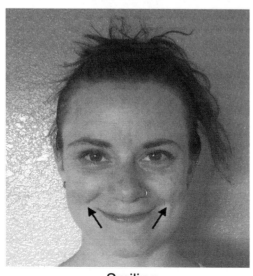

Smiling

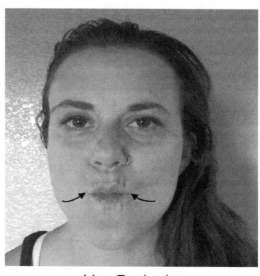

Lips Puckering

125

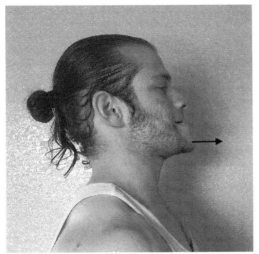

Jaw Protraction

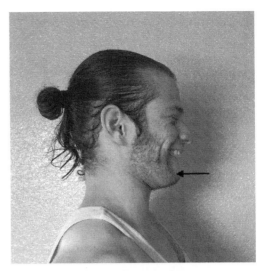

Jaw Retraction

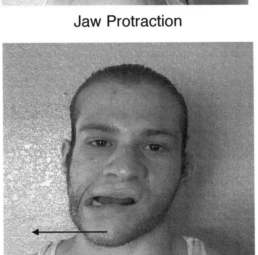

Jaw Lateral Deviation

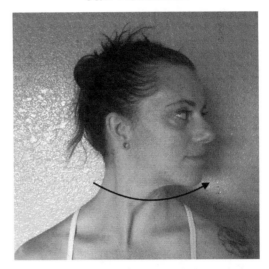

Neck Rotation

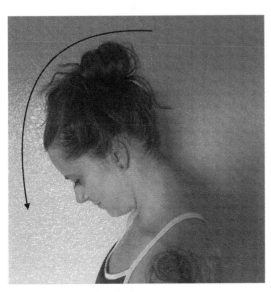

Neck Flexion

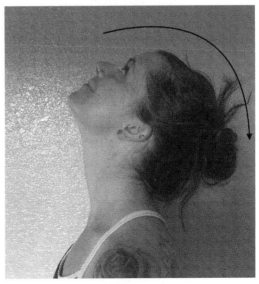

Neck Extension

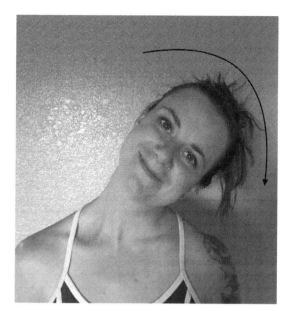

Neck Lateral Flexion

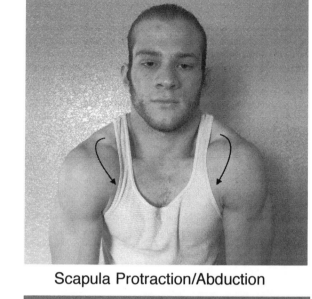

Scapula Protraction/Abduction

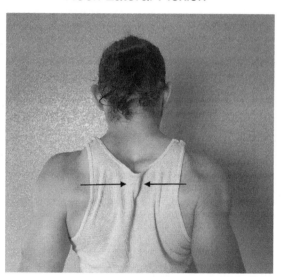

Scapula Retraction/Adduction

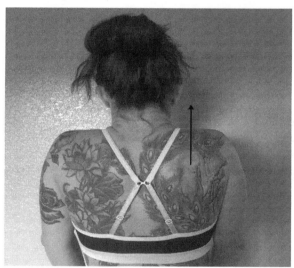

Scapula Elevation

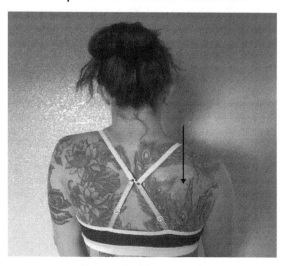

Scapula Depression

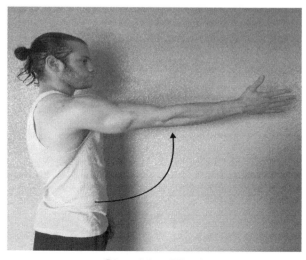

Shoulder Flexion

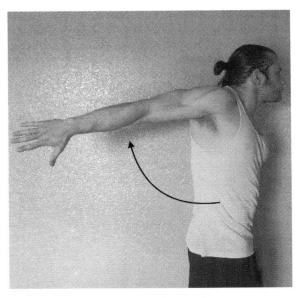

Shoulder Extension

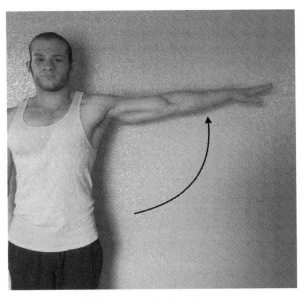

Shoulder Abduction

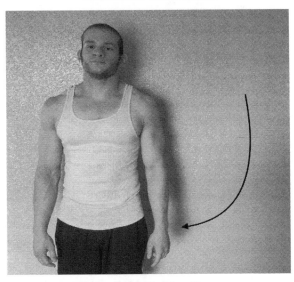

Shoulder Adduction

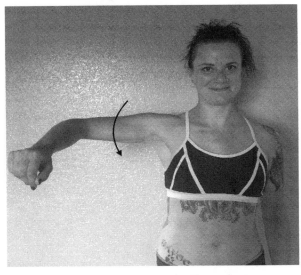

Shoulder Medial Rotation

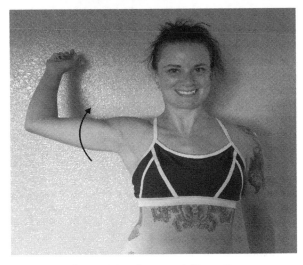

Shoulder Lateral Rotation

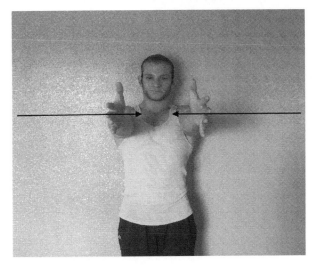

Shoulder Horizontal Adduction

128

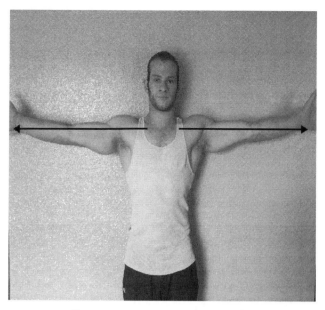

Shoulder Horizontal Abduction

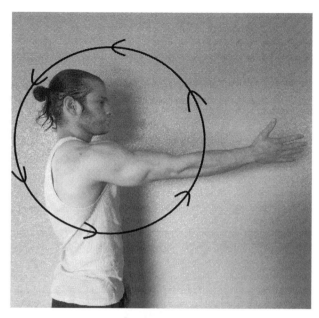

Circumduction

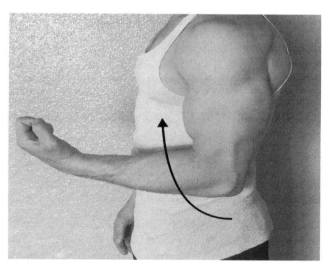

Elbow Flexion

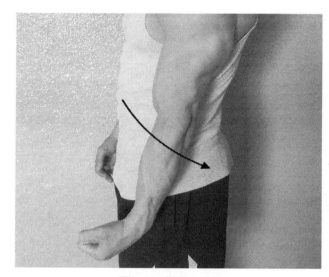

Elbow Extension

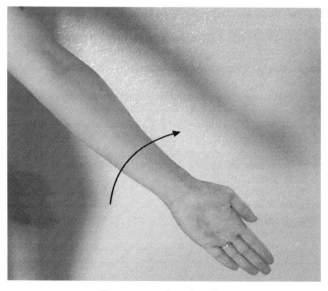

Forearm Supination

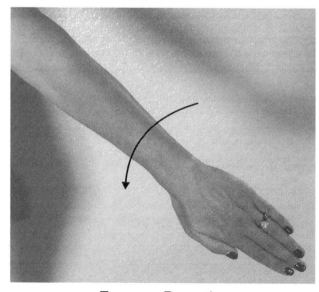

Forearm Pronation

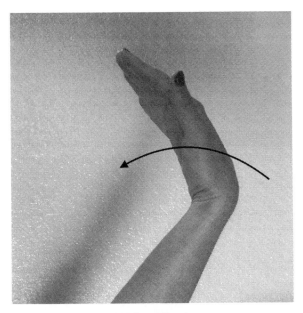

Wrist Flexion

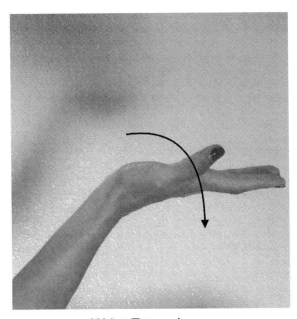

Wrist Extension

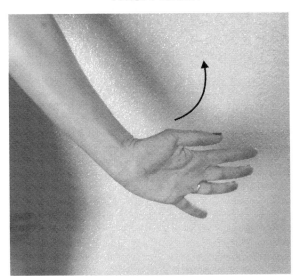

Wrist Abduction

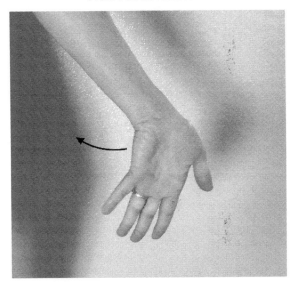

Wrist Adduction

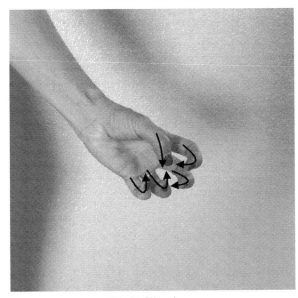

Digit Flexion

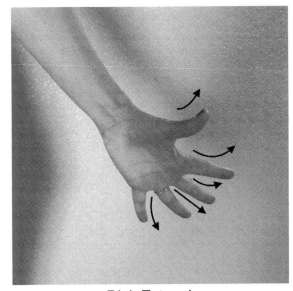

Digit Extension

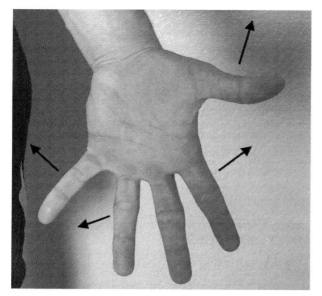

Digit Abduction

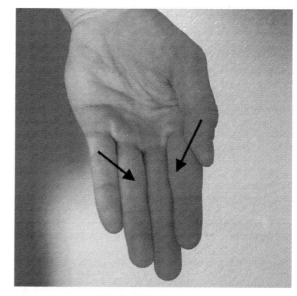

Digit Adduction

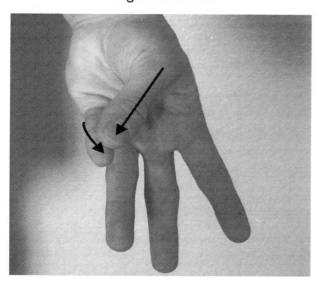

Opposition

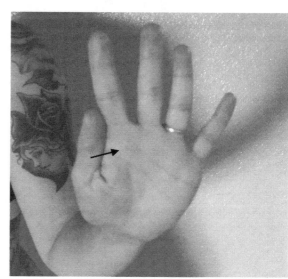

Thumb Adduction

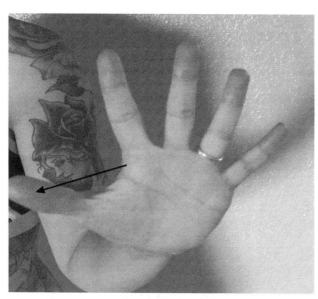

Thumb Abduction

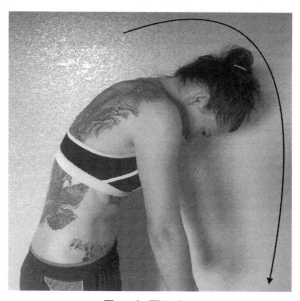

Trunk Flexion

131

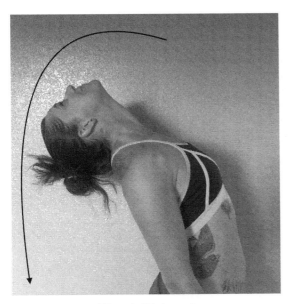

Trunk Extension

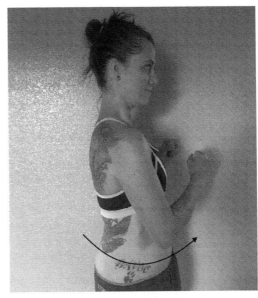

Trunk Rotation

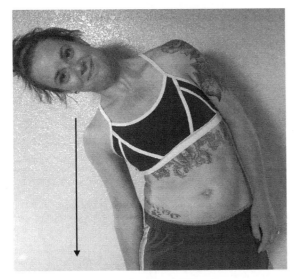

Trunk Lateral Flexion

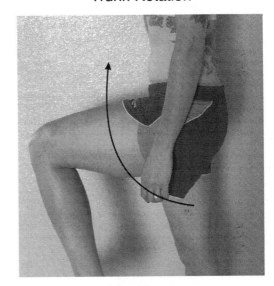

Hip Flexion

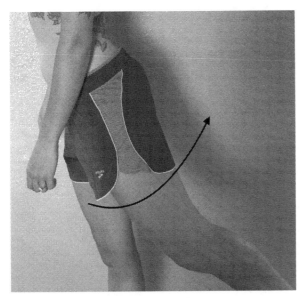

Hip Extension

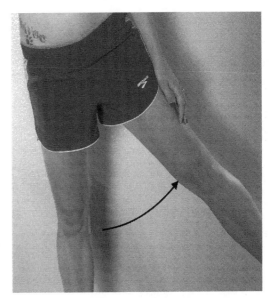

Hip Abduction

132

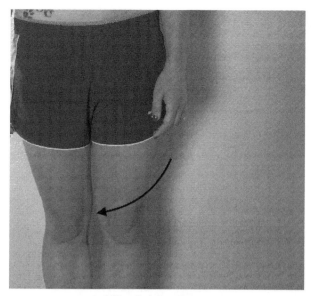

Hip Adduction

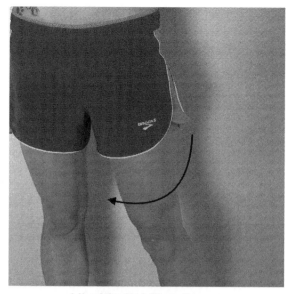

Hip Medial Rotation

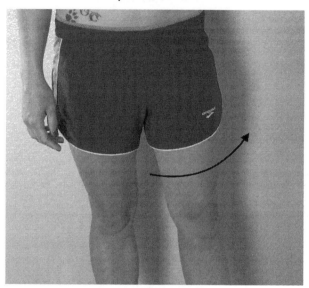

Hip Lateral Rotation

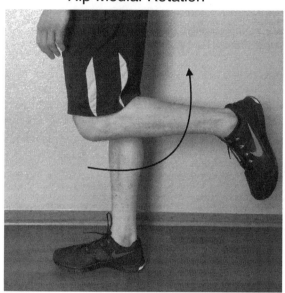

Knee Flexion

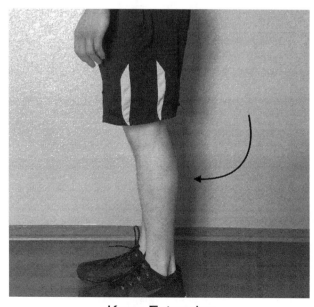

Knee Extension

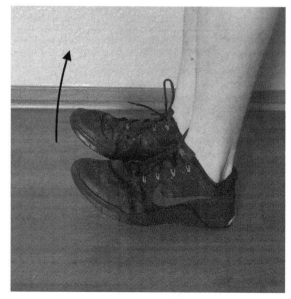

Dorsifexion

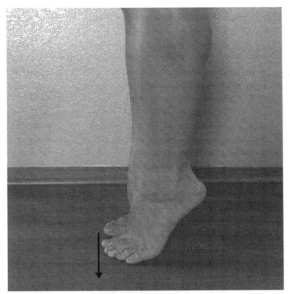

Plantarfexion

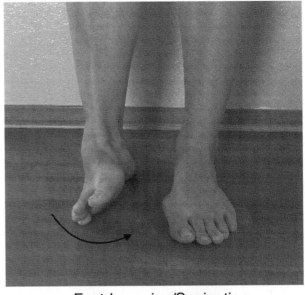

Foot Inversion/Supination

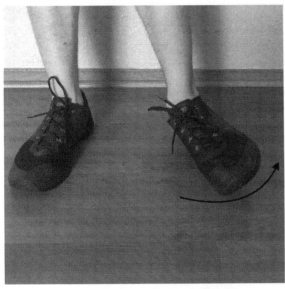

Foot Eversion/Pronation

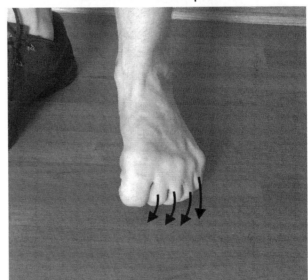

Digit Flexion

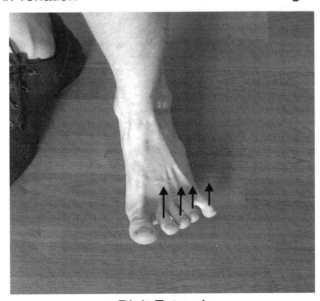

Digit Extension

Bony Landmarks

The bony landmarks are specific locations on bones where muscles attach to. There are many different kinds of landmarks, from tubercles and tuberosities, to condyles and epicondyles.

A condyle is a rounded projection coming off a bone at an articulation.
An epicondyle is the part of the bone located superior to the condyle.
A crest is a thin ridge of a bone.
A facet is a smooth articular surface of a bone.
A fissure is a narrow opening, resembling a crack.
A foramina(foramen) is a hole or opening in a bone.
A fossa is a shallow depression in a bone.
A linea is a narrow ridge, less pronounced than a crest.
A meatus is a canal-like passage.
A process is a prominent structure on a bone.
A ramus is an elongated, seemingly stretched-out part of a bone.
A sinus is a cavity created by bones.
A suture is a type of synarthrotic joint that doesn't allow movement.
A trochanter is a very large process, only found on the femur.
A tubercle is a small, rounded projection.
A tuberosity is a large, rounded, often rough projection.

Bones have numerous different types of landmarks. Landmarks are not only named after their type(above), but often times what they look like(example, "coracoid" means "resembling a crow's beak"), what muscles attach to them(example, deltoid tuberosity), or even where they're located in the body(example, anterior superior iliac spine).

Head

Temporal Fossa
O: Temporalis

Zygomatic Arch

Mastoid Process
I: Sternocleidomastoid

Angle of Mandible

External Occipital Protuberance
O: Trapezius

Superior Nuchal Line
O: Trapezius

136

Vertebrae

Spinous Process

Superior Articular Process

Vertebral Body

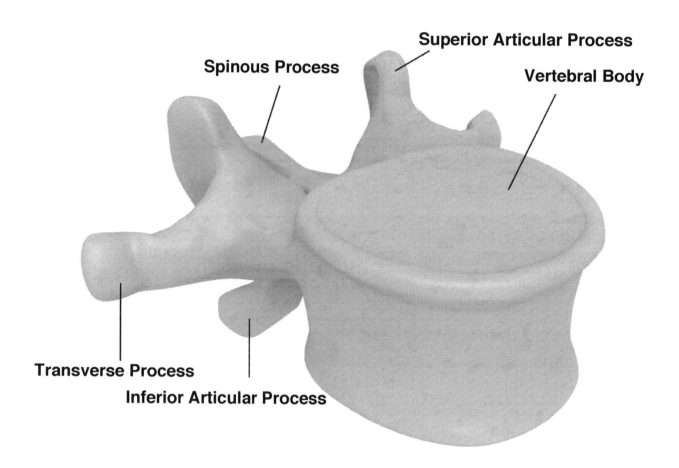

Transverse Process

Inferior Articular Process

Back

Anterior Scapula

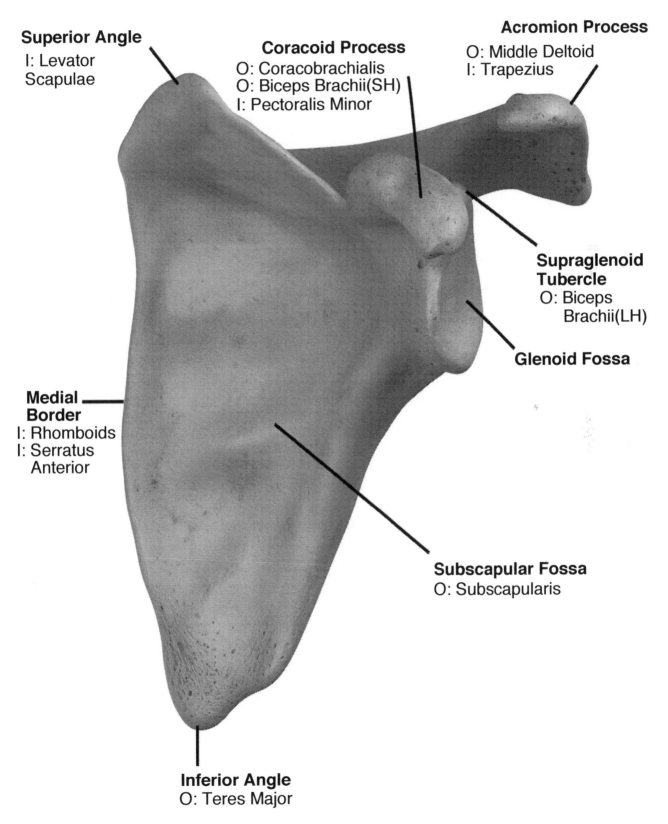

Superior Angle
I: Levator Scapulae

Coracoid Process
O: Coracobrachialis
O: Biceps Brachii(SH)
I: Pectoralis Minor

Acromion Process
O: Middle Deltoid
I: Trapezius

Supraglenoid Tubercle
O: Biceps Brachii(LH)

Glenoid Fossa

Medial Border
I: Rhomboids
I: Serratus Anterior

Subscapular Fossa
O: Subscapularis

Inferior Angle
O: Teres Major

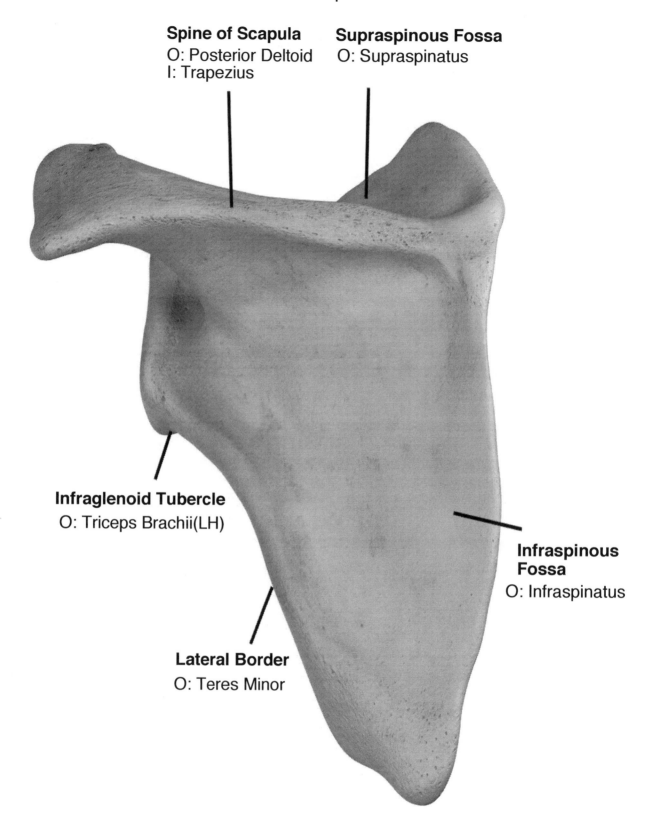

Spine of Scapula
O: Posterior Deltoid
I: Trapezius

Supraspinous Fossa
O: Supraspinatus

Infraglenoid Tubercle
O: Triceps Brachii(LH)

**Infraspinous
Fossa**
O: Infraspinatus

Lateral Border
O: Teres Minor

Chest

Clavicle

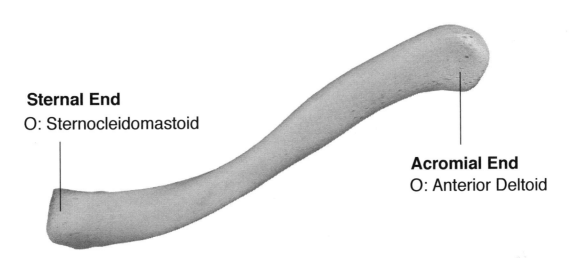

Sternal End
O: Sternocleidomastoid

Acromial End
O: Anterior Deltoid

Sternum

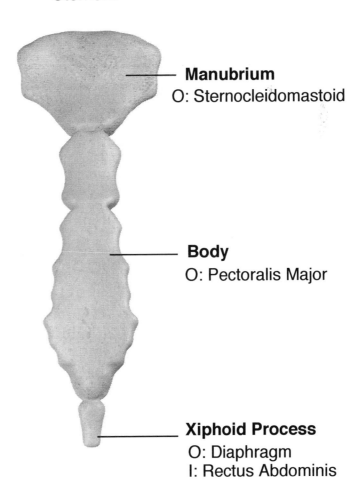

Manubrium
O: Sternocleidomastoid

Body
O: Pectoralis Major

Xiphoid Process
O: Diaphragm
I: Rectus Abdominis

Arm

Anterior Humerus

Posterior Humerus

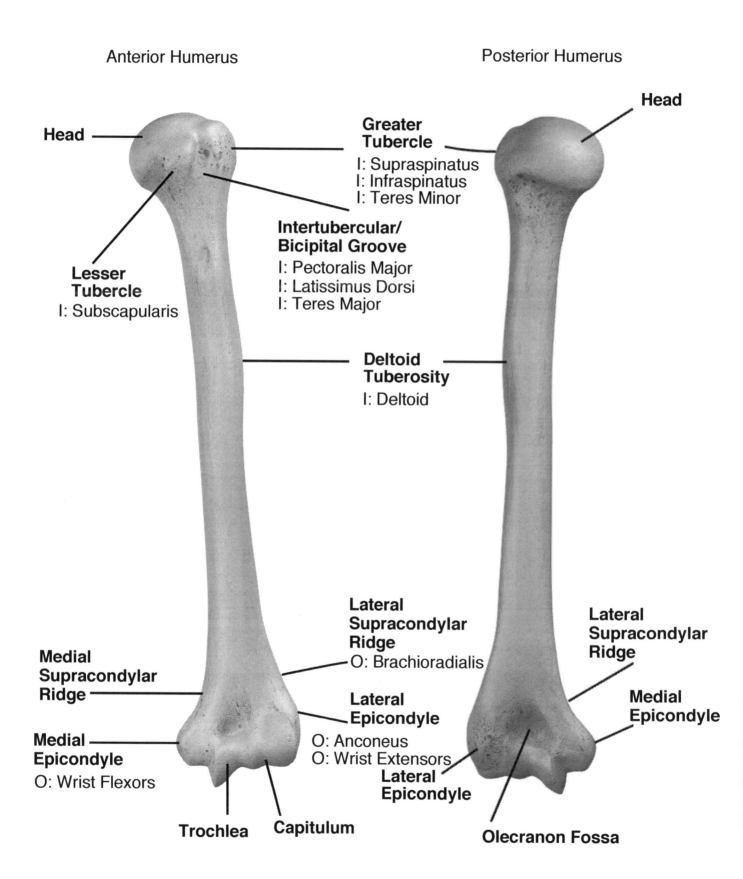

Head

Greater Tubercle
I: Supraspinatus
I: Infraspinatus
I: Teres Minor

Head

Lesser Tubercle
I: Subscapularis

Intertubercular/ Bicipital Groove
I: Pectoralis Major
I: Latissimus Dorsi
I: Teres Major

Deltoid Tuberosity
I: Deltoid

Lateral Supracondylar Ridge
O: Brachioradialis

Lateral Supracondylar Ridge

Medial Supracondylar Ridge

Lateral Epicondyle
O: Anconeus
O: Wrist Extensors

Medial Epicondyle

Medial Epicondyle
O: Wrist Flexors

Lateral Epicondyle

Trochlea   **Capitulum**

Olecranon Fossa

Forearm

Radius

Ulna

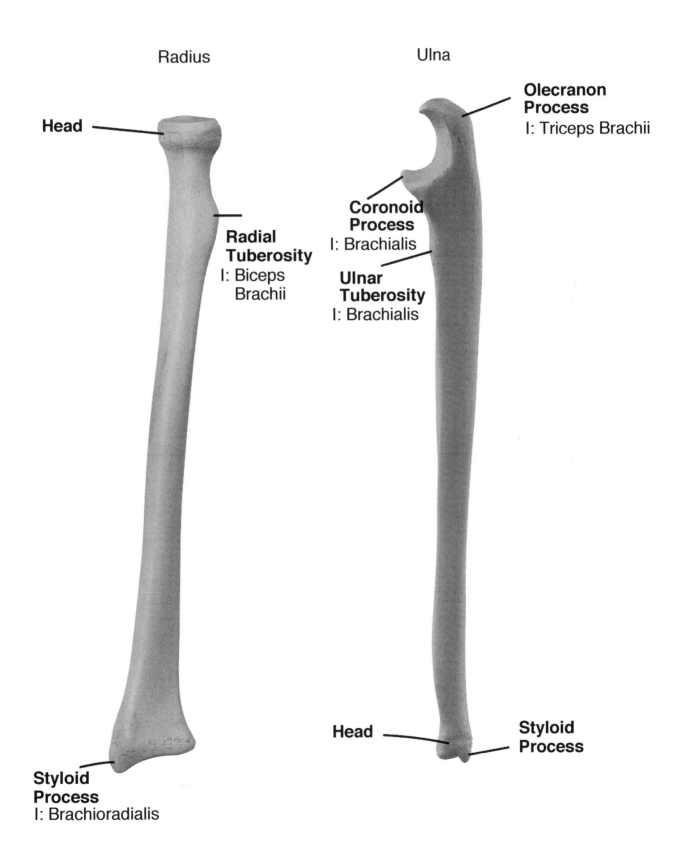

Head

Olecranon Process
I: Triceps Brachii

Coronoid Process
I: Brachialis

Radial Tuberosity
I: Biceps Brachii

Ulnar Tuberosity
I: Brachialis

Head

Styloid Process

Styloid Process
I: Brachioradialis

Wrist

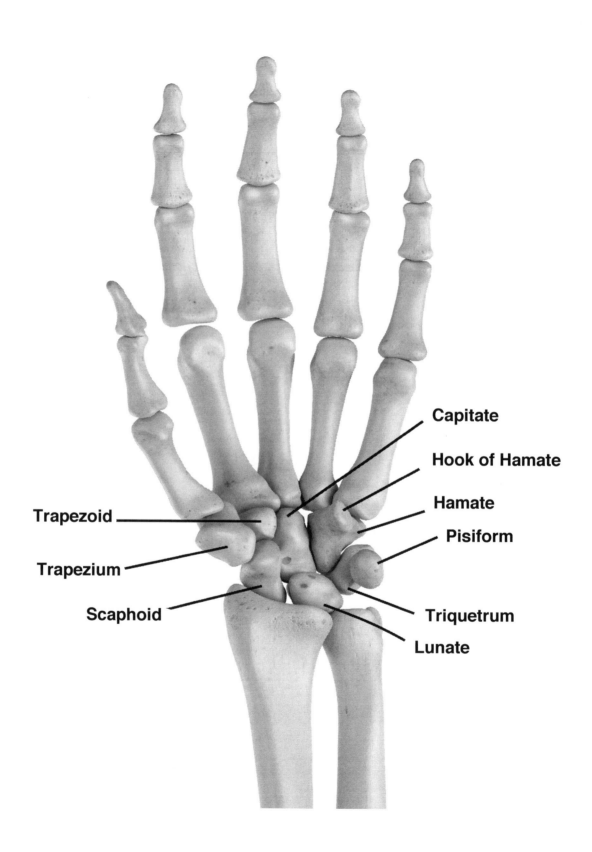

Capitate

Hook of Hamate

Hamate

Pisiform

Trapezoid

Trapezium

Triquetrum

Scaphoid

Lunate

Pelvis

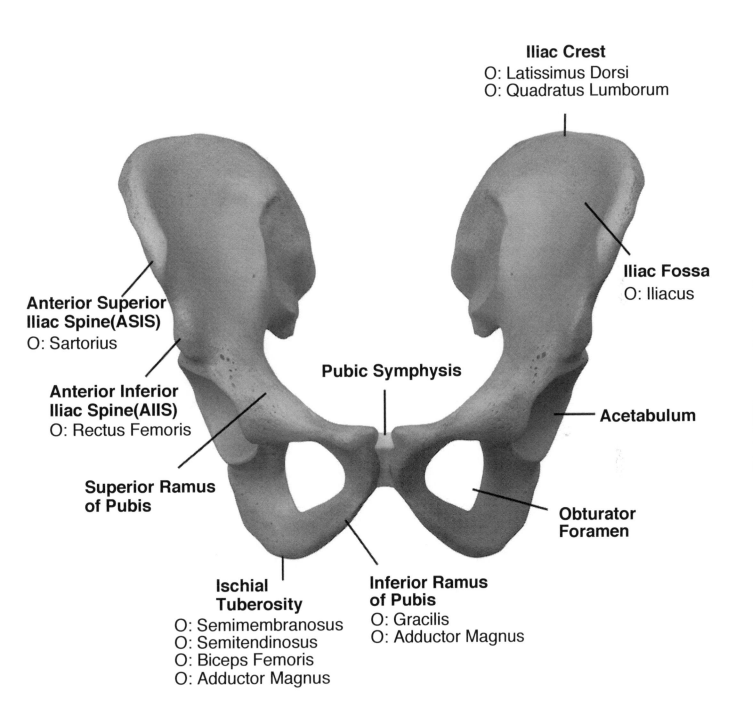

Iliac Crest
O: Latissimus Dorsi
O: Quadratus Lumborum

Iliac Fossa
O: Iliacus

Anterior Superior Iliac Spine(ASIS)
O: Sartorius

Anterior Inferior Iliac Spine(AIIS)
O: Rectus Femoris

Pubic Symphysis

Acetabulum

Superior Ramus of Pubis

Obturator Foramen

Ischial Tuberosity
O: Semimembranosus
O: Semitendinosus
O: Biceps Femoris
O: Adductor Magnus

Inferior Ramus of Pubis
O: Gracilis
O: Adductor Magnus

Thigh

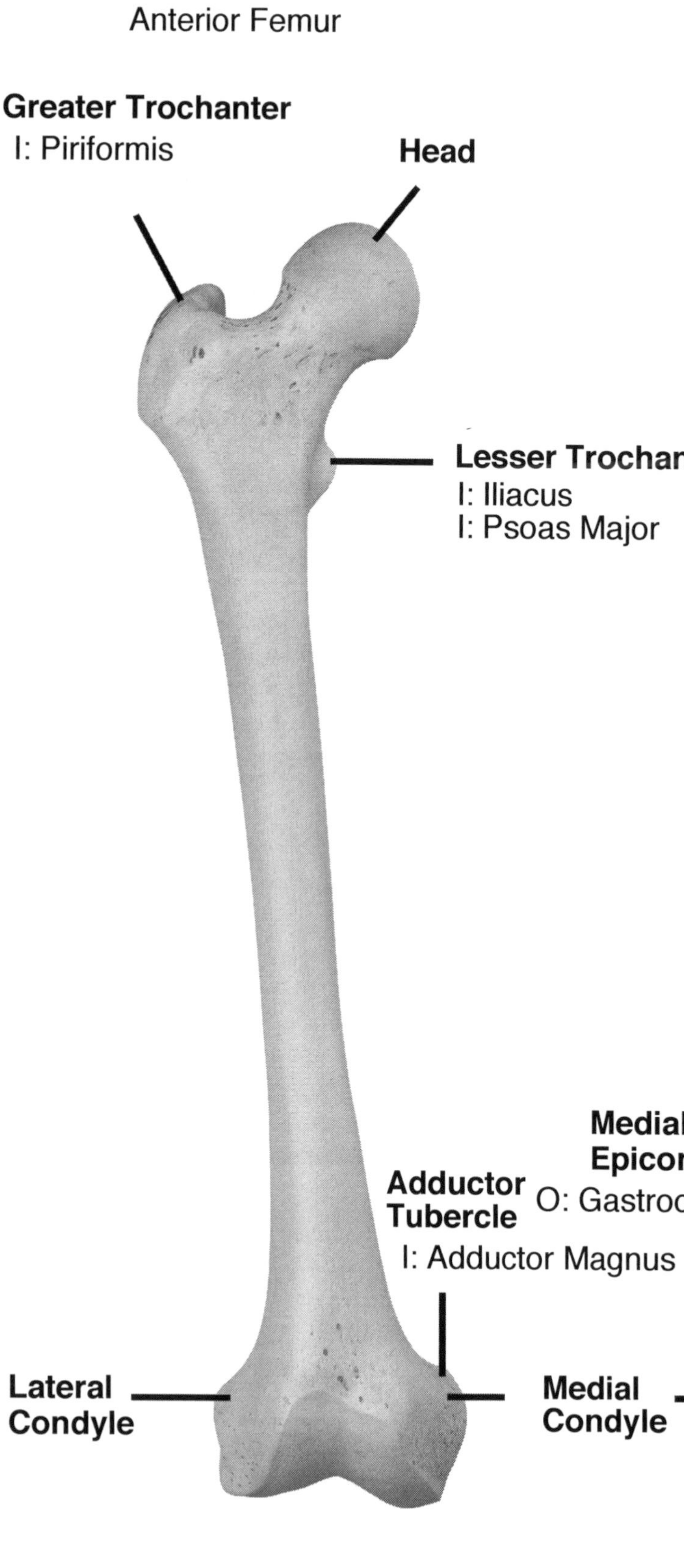

Anterior Femur
Greater Trochanter
I: Piriformis
Head
Lesser Trochanter
I: Iliacus
I: Psoas Major
Adductor Tubercle
I: Adductor Magnus
Lateral Condyle
Medial Condyle

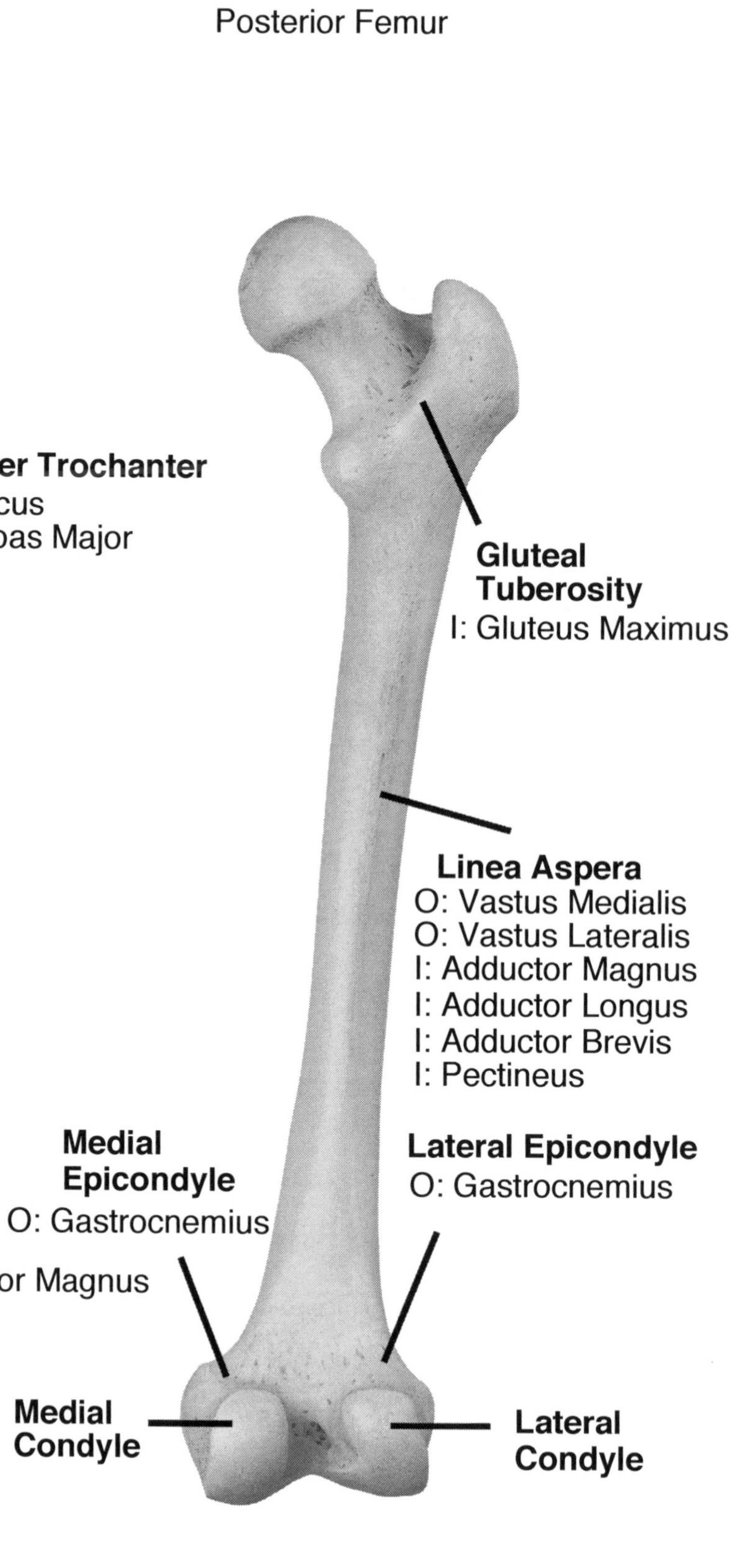

Posterior Femur
Gluteal Tuberosity
I: Gluteus Maximus
Linea Aspera
O: Vastus Medialis
O: Vastus Lateralis
I: Adductor Magnus
I: Adductor Longus
I: Adductor Brevis
I: Pectineus
Medial Epicondyle
O: Gastrocnemius
Lateral Epicondyle
O: Gastrocnemius
Medial Condyle
Lateral Condyle

Leg

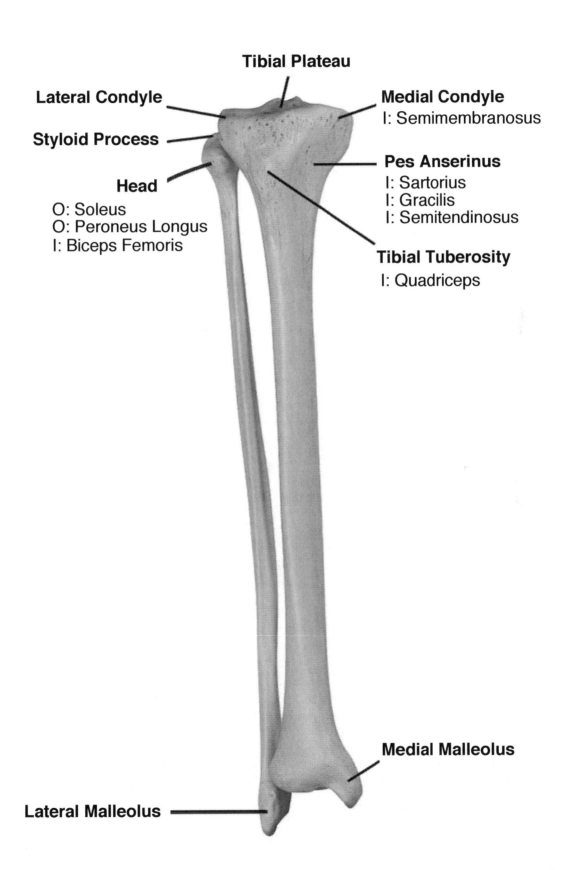

Tibial Plateau

Lateral Condyle

Styloid Process

Medial Condyle
I: Semimembranosus

Pes Anserinus
I: Sartorius
I: Gracilis
I: Semitendinosus

Head
O: Soleus
O: Peroneus Longus
I: Biceps Femoris

Tibial Tuberosity
I: Quadriceps

Medial Malleolus

Lateral Malleolus

146

Ankle

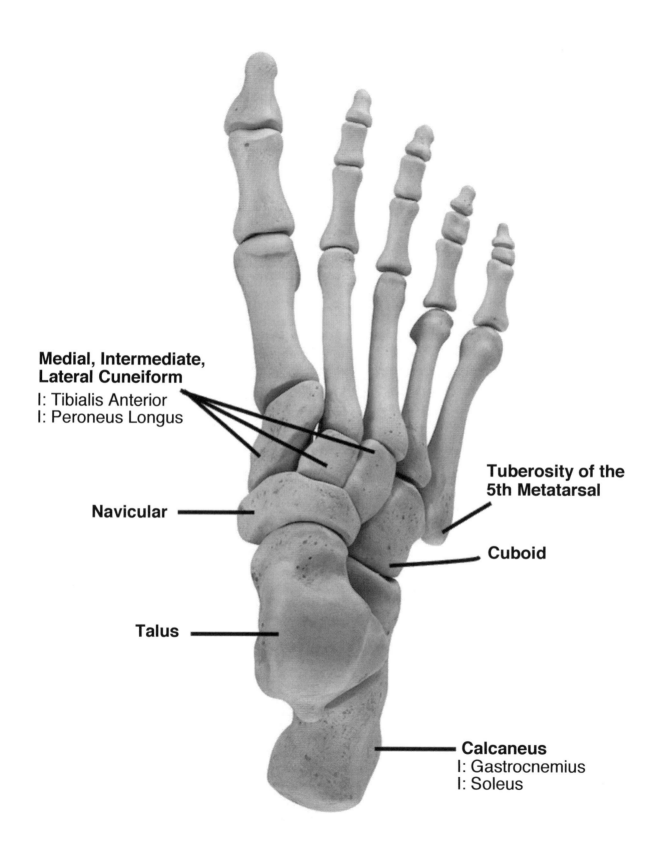

Medial, Intermediate, Lateral Cuneiform

I: Tibialis Anterior
I: Peroneus Longus

Navicular

Talus

Tuberosity of the 5th Metatarsal

Cuboid

Calcaneus
I: Gastrocnemius
I: Soleus

Muscles of the Head

Muscles to Know:
Buccinator
Masseter
Temporalis

Terms to Know:
Bucc/o: Cheek

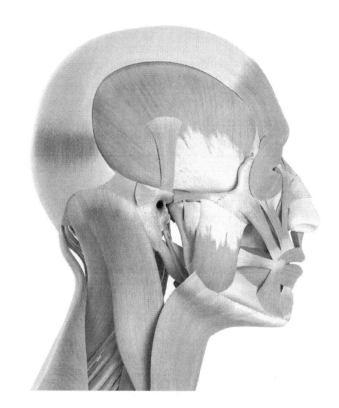

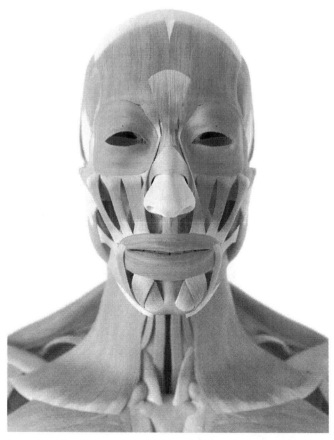

148

Buccinator

Buccinator is a muscle of the face located in the area of the cheek, also known as the "buccal" region. The term "bucc/o" means "cheek".

Buccinator originates on the Alveolar Processes of the Mandible and Maxilla, and inserts onto the angle of the mouth and the Orbicularis Oris muscle.

Buccinator primarily assists in chewing by squeezing the cheeks closer together while the jaw is depressed. This forces the food back in towards the teeth, allowing proper mastication to take place upon elevation of the mandible. Buccinator is also the muscle primarily used for whistling, again by squeezing the cheeks together.

If a person is affected by Bell's Palsy, the Buccinator becomes paralyzed, which produces slurred speech.

Origin: Alveolar Processes of Mandible and Maxilla
Insertion: Angle of the Mouth, Orbicularis Oris
Action(s): Elevation of Mandible, Compresses Cheeks against Teeth
Innervation: Buccal Branch of Facial Nerve
Synergist: Masseter
Antagonist: Lateral Pterygoid

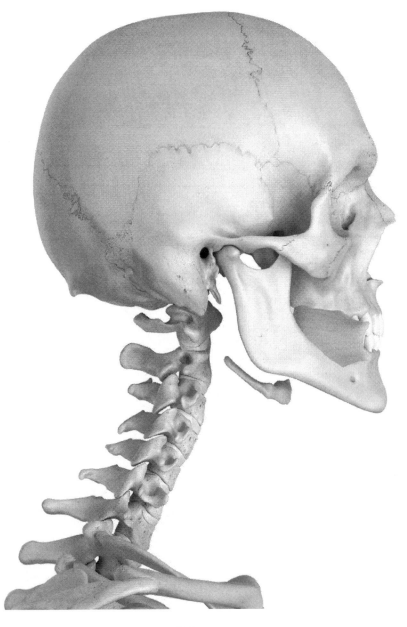

Masseter

Masseter, named after its primary action of mastication, is a muscle of the face that attaches to the mandible. When it contracts, it allows for chewing to take place. It works with other muscles, such as Buccinator, to perform mastication.

Masseter is the strongest muscle in the body by proportional size.

Masseter is one muscle primarily involved in TMJ(Temporomandibular Joint) Dysfunction, along with Temporalis and Pterygoid.

Origin: Zygomatic Arch, Maxilla
Insertion: Coronoid Process and Ramus of Mandible
Action(s): Elevation, Protraction of Mandible
Innervation: Mandibular Nerve
Synergist: Buccinator
Antagonist: Lateral Pterygoid

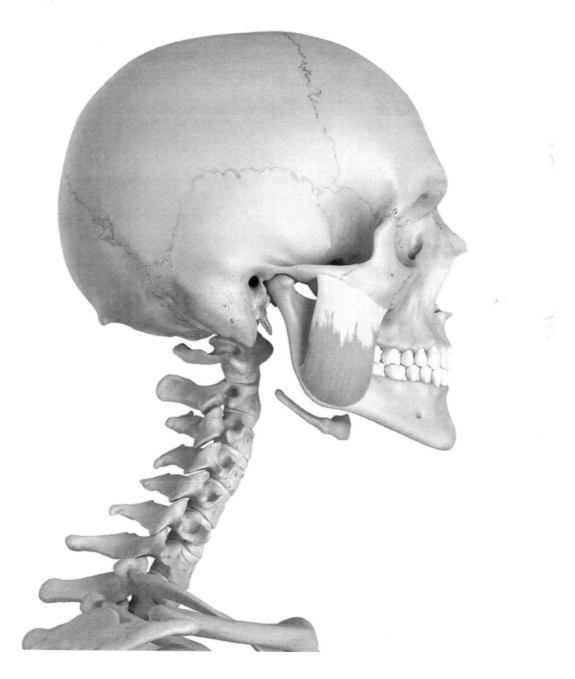

Temporalis

Temporalis is a muscle of the cranium, named after the Temporal bone, which is its origin.

Temporalis inserts onto the Coronoid Process of the Mandible. "Coronoid" means "resembling a crown". Inserting onto the Mandible allows the Temporalis to assist in mastication, along with Masseter.

If a person is affected by TMJ(Temporomandibular Joint) Dysfunction, Temporalis may be involved.

Origin: Temporal Fossa
Insertion: Coronoid Process of Mandible
Action(s): Elevation, Retraction of Mandible
Innervation: Facial Nerve
Synergist: Masseter
Antagonist: Lateral Pterygoid

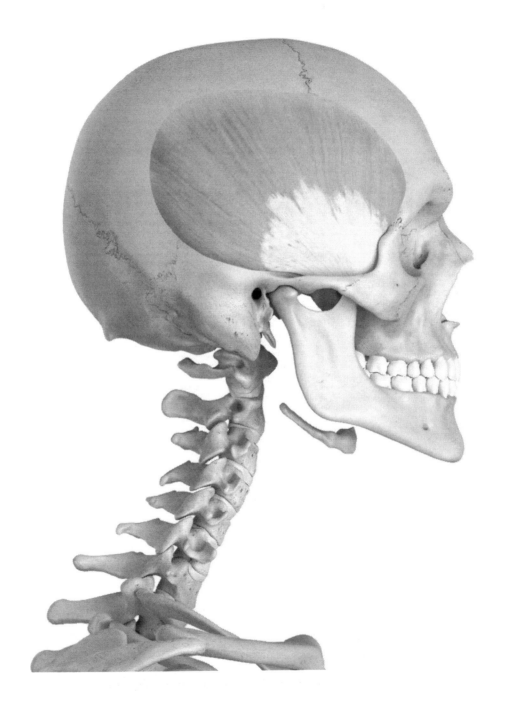

Muscles of the Neck

Muscles to Know:
Levator Scapulae
Scalenes
Sternocleidomastoid

Terms to Know:
Skalenos: Uneven
Stern/o: Sternum
Cleid/o: Clavicle
Mast/o: Breast
-oid: Resembling

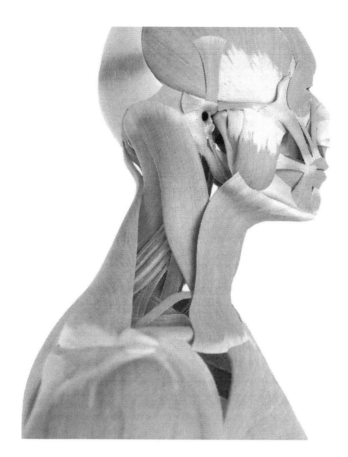

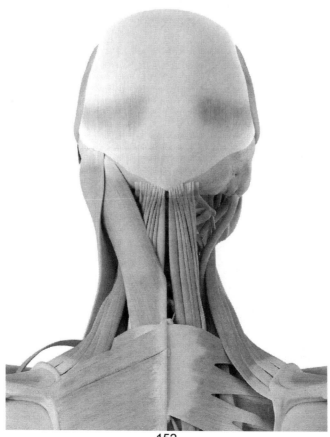

Levator Scapulae

Levator Scapulae is a muscle of the posterior neck, named after its action(elevation), and insertion(scapula).

Levator Scapulae originates on the Transverse Processes of C1-C4, and inserts onto the Superior Angle of the Scapula.

Levator Scapulae is one of the prime movers of scapular elevation, such as shrugging the shoulders. It also may slightly downwardly rotate the scapula.

Origin: Transverse Processes of C1-C4
Insertion: Superior Angle of Scapula
Action(s): Elevation of Scapula
Innervation: Dorsal Scapular Nerve
Synergist: Upper Trapezius
Antagonist: Lower Trapezius, Serratus Anterior

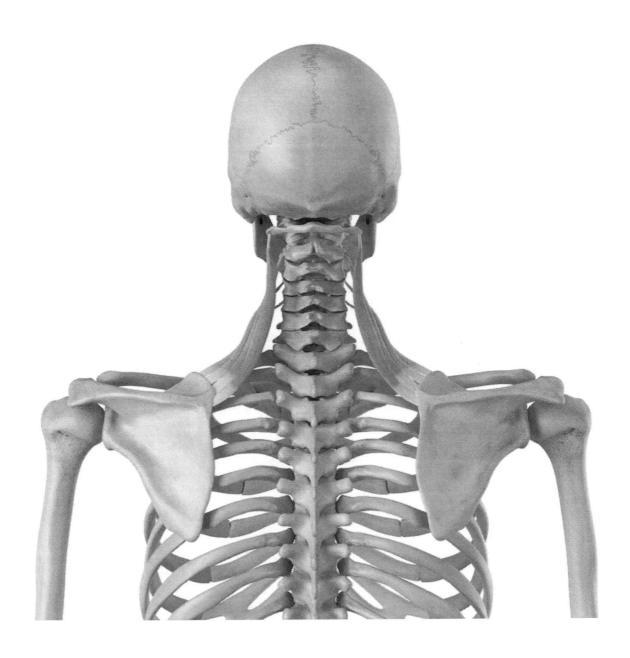

Scalenes

The Scalenes are muscles of the anterior neck. The Scalenes are split into three parts: Anterior Scalene, Middle Scalene, and Posterior Scalene. The name "Scalene" comes from the Greek word "skalenos", which means uneven. All three Scalene muscles are a different size.

The Scalenes originate on the Transverse Processes of C1-C7, and insert onto Ribs 1 and 2.

The Scalenes, unilaterally, laterally flex the cervical vertebrae, bringing the ear to the shoulder. The Scalenes also elevate the ribs.

The Scalenes are neurovascular entrappers. Conditions such as Thoracic Outlet Syndrome, where the Brachial plexus, Subclavian artery, and Subclavian vein are compressed, can be caused by hypertonic Scalenes. This condition may result in loss of sensation in the upper limb and reduced blood flow.

Origin: Transverse Processes of C1-C7
Insertion: Ribs 1 and 2
Action(s): Unilaterally: Lateral Flexion of Cervical Vertebrae; Elevation of Ribs
Innervation: Branches of Cervical Plexus and Brachial Plexus
Synergist: Sternocleidomastoid
Antagonist: Spinalis Cervicis, Splenius Capitis

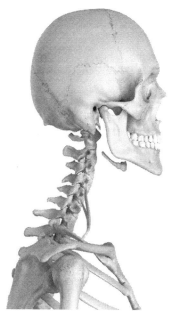

Anterior Scalene

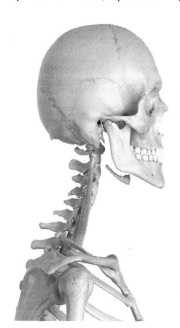

Middle Scalene

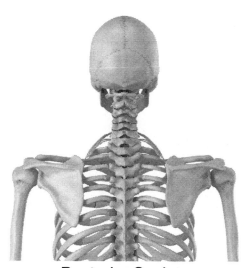

Posterior Scalene

Sternocleidomastoid

Sternocleidomastoid is a muscle of the anterior neck, named after its origins(Sternum, Clavicle) and insertion(Mastoid Process). This muscle may also be known as "Sternomastoid".

Sternocleidomastoid has numerous actions. Unilaterally, it rotates the cervical vertebrae to the opposite side of the contracting muscle. It also laterally flexes the cervical vertebrae to the side side of the contracting muscle. Bilaterally, it flexes the cervical vertebrae, allowing the chin to come to the chest.

Sternocleidomastoid establishes the borders of the anterior triangle of the neck, creating a V shape.

Origin: Manubrium, Medial Third of Clavicle
Insertion: Mastoid Process of Temporal bone
Action(s): Unilaterally: Rotation of Cervical Vertebrae to opposite side, Lateral Flexion of Cervical Vertebrae to same side; Bilaterally: Flexion of Cervical Vertebrae
Innervation: Accessory Nerve
Synergist: Scalenes
Antagonist: Splenius Capitis, Trapezius

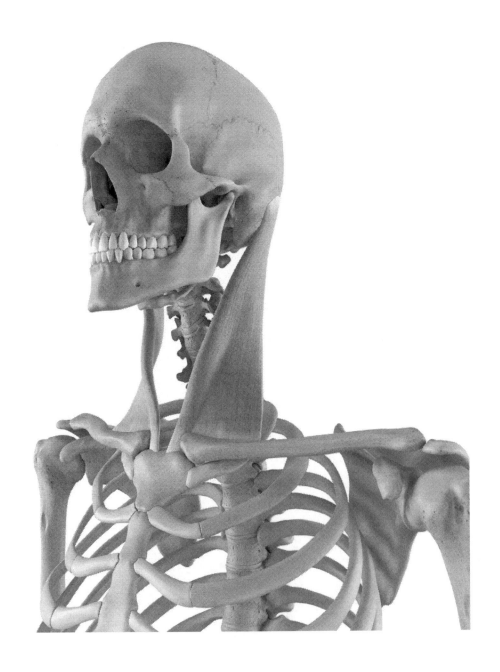

Muscles of the Back

Muscles to Know:
Infraspinatus
Latissimus Dorsi
Longissimus
Multifidus
Quadratus Lumborum
Rhomboids
Rotatores
Spinalis
Subscapularis
Supraspinatus
Teres Major
Teres Minor
Trapezius

Terms to Know:
Infra-: Below
Latissimus: Wide
Dorsi: Back
Quadr/o: Four
Lumb/o: Lumbar
Sub-: Under
Supra-: Above
Teres: Round and Long

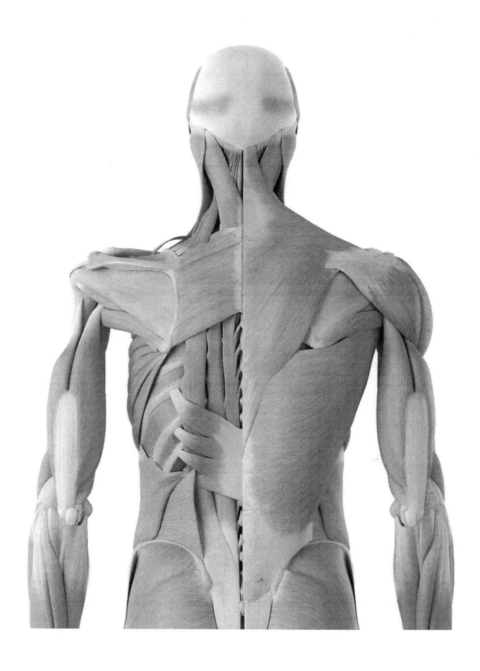

Infraspinatus

Infraspinatus is a muscle of the back, named after its location(inferior to the Spine of Scapula).

Infraspinatus is a member of the rotator cuff muscle group, along with Supraspinatus, Teres Minor, and Subscapularis. Infraspinatus originates on the Infraspinous Fossa, located on the posterior surface of the Scapula. Infraspinatus inserts onto the Greater Tubercle(sometimes also known as the Greater Tuberosity) of the Humerus.

Infraspinatus is primarily responsible for lateral rotation, extension, and horizontal abduction of the shoulder. Infraspinatus and Teres Minor have the same actions.

Origin: Infraspinous Fossa
Insertion: Greater Tubercle of Humerus
Action(s): Lateral Rotation, Horizontal Abduction of Shoulder
Innervation: Suprascapular Nerve
Synergist: Teres Minor, Latissimus Dorsi, Posterior Deltoid
Antagonist: Anterior Deltoid, Subscapularis, Pectoralis Major

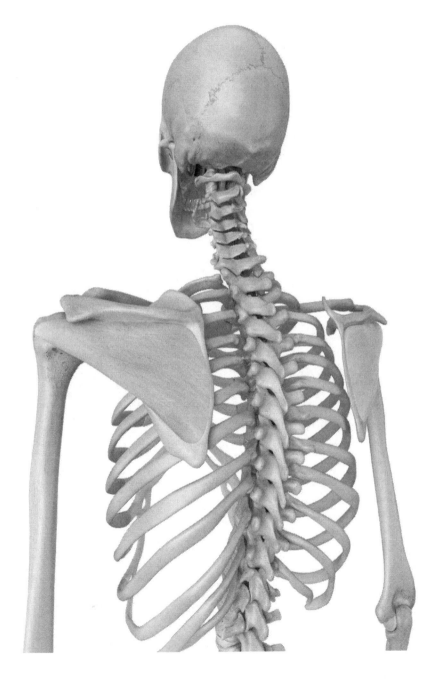

Latissimus Dorsi

Latissimus Dorsi is a muscle of the back, named after its size("Latissimus" means "wide") and location("Dorsi" refers to the back). Latissimus Dorsi is the widest muscle in the body.

Latissimus Dorsi originates on the Iliac Crest, Thoracolumbar Aponeurosis, and the Spinous Processes of T7-T12. Latissimus Dorsi inserts onto the Medial Lip of the Intertubercular Groove(also may be known as the Bicipital Groove).

Latissimus Dorsi is the muscle primarily responsible for performing adduction of the shoulder. If a person were to perform pull-up exercises, it would be Latissimus Dorsi contracting strongest. Latissimus Dorsi also medially rotates and extends the shoulder. Latissimus Dorsi, Teres Major, and Subscapularis all perform the same actions. When the insertion is fixed in place, Latissimus Dorsi may elevate the hip.

Latissimus Dorsi is often referred to as the "Swimmer's Muscle" due to its actions, which are used when swimming.

Origin: Iliac Crest, Thoracolumbar Aponeurosis, Spinous Processes of T7-T12
Insertion: Medial Lip of Intertubercular Groove
Action(s): Extension, Adduction, Medial Rotation of Shoulder
Innervation: Thoracodorsal Nerve
Synergist: Teres Major, Subscapularis
Antagonist: Pectoralis Major, Coracobrachialis

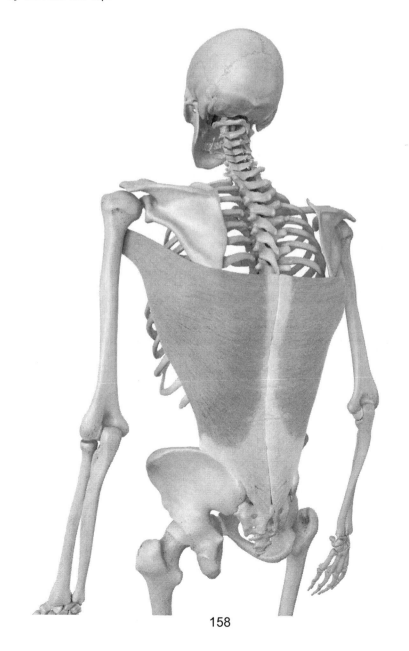

158

Longissimus

Longissimus is a group of three muscles, Longissimus Cervicis, Longissimus Capitis, and Longissimus Thoracis, which are all part of the Erector Spinae muscle group. Each muscle is named after the region of the body it is located on or attaches to.

Longissimus Thoracis originates on the Transverse Processes of L1-L5, the Iliac Crest, and the Sacrum. Longissimus Cervicis originates on the Transverse Processes of T1-T5. Longissimus Capitis originates on the Articular Surfaces of C4-C7.

Longissimus Thoracis inserts onto the Transverse Processes of T1-T12. Longissimus Cervicis inserts onto the Transverse Processes of C2-C6. Longissimus Capitis inserts onto the Mastoid Process.

Unilaterally, the Longissimus laterally flexes the trunk. Bilaterally, Longissimus extends the trunk.

Origin: Transverse and Spinous Processes of L1-L5, Iliac Crest, Sacrum, Transverse Processes of T1-T5, Articular Surfaces of C4-C7
Insertion: Transverse Processes of T1-T12, Transverse Processes of C2-C6, Mastoid Process
Action(s): Unilaterally: Lateral Flexion of Trunk; Bilaterally: Extension of Trunk
Innervation: Dorsal Primary Rami of T1-L5
Synergist: Spinalis
Antagonist: Rectus Abdominis

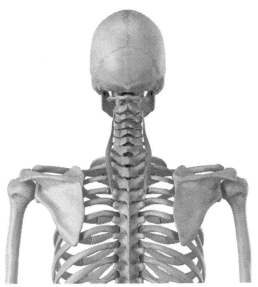

Longissimus Cervicis

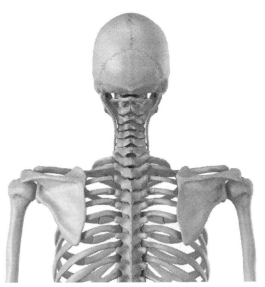

Longissimus Capitis

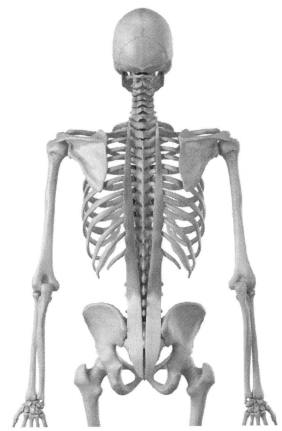

Longissimus Thoracis

159

Multifidus

Multifidus is a muscle of the back, often grouped together with other multifidus muscles to create the Multifidi.

The Multifidi as a group originate on the Posterior Surface of the Sacrum, the Posterior Superior Iliac Spine(PSIS), Mamillary Processes of L1-L5, the Transverse Processes of T1-T12, and the Articular Processes of C4-C7. The Multifidi insert on the Transverse Processes of C2-L5, spanning essentially the entire vertebral column.

Unilaterally, the Multifidi will laterally flex the trunk, and rotate the trunk. Bilaterally, the Multifidi extend the trunk.

The Multifidi span the most number of vertebrae of any muscle.

Origin: Posterior Surface of Sacrum, Posterior Superior Iliac Spine, Mamillary Processes of L1-L5, Transverse Processes of T1-T12, Articular Processes of C4-C7
Insertion: Spinous Processes of C2-L5
Action(s): Unilaterally: Lateral Flexion of Trunk, Rotation of Trunk; Bilaterally: Extension of Trunk
Innervation: Dorsal Rami of Spinal Nerves
Synergist: Longissimus, Spinalis
Antagonist: Rectus Abdominis

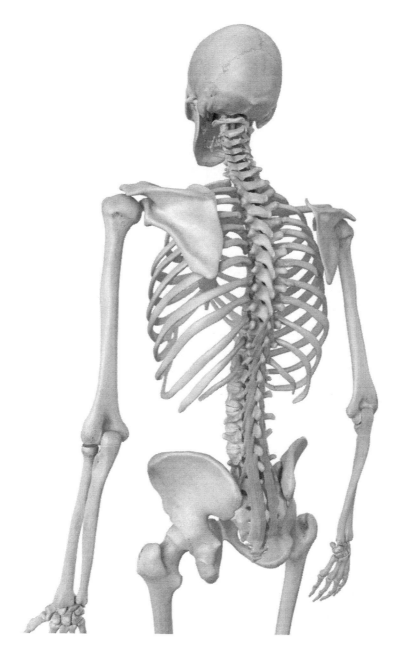

Quadratus Lumborum

Quadratus Lumborum is a muscle of the lower back, named after its shape(four sides), and its location(in the lumbar region).

Quadratus Lumborum originates on the Iliac Crest, and inserts onto the 12th Rib, and the Transverse Processes of L1-L4.

Quadratus Lumborum, unilaterally, will assist in lateral flexion of the trunk. Bilaterally, it will assist in extension of the trunk.

If a person suffers from Lordosis(also known as Swayback), it may be caused by hypertonicity in the Quadratus Lumborum, pulling the pelvis anteriorly, thus increasing the curvature of the Lumbar vertebrae.

Origin: Iliac Crest
Insertion: 12th Rib, Transverse Processes of L1-L4
Action(s): Unilaterally: Lateral Flexion of Trunk;
Bilaterally: Extension of Trunk
Innervation: Ventral Primary Rami of T12-L3
Synergist: Longissimus, Spinalis
Antagonist: Rectus Abdominis

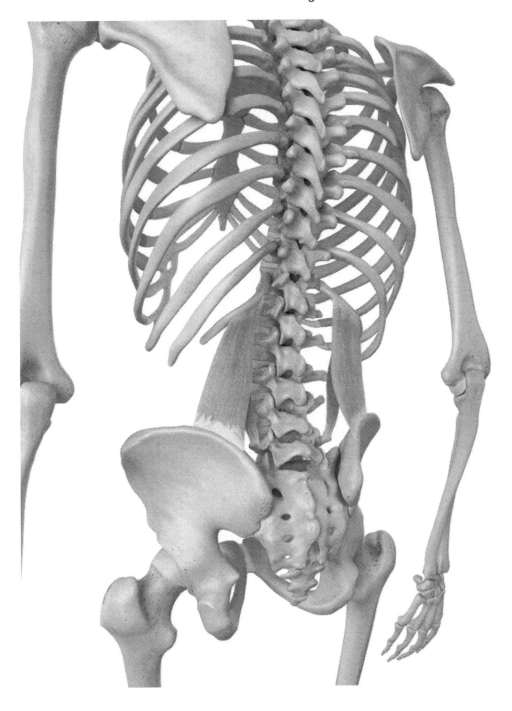

Rhomboids

The Rhomboids(Rhomboid Major and Rhomboid Minor) are two muscles located on the back. They are named after their shape(rhombus).

Rhomboid Major originates on the Spinous Processes of T3-T5. Rhomboid Minor originates on the Spinous Processes of C7-T2. Together, the Rhomboids insert onto the Medial/Vertebral Border of the Scapula.

When the Rhomboids contract, they pull the Scapula towards the vertebrae. This action is known as retraction/adduction. Two primary antagonists to the Rhomboids are Serratus Anterior and Pectoralis Minor. Both of these muscles protract/abduct the Scapula.

If the Rhomboids are hypertonic on one side, it may contribute to the development of Scoliosis.

Origin: Rhomboid Minor: Spinous processes of C7-T2; Rhomboid Major: Spinous processes of T3-T5
Insertion: Medial/Vertebral Border of Scapula
Action(s): Retraction/Adduction of Scapula
Innervation: Dorsal Scapular Nerve C5
Synergist: Middle Trapezius
Antagonist: Serratus Anterior, Pectoralis Minor

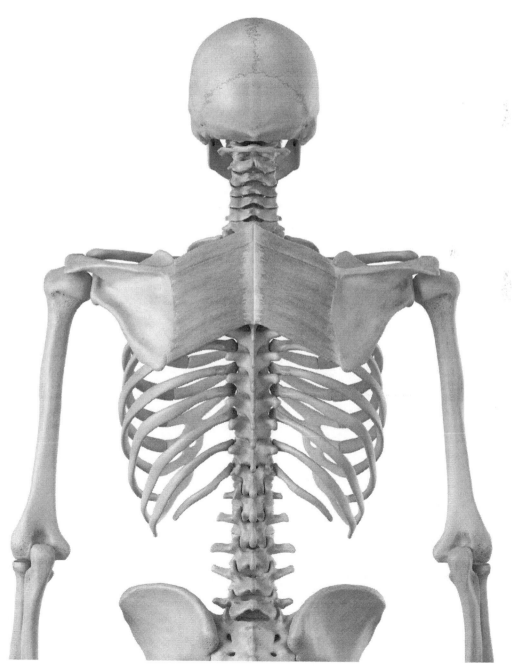

Rotatores

The Rotatores are a group of muscles that span the entire vertebral column. They are named after their action.

The Rotatores originate on the Transverse Processes of C1-L5, and insert onto the Spinous Processes of the vertebrae just superior. An example, the Rotator muscle that originates on the Transverse Process of C2 would insert onto the Spinous Process of C1.

Unilaterally, the Rotatores will rotate the trunk to the opposite side. Bilaterally, the Rotatores assist in extension of the trunk.

Origin: Transverse Processes of C1-L5
Insertion: Spinous Processes of Vertebrae just superior
Action(s): Unilaterally: Rotate Trunk to opposite side; Bilaterally: Extension of Trunk
Innervation: Dorsal Primary Rami of Spinal Nerves C1-T12
Synergist: Spinalis, Longissimus
Antagonist: Rectus Abdominis

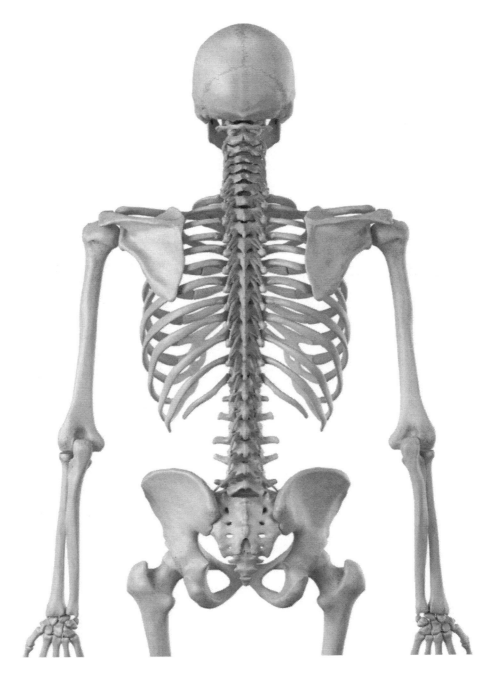

Spinalis

Spinalis is a pair of two muscles, both located on the back. Each muscle is named after its location: Spinalis Thoracis (in the Thoracic region), Spinalis Cervicis (in the Cervical region).

Spinalis Thoracis originates on the Spinous Processes of T11-L2. There may be slight variation of the origin, however, ranging from T10-L3. Spinalis Cervicis originates on the Nuchal Ligament, and Spinous Process of C7. Spinalis Thoracis inserts onto the Spinous Processes of T3-T8. Spinalis Cervicis inserts onto the Spinous Process of C2.

Unilaterally, the Spinalis muscles laterally flex and rotate the trunk to the same side. Bilaterally, they work with other muscles such as Longissimus to extend the trunk.

Origin: Spinalis Thoracis: Spinous Processes of T11-L2; Spinalis Cervicis: Nuchal Ligament, Spinous Process of C7
Insertion: Spinalis Thoracis: Spinous Processes of T3-T8; Spinalis Cervicis: Spinous Process of C2
Action(s): Unilaterally: Flex and Rotate Spine to the same side; Bilaterally: Extend the Trunk
Innervation: Dorsal Rami of Cervical and Thoracic Spinal Nerves
Synergist: Longissimus
Antagonist: Rectus Abdominis

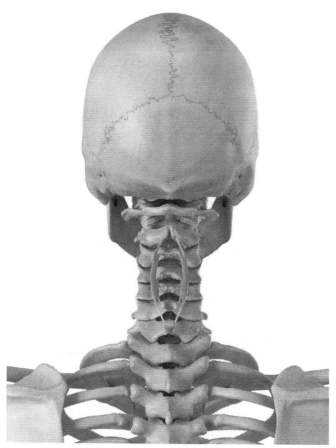

Spinalis Cervicis

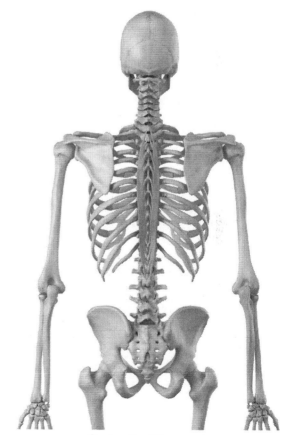

Spinalis Thoracis

Subscapularis

Subscapularis is a muscle of the back, named after it's location(under the scapula).

Subscapularis originates on the Subscapular Fossa, located on the anterior surface of the Scapula. Subscapularis inserts onto the Lesser Tubercle(sometimes also called the Lesser Tuberosity of the Humerus). It is part of the rotator cuff muscle group, along with Infraspinatus, Teres Minor, and Supraspinatus.

Subscapularis is a synergist to Latissimus Dorsi, performing the same actions on the shoulder. These actions are adduction, extension, and medial rotation.

If a person is affected by Adhesive Capsulitis(Frozen Shoulder), there may be hypertonicity in the Subscapularis, reducing the range-of-motion during actions such as shoulder flexion.

Origin: Subscapular Fossa
Insertion: Lesser Tubercle of Humerus
Action(s): Medial Rotation, Adduction, Extension of the Shoulder
Innervation: Upper and Lower Subscapular Nerves
Synergist: Latissimus Dorsi, Teres Major
Antagonist: Pectoralis Major, Coracobrachialis

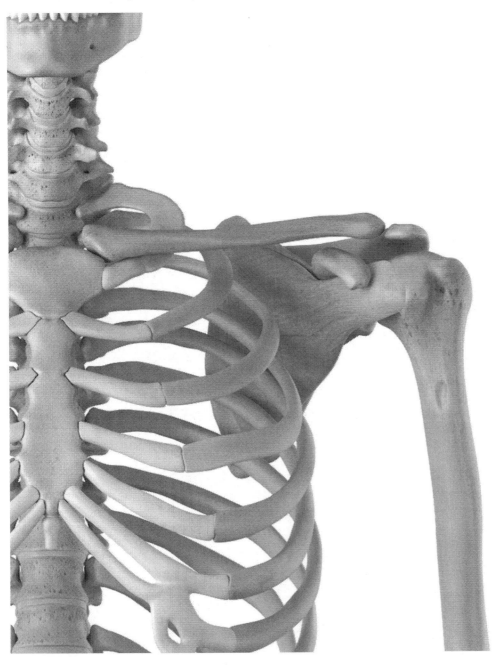

Supraspinatus

Supraspinatus is a muscle of the back, named after it's location(superior to the Spine of the Scapula).

Supraspinatus originates on the Supraspinous Fossa, just above the Spine of the Scapula. Supraspinatus inserts onto the Greater Tubercle(sometimes called the Greater Tuberosity of the Humerus). It is part of the rotator cuff muscle group, along with Infraspinatus, Teres Minor, and Subscapularis.

Supraspinatus primarily has one action: abduction of the shoulder. It is a synergist to the Deltoid in performing this action. Supraspinatus also helps hold the Humerus in place against the Glenoid Fossa, providing stability to the shoulder joint.

Most commonly, if a person suffers from a torn rotator cuff, it likely involves the Supraspinatus more than other muscles. A torn rotator cuff might require surgery to repair, depending on the severity.

Origin: Supraspinous Fossa
Insertion: Greater Tubercle of Humerus
Action(s): Abduction of Shoulder
Innervation: Suprascapular Nerve
Synergist: Deltoid
Antagonist: Latissimus Dorsi, Teres Major

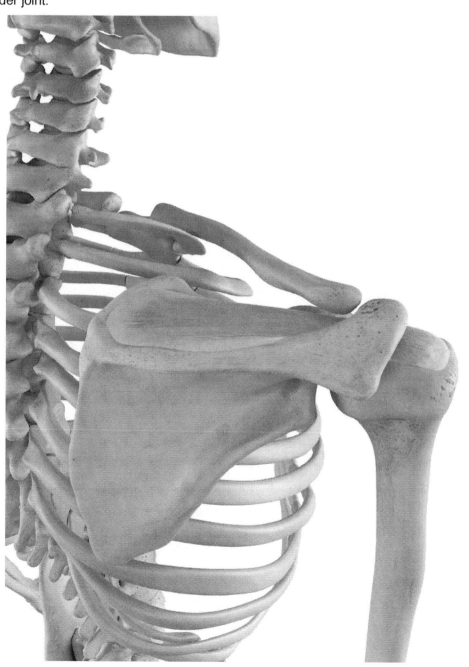

Teres Major

Teres Major is a muscle of the back. The name "Teres" means "round and long". Teres Major has a long, round shape.

Teres Major originates on the Inferior Angle of the Scapula, and inserts onto the Medial Lip of the Intertubercular Groove. It shares its insertion with Latissimus Dorsi.

Teres Major and Latissimus Dorsi both perform the same actions: medial rotation, extension, and adduction of the shoulder.

Origin: Inferior Angle of Scapula
Insertion: Medial Lip of Intertubercular Groove
Action(s): Medial Rotation, Adduction, Extension of Shoulder
Innervation: Lower Subscapular Nerve
Synergist: Latissimus Dorsi, Subscapularis
Antagonist: Pectoralis Major, Coracobrachialis

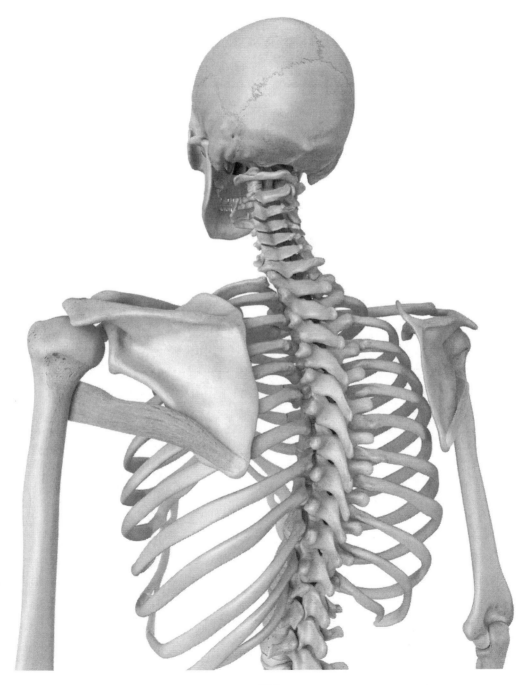

167

Teres Minor

Teres Minor is a muscle of the back. The word "Teres" means "round and long". Teres Minor has a long, round shape.

Teres Minor originates on the Lateral/Axillary Border of the Scapula. The term "Axillary" refers to the armpit, which Teres Minor is located next to. Teres Minor inserts onto the Greater Tubercle(sometimes known as the Greater Tuberosity) of the Humerus. Teres Minor is a member of the rotator cuff muscle group, along with Infraspinatus, Subscapularis, and Supraspinatus.

Teres Minor and Infraspinatus are located immediately next to one another, and sometimes may even fuse together. These muscles perform the same actions: lateral rotation, extension, and horizontal abduction of the shoulder.

Origin: Lateral/Axillary Border of Scapula
Insertion: Greater Tubercle of Humerus
Action(s): Lateral Rotation, Horizontal Abduction of Shoulder
Innervation: Axillary Nerve
Synergist: Infraspinatus
Antagonist: Pectoralis Major

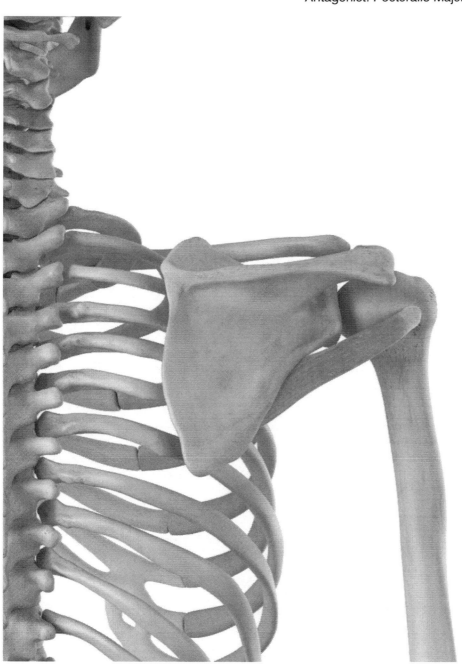

168

Trapezius

Trapezius is a large muscle of the back, named after its shape(trapezoid). Trapezius is the most superficial muscle of the back.

Trapezius originates on the External Occipital Protuberance of the Occipital bone, and the Spinous Processes of T1-T12. Trapezius inserts on the Acromion Process, the Spine of the Scapula, and the Lateral 1/3 of the Clavicle.

The Trapezius can be divided into three sections: Upper Trapezius, Middle Trapezius, and Lower Trapezius. When contracting, Upper Trapezius assists in elevation of the scapula. When contracting, Middle Trapezius assists in retraction/adduction of the scapula. When contracting, Lower Trapezius depresses the scapula.

Origin: External Occipital Protuberance, Spinous Processes of T1-T12
Insertion: Lateral 1/3 of Clavicle, Acromion Process, Spine of Scapula
Action(s): Elevation, Retraction/Adduction, Depression of Scapula
Innervation: Accessory Nerve, Cervical Nerves C3 and C4
Synergist: Levator Scapulae(elevation), Rhomboids(retraction), Serratus Anterior(depression)
Antagonist: Serratus Anterior(elevation), Pectoralis Minor(retraction), Levator Scapulae(depression)

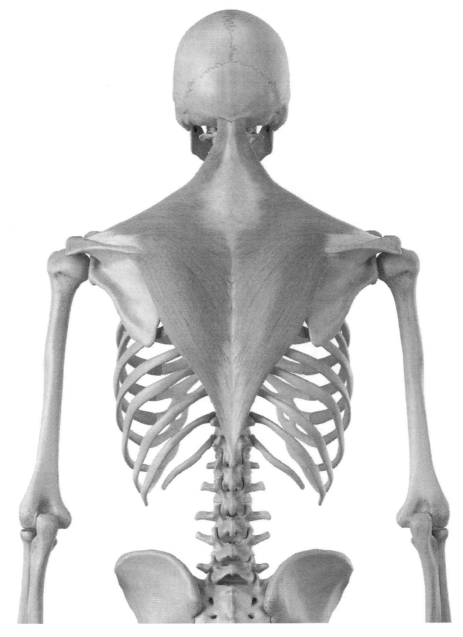

Muscles of the Chest

Muscles to Know:
Pectoralis Major
Pectoralis Minor
Serratus Anterior

Terms to Know:
Pector/o: Chest
Serratus: Finely Notched Edge

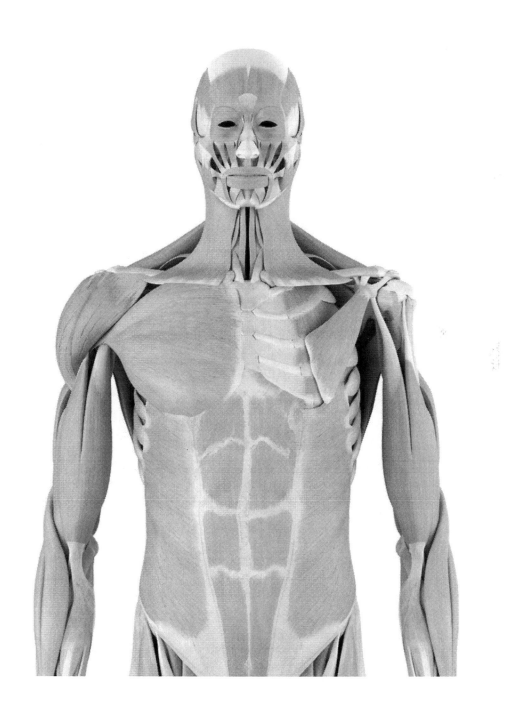

Pectoralis Major

Pectoralis Major is a large muscle of the chest. The term "pector/o" means "breast" or "chest".

Pectoralis Major originates on the Medial Half of the Clavicle, the Anterior Surface of the Sternum, and the Costal Cartilage of Ribs 1-6. Pectoralis Major inserts onto the Lateral Lip of the Intertubercular Groove.

When contracting, the Pectoralis Major has multiple actions: Flexion, medial rotation, and horizontal adduction of the shoulder. Pectoralis Major also performs extension of the shoulder when the shoulder is already flexed, making it an antagonist to itself.

Origin: Medial Half of Clavicle, Anterior Surface of Sternum, Costal Cartilage 1-6
Insertion: Lateral Lip of Intertubercular Groove
Action(s): Flexion, Medial Rotation, Horizontal Adduction, Extension of Shoulder
Innervation: Lateral and Medial Pectoral Nerves
Synergist: Coracobrachialis, Biceps Brachii, Anterior Deltoid
Antagonist: Latissimus Dorsi, Teres Major, Subscapularis, Posterior Deltoid

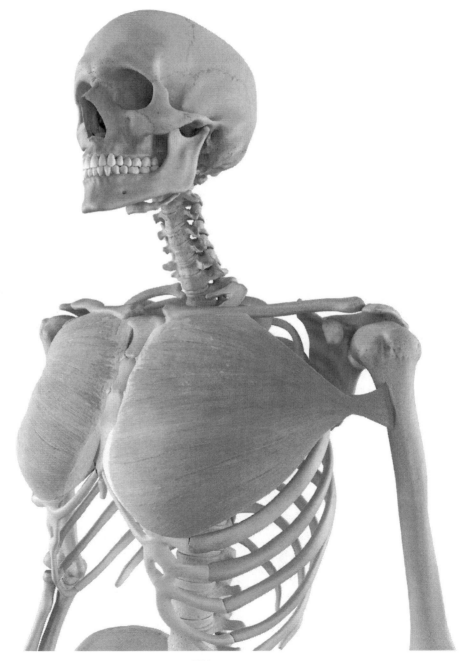

Pectoralis Minor

Pectoralis Minor is a muscle of the chest, lying deep to the Pectoralis Major.

Pectoralis Minor originates on the Anterior Surface of Ribs 3-5. Pectoralis Minor inserts onto the Coracoid Process.

When Pectoralis Minor contracts, it protracts/abducts the scapula. Along with Serratus Anterior, it is an antagonist to the Rhomboids.

Pectoralis Minor is often associated with Thoracic Outlet Syndrome. When hypertonic, Pectoralis Minor may compress the Brachial plexus, Subclavian artery, and Subclavian nerve, which may cause a lack of sensation in the upper limb, or restrict blood supply.

Pectoralis Minor is very commonly associated with Kyphosis, a rounding of the back in the Thoracic region of the vertebrae(hunch back), caused by Pectoralis Minor being hypertonic, pulling the scapulae anteriorly.

Origin: Anterior Surface of Ribs 3-5
Insertion: Coracoid Process of Scapula
Action(s): Protraction/Abduction of Scapula
Innervation: Medial Pectoral Nerve
Synergist: Serratus Anterior
Antagonist: Rhomboids

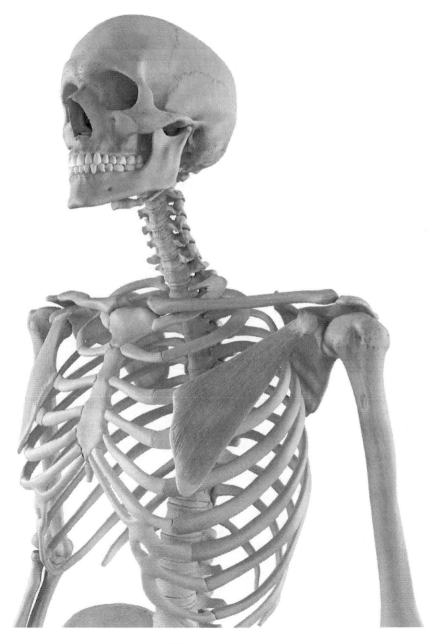

Serratus Anterior

Serratus Anterior is a muscle of the chest. "Serratus" means "finely notched edge", such as a serrated knife.

Serratus Anterior originates on the Anterior Surface of Ribs 1-8. Serratus Anterior inserts onto the Anterior Surface of the Medial/Vertebral Border of the Scapula.

When Serratus Anterior contracts, it moves the scapula anteriorly, producing protraction/abduction. Serratus Anterior also may assist in depression of the scapula.

If Serratus Anterior is hypertonic, it may pull the scapulae too far into protraction/abduction, which would produce Kyphosis, a rounding of the vertebrae in the Thoracic region.

Origin: Anterior Surface of Ribs 1-8
Insertion: Medial/Vertebral Border of Scapula
Action(s): Protraction/Abduction, Depression of Scapula
Innervation: Long Thoracic Nerve
Synergist: Pectoralis Minor, Lower Trapezius
Antagonist: Rhomboids, Levator Scapulae

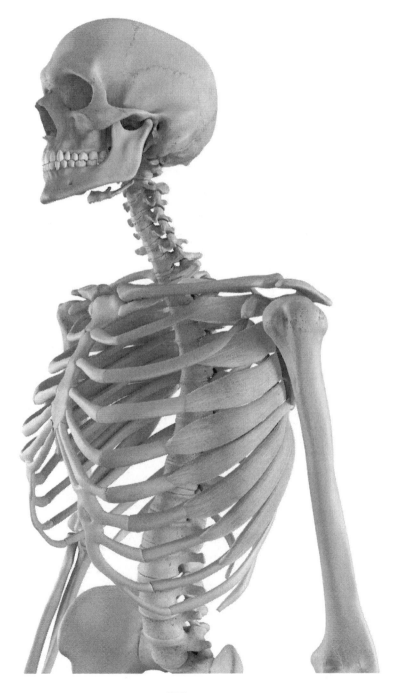

Muscles of the Abdomen

Muscles to Know:
Rectus Abdominis

Terms to Know:
Rectus: Straight

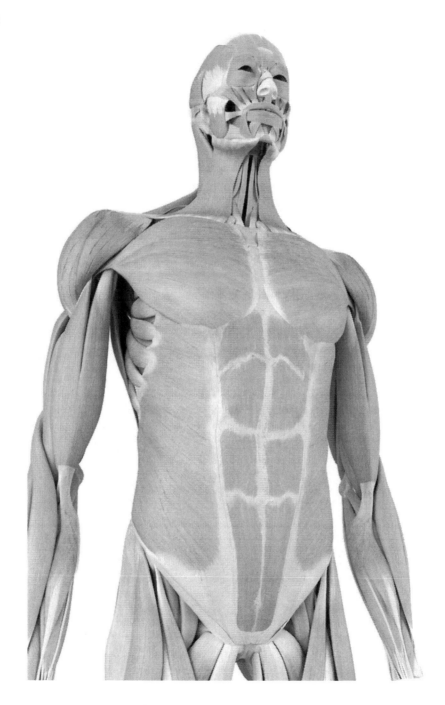

Rectus Abdominis

Rectus Abdominis is a muscle of the abdomen. Rectus Abdominis is the most superficial muscle of the abdomen.

Rectus Abdominis originates on the Pubic Symphysis and the Pubic Crest. Rectus Abdominis inserts onto the Xiphoid Process of the Sternum and the Costal Cartilage of Ribs 5-7.

When Rectus Abdominis contracts, is allows the trunk to flex.

If Rectus Abdominis is too weak, it may lead to a condition known as Lordosis, or Swayback. This causes an increased anterior tilt to the pelvis and Lumbar vertebrae. Strengthening of the Rectus Abdominis may help return the pelvis and vertebrae to their natural state.

Origin: Pubic Symphysis, Pubic Crest
Insertion: Xiphoid Process, Costal Cartilage of Ribs 5-7
Action(s): Flexion of Trunk
Innervation: Anterior Primary Rami T7-T12
Synergist: External Obliques, Internal Obliques
Antagonist: Spinalis, Longissimus

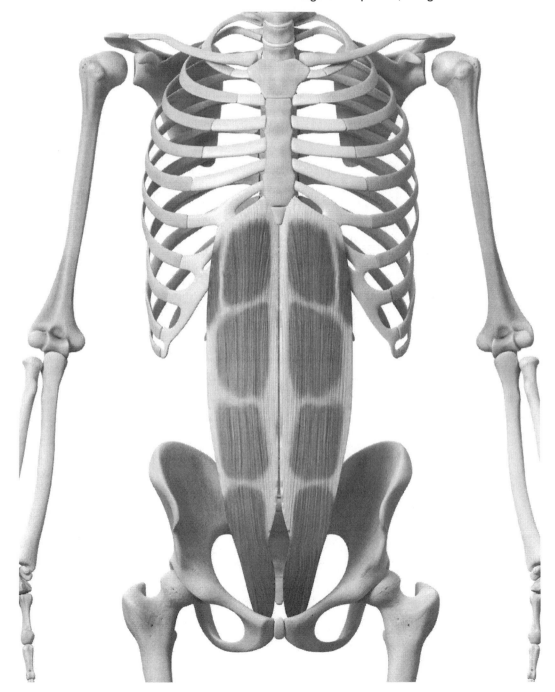

Muscles of the Arm

Muscles to Know:
Biceps Brachii
Brachialis
Coracobrachialis
Deltoid
Triceps Brachii

Terms to Know:
Bi-: Two
-cep: Head
Brachi/o: Arm
Corac/o: Coracoid
Tri-: Three

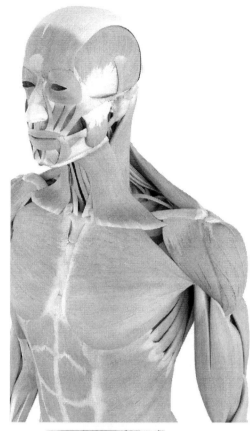

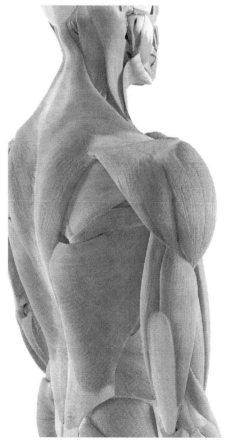

Biceps Brachii

Biceps Brachii is a muscle of the arm. The term "Biceps" means "two head", and "Brachii" refers to the arm.

Biceps Brachii has two heads. The Short Head of the Biceps Brachii originates on the Coracoid Process. The Long Head of the Biceps Brachii originates on the Supraglenoid Tubercle. Both heads join together in the arm, and together, insert onto the Radial Tuberosity.

When Biceps Brachii contracts, it helps produce flexion of the shoulder, flexion of the elbow, and supination of the forearm. Biceps Brachii is the prime mover of supination.

Origin: Long Head: Supraglenoid Tubercle; Short Head: Coracoid Process
Insertion: Radial Tuberosity
Action(s): Flexion of Shoulder, Flexion of Elbow, Supination of Forearm
Innervation: Musculocutaneous Nerve
Synergist: Pectoralis Major, Brachialis, Supinator
Antagonist: Triceps Brachii, Pronator Teres

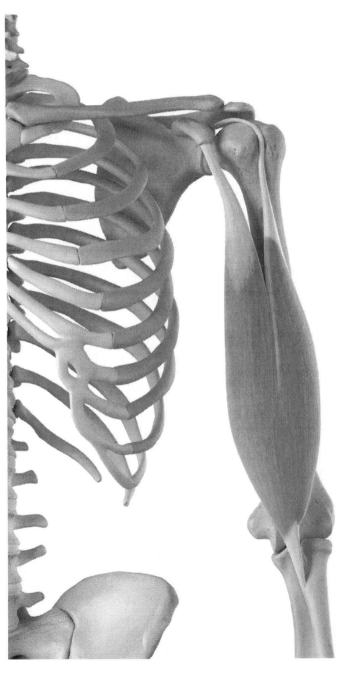

Brachialis

Brachialis is a muscle of the arm. It is named after it's location, the "brachial" region.

Brachialis originates on the Anterior Distal Shaft of the Humerus, and inserts onto both the Coronoid Process of the Ulna, and the Ulnar Tuberosity.

Brachialis is a powerful muscle. It is the prime mover of elbow flexion. It is located deep to the Biceps Brachii. When Brachialis contracts, it pushes the Biceps Brachii up, allowing Biceps Brachii to be more visible during this action.

Origin: Anterior Distal Shaft of Humerus
Insertion: Coronoid Process and Ulnar Tuberosity
Action(s): Flexion of Elbow
Innervation: Musculocutaneous Nerve
Synergist: Biceps Brachii
Antagonist: Triceps Brachii

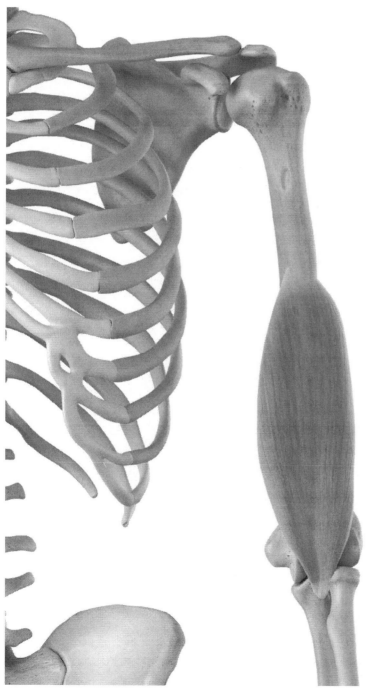

Coracobrachialis

Coracobrachialis is a muscle of the arm, named after it's origin and location.

Coracobrachialis originates on the Coracoid Process, and inserts onto the Medial Proximal Shaft of the Humerus.

Coracobrachialis is primarily a synergist to Pectoralis Major. When Coracobrachialis contracts, it flexes and horizontally adducts the shoulder.

Origin: Coracoid Process
Insertion: Medial Proximal Shaft of Humerus
Action(s): Flexion, Horizontal Adduction of Shoulder
Innervation: Musculocutaneous Nerve
Synergist: Pectoralis Major, Biceps Brachii
Antagonist: Infraspinatus, Teres Minor

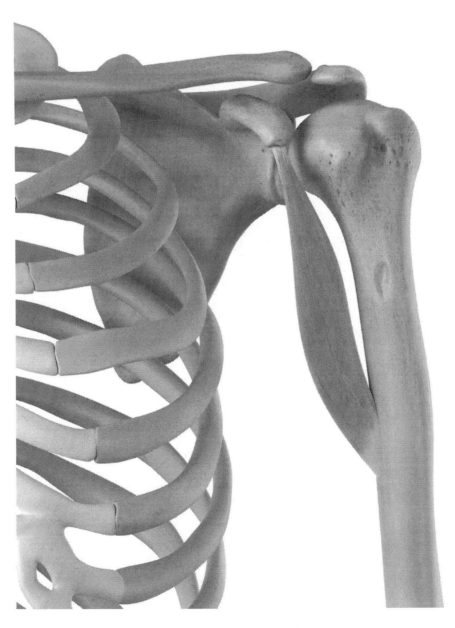

179

Deltoid

Deltoid is a muscle of the arm/shoulder, named after the Greek letter "delta", which is shaped like an equilateral triangle(all sides are the same length).

Deltoid has three different portions that make up the muscle: Anterior Deltoid, Middle Deltoid, and Posterior Deltoid. All three combined create the Deltoid muscle.

Anterior Deltoid originates on the lateral third of the clavicle. Middle Deltoid originates on the Acromion Process. Posterior Deltoid originates on the Spine of the Scapula. All three join together distally and insert onto the Deltoid Tuberosity.

The Deltoid has many different actions, depending on which fibers of the muscle are contracting. Anterior Deltoid assists in flexion, horizontal adduction, and medial rotation of the shoulder. Posterior Deltoid assists in extension, horizontal abduction, and lateral rotation of the shoulder. Middle Deltoid, in conjunction with the two other Deltoid fibers, abducts the shoulder.

Origin: Anterior Deltoid: Lateral Third of Clavicle; Middle Deltoid: Acromion Process; Posterior Deltoid: Spine of Scapula
Insertion: Deltoid Tuberosity
Action(s): Abduction, Medial Rotation, Lateral Rotation, Horizontal Adduction, Horizontal Abduction, Flexion, Extension of Shoulder
Innervation: Axillary Nerve
Synergist: Supraspinatus(abduction), Pectoralis Major(flexion, horizontal adduction, medial rotation), Infraspinatus(extension, horizontal abduction, lateral rotation)
Antagonist: Latissimus Dorsi(abduction), Infraspinatus(flexion, horizontal adduction, medial rotation), Pectoralis Major(extension, horizontal abduction, lateral rotation)

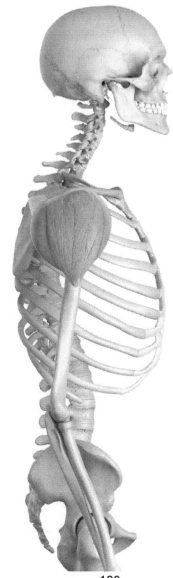

180

Triceps Brachii

Triceps Brachii is a muscle of the posterior arm. The name "Triceps" means "three heads", and "Brachii" refers to the arm.

Triceps Brachii has three heads. The Long Head originates on the Infraglenoid Tubercle of the Humerus. The Medial Head originates on the Posterior Shaft of the Humerus, on the medial side. The Lateral Head originates on the Posterior Shaft of the Humerus, on the lateral side. All three heads join together and insert on the Olecranon Process.

Triceps Brachii, when it contracts, extends the shoulder and extends the elbow.

Origin: Long Head: Infraglenoid Tubercle; Medial Head: Posterior Shaft of Humerus; Lateral Head: Posterior Shaft of Humerus
Insertion: Olecranon Process
Action(s): Extension of Shoulder, Extension of Elbow
Innervation: Radial Nerve
Synergist: Latissimus Dorsi, Anconeus
Antagonist: Pectoralis Major, Biceps Brachii

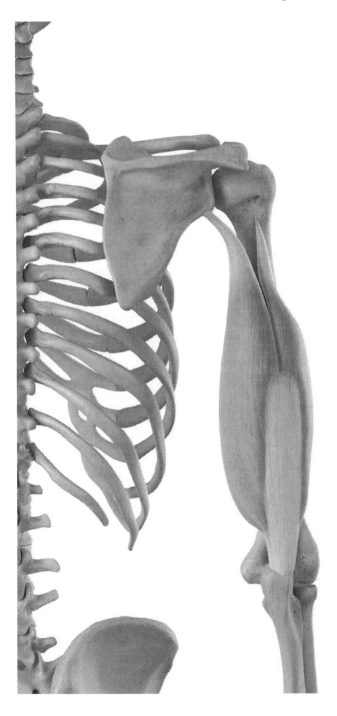

Muscles of the Forearm

Muscles to Know:
Anconeus
Brachioradialis
Pronator Teres

Terms to Know:
Agkon: Elbow
Brachi/o: Arm
Teres: Round and Long

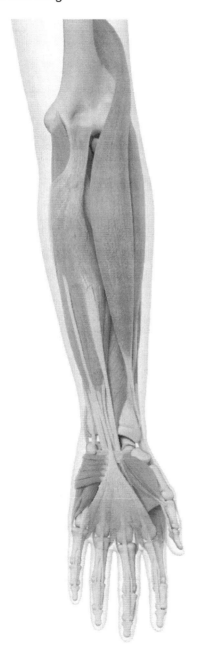
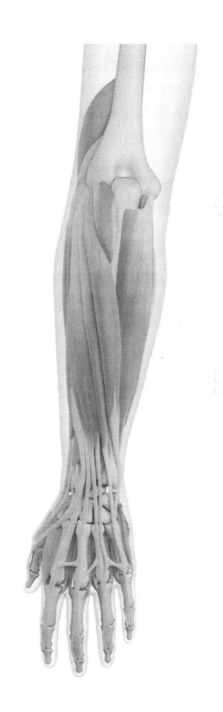

Anconeus

Anconeus is a muscle of the forearm. It's name derives from the Greek "agkon", which means "elbow".

Anconeus originates on the Lateral Epicondyle of the Humerus, and inserts onto the Olecranon Process.

Anconeus is primarily only a synergist to the Triceps Brachii, assisting to perform elbow extension.

Because Anconeus originates on the Lateral Epicondyle of the Humerus, it may be affected if a person is suffering from Tennis Elbow, a type of tendonitis which causes inflammation at the Lateral Epicondyle of the Humerus.

Origin: Lateral Epicondyle of Humerus
Insertion: Olecranon Process
Action(s): Extension of Elbow
Innervation: Radial Nerve
Synergist: Triceps Brachii
Antagonist: Brachialis

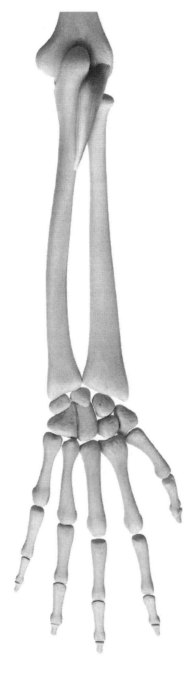

Brachioradialis

Brachioradialis is a muscle of the forearm, named after its location and insertion. "Brachio" refers to the arm, and "radialis" refers to the Radius.

Brachioradialis originates on the Lateral Supracondylar Ridge of the Humerus, the ridge just superior to the Lateral Epicondyle. Brachioradialis inserts onto the Styloid Process of the Radius.

Brachioradialis primarily performs flexion of the elbow with the hand in the neutral position(neither in pronation or supination).

Origin: Lateral Supracondylar Ridge of Humerus
Insertion: Styloid Process of Radius
Action(s): Flexion of Elbow
Innervation: Radial Nerve
Synergist: Biceps Brachii
Antagonist: Triceps Brachii

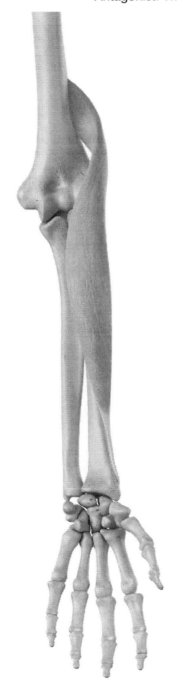

Pronator Teres

Pronator Teres is a muscle of the forearm, named for its action and shape("Teres" means "round and long". Pronator Teres has a long, round shape).

Pronator Teres originates on the Medial Epicondyle of the Humerus and the Coronoid Process of the Ulna. Pronator Teres inserts onto the Middle of the Lateral Surface of the Radius.

Pronator Teres, as the name suggests, is the strongest pronator of the forearm. Because Pronator Teres crosses the elbow joint, it also assists in flexion of the elbow.

Origin: Medial Epicondyle of Humerus, Coronoid Process of Ulna
Insertion: Middle of Lateral Surface of Radius
Action(s): Pronation of Forearm, Flexion of Elbow
Innervation: Median Nerve
Synergist: Pronator Quadratus, Brachialis
Antagonist: Biceps Brachii, Triceps Brachii

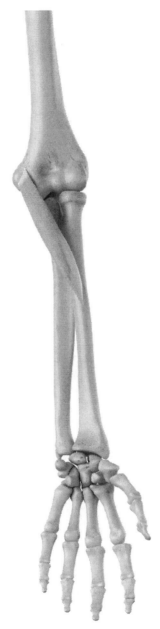

Muscles of the Pelvis

Muscles to Know:
Gluteus Maximus
Iliacus
Piriformis
Psoas Major

Terms to Know:
Iliac: Ilium
Pirum: Pear
Psoa: Loin Region

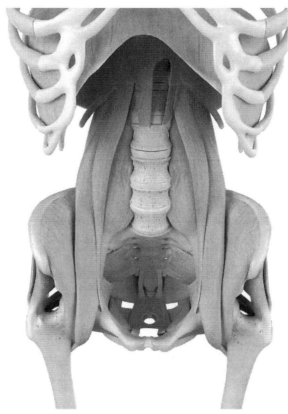

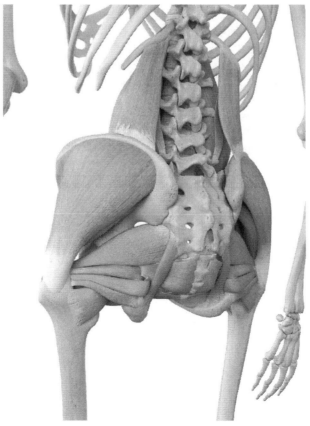

Gluteus Maximus

Gluteus Maximus is a muscle of the pelvis, named for its location and size.

Gluteus Maximus originates on the Posterior Iliac Crest, the Posterior Sacrum and Coccyx, and the Sacrotuberous Ligament. Gluteus Maximus inserts partially onto the Gluteal Tuberosity, and into the Iliotibial Band.

Gluteus Maximus is primarily responsible for assisting in extension of the hip, and abduction of the hip.

The Gluteus Maximus is the largest muscle in the human body. It is also the most superficial of the gluteus muscle group.

Origin: Posterior Iliac Crest, Posterior Sacrum and Coccyx, Sacrotuberous Ligament
Insertion: Gluteal Tuberosity, Iliotibial Band
Action(s): Extension, Abduction of Hip
Innervation: Inferior Gluteal Nerve
Synergist: Hamstrings, Piriformis
Antagonist: Rectus Femoris, Adductor Magnus

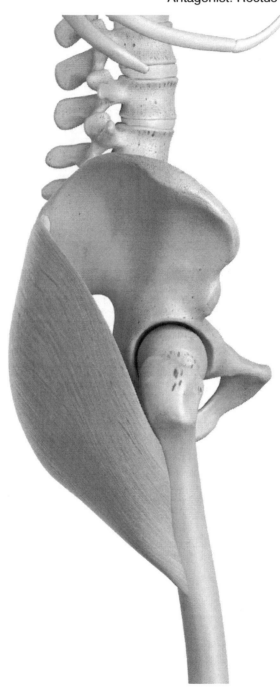

Iliacus

Iliacus is a muscle of the pelvis, named for its origin.

Iliacus originates in the Iliac Fossa, and crosses the hip joint to insert onto the Lesser Trochanter.

Iliacus is one of the prime movers of hip flexion. It often is joined with the Psoas Major, which also aids in hip flexion, to make a single muscle named the Iliopsoas.

If the Iliacus is hypertonic, it may pull the pelvis anteriorly. This shift of the pelvis results in a hypercurvature in the lumbar vertebrae, a condition known as Lordosis(Swayback).

Origin: Iliac Fossa
Insertion: Lesser Trochanter
Action(s): Flexion of Hip
Innervation: Femoral Nerve
Synergist: Psoas Major
Antagonist: Hamstrings

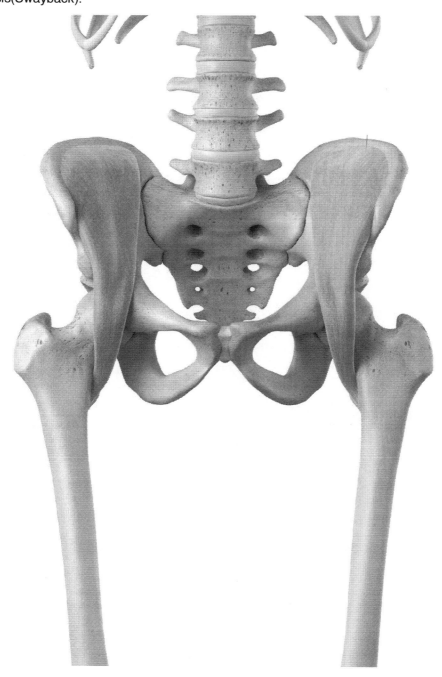

Piriformis

Piriformis is a muscle of the pelvis, named for its shape("piri" refers to "pirum", which means "pear" in Latin. Piriformis is shaped like a pear).

Piriformis originates on the Anterior Surface of the Sacrum, and inserts onto the Greater Trochanter.

Piriformis works with the Gluteus Maximus to perform abduction and lateral rotation of the hip.

Piriformis is part of the Deep Six muscle group.

Piriformis, when hypertonic, may place substantial pressure on the Sciatic Nerve, which passes by, and sometimes through, the muscle itself. This is known as Piriformis Syndrome. This can result in pain in the hip, posterior thigh, posterior leg, and plantar surface of the foot.

Origin: Anterior Surface of Sacrum
Insertion: Greater Trochanter
Action(s): Abduction, Lateral Rotation of Hip
Innervation: Piriformis Nerve
Synergist: Gluteus Maximus, Sartorius
Antagonist: Adductor Magnus, Pectineus

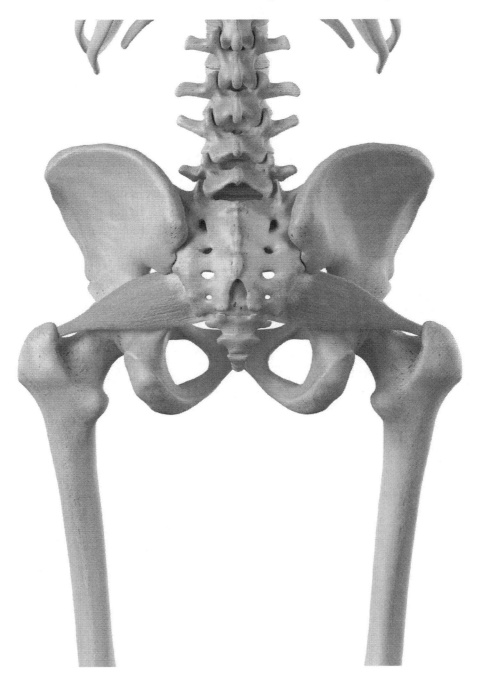

Psoas Major

Psoas Major is a muscle of the abdomen and pelvis, named for its location("psoas" comes from the Greek word "psoa", which means "loin region") and size.

Psoas Major originates on the Anterior Surface of the Lumbar Vertebrae. Psoas Major inserts onto the Lesser Trochanter.

Psoas Major is responsible for flexion of the hip, along with Iliacus. Psoas Major often joins with Iliacus to form one muscle known as the Iliopsoas.

If the Psoas Major is hypertonic, it pulls the Lumbar Vertebrae anteriorly, which may also force the pelvis anteriorly. This is a condition known as Lordosis(Swayback).

Origin: Anterior Surface of Lumbar Vertebrae
Insertion: Lesser Trochanter
Action(s): Flexion of Hip, Flexion of Trunk
Innervation: Lumbar Plexus
Synergist: Iliacus, Rectus Abdominis
Antagonist: Hamstrings, Spinalis

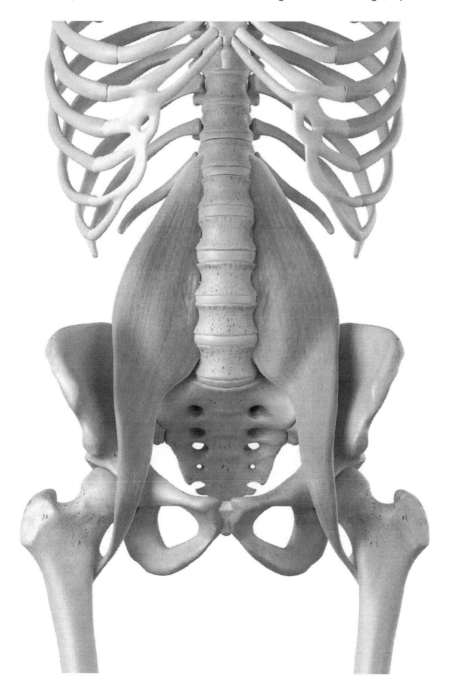

Muscles of the Thigh

Muscles to Know:
Adductor Magnus
Biceps Femoris
Gracilis
Rectus Femoris
Sartorius
Semimembranosus
Semitendinosus
Tensor Fasciae Latae

Terms to Know:
Magnus: Great
Bi-: Two
-cep: Head
Gracilis: Slender
Rectus: Straight
Sartor: Tailor
Semi-: Half
Membranosus: Skin
Tendere: To Stretch
Fasciae: Band
Latae: Side

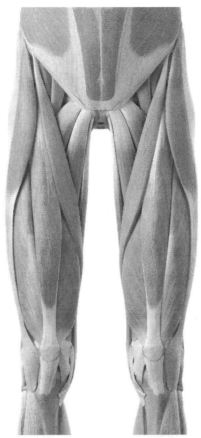

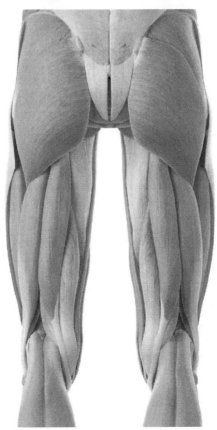

Adductor Magnus

Adductor Magnus is a muscle of the thigh, named after its action(adduction) and size("Magnus" means "great" in Latin).

Adductor Magnus has multiple origins. It originates on the Inferior Ramus of the Pubis and Ischial Tuberosity. Adductor Magnus inserts onto the Medial Lip of the Linea Aspera, and the Adductor Tubercle.

Adductor Magnus is an antagonist to itself. It can flex and extend the hip. It also, as the name implies, adducts the hip.

Adductor Magnus is the largest muscle of the Adductor muscle group, which also consists of Adductor Longus, Adductor Brevis, Gracilis, and Pectineus.

Origin: Inferior Ramus of Pubis, Ischial Tuberosity
Insertion: Linea Aspera, Adductor Tubercle
Action(s): Adduction, Flexion, Extension of Hip
Innervation: Obturator Nerve, Sciatic Nerve(Tibial branch)
Synergist: Adductor Longus(adduction), Iliacus(flexion), Gluteus Maximus(extension)
Antagonist: Piriformis(adduction), Hamstrings(flexion), Rectus Femoris(extension)

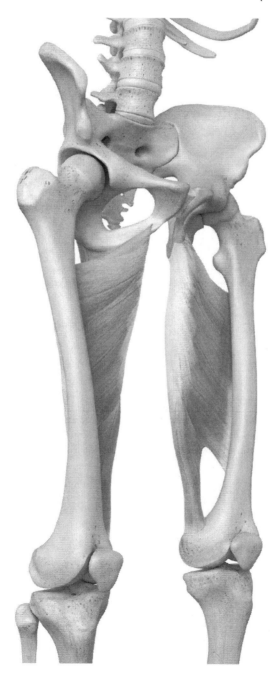

Biceps Femoris

Biceps Femoris is a muscle of the posterior thigh, named after the number of heads if has("Biceps" means "two heads") and its location(Femur).

Biceps Femoris has two origins: The Long Head of Biceps Femoris originates on the Ischial Tuberosity. The Short Head of Biceps Femoris originates on the Lateral Lip of the Linea Aspera, on the distal end of the femur. Biceps Femoris inserts onto the Head of the Fibula.

Biceps Femoris crosses the hip and the knee. When it contracts, it extends the hip, and flexes the knee.

Biceps Femoris is a member of the Hamstrings muscle group. It is the most lateral Hamstring muscle, the only Hamstring muscle that attaches to the Fibula.

Origin: Long Head: Ischial Tuberosity; Short Head: Lateral Lip of Linea Aspera
Insertion: Head of Fibula
Action(s): Extension of Hip, Flexion of Knee
Innervation: Sciatic Nerve(Tibial branch)
Synergist: Semimembranosus, Semitendinosus
Antagonist: Rectus Femoris

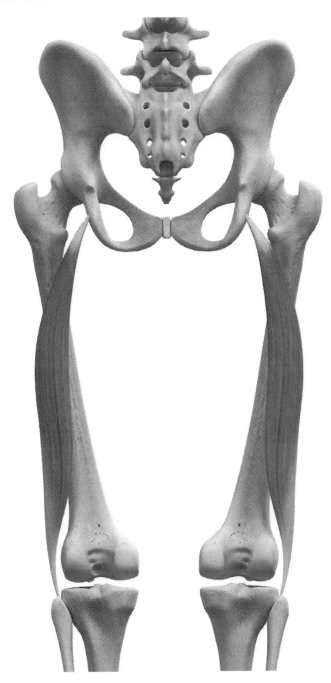

Gracilis

Gracilis is a muscle of the medial thigh. The word "Gracilis" means "slender" in Latin. The Gracilis is a thin, slender, long muscle.

Gracilis originates on the Inferior Ramus of the Pubis, along with Adductor Magnus. Gracilis inserts onto the Pes Anserinus, located on the Medial Proximal Shaft of the Tibia, just medial to the Tibial Tuberosity.

Gracilis performs adduction and flexion of the hip. Gracilis also crosses the knee, and will assist in flexion of the knee.

Gracilis is a member of the Adductor muscle group, the most medial muscle of the group. The Gracilis is the only Adductor muscle that crosses two joints. All the other Adductor muscles(Adductor Magnus, Adductor Longus, Adductor Brevis, Pectineus) only cross the hip.

Origin: Inferior Ramus of Pubis
Insertion: Pes Anserinus
Action(s): Adduction, Flexion of Hip, Flexion of Knee
Innervation: Obturator Nerve
Synergist: Adductor Magnus, Gastrocnemius
Antagonist: Gluteus Maximus, Hamstrings, Rectus Femoris

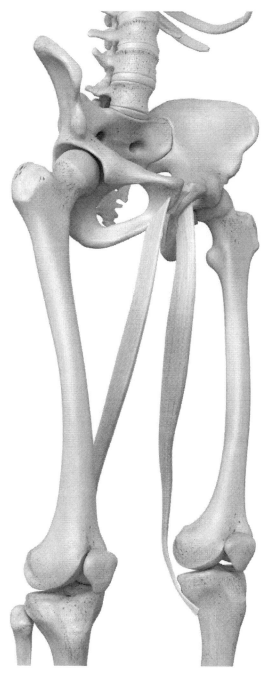

Rectus Femoris

Rectus Femoris is a muscle of the thigh, named after its function("rectus" in Latin means "straight", referring to ones ability to stand straight) and location.

Rectus Femoris originates on the Anterior Inferior Iliac Spine(AIIS), and inserts onto the Tibial Tuberosity.

Rectus Femoris is the prime mover of both hip flexion and knee extension.

Rectus Femoris is the most anterior muscle of the Quadriceps muscle group. Rectus Femoris is also the only Quadriceps muscle that crosses two joints(hip and knee). The rest of the Quadriceps muscles only cross the knee.

Origin: Anterior Inferior Iliac Spine
Insertion: Tibial Tuberosity
Action(s): Flexion of Hip, Extension of Knee
Innervation: Femoral Nerve
Synergist: Sartorius, Vastus Lateralis
Antagonist: Hamstrings

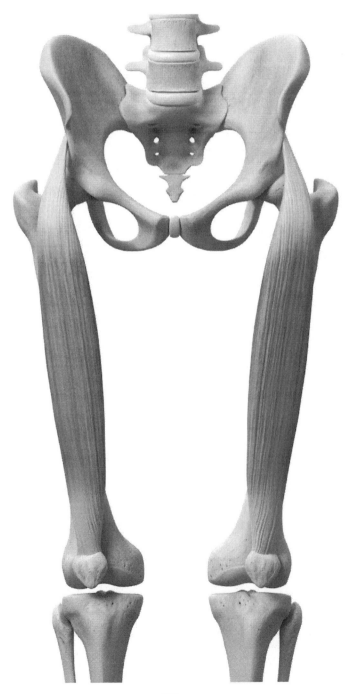

Sartorius

Sartorius is a muscle of the thigh, named for its action("sartor" is Latin for "tailor". It is named as such due to the actions of the muscle, which are the position a tailor places their leg into while working).

Sartorius originates on the Anterior Superior Iliac Spine(ASIS), and inserts onto the Pes Anserinus, located just medial to the Tibial Tuberosity.

Sartorius is responsible for flexion and lateral rotation of the hip, and flexion of the knee.

Sartorius is the longest muscle in the human body.

Origin: Anterior Superior Iliac Spine
Insertion: Pes Anserinus
Action(s): Flexion, Abduction, Lateral Rotation of Hip, Flexion of Knee
Innervation: Femoral Nerve
Synergist: Rectus Femoris(hip flexion), Gluteus Maximus(abduction), Piriformis(lateral rotation), Gastrocnemius(knee flexion)
Antagonist: Biceps Femoris(hip flexion), Adductor Magnus(abduction), Pectineus(lateral rotation), Rectus Femoris(knee flexion)

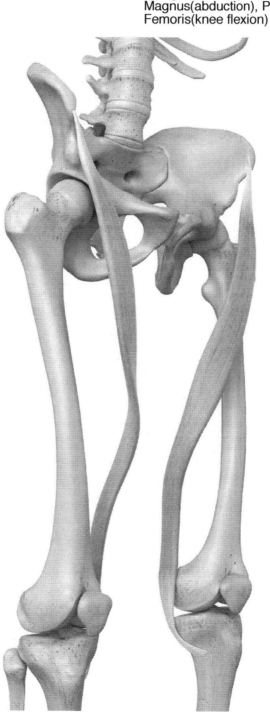

196

Semimembranosus

Semimembranosus is a muscle of the thigh, named after its appearance("semi" means "half", "membranosus" means "skin". Semimembranosus is about half muscle, half membranous tendon).

Semimembranosus originates on the Ischial Tuberosity, and inserts onto the Posterior Medial Condyle of the Tibia.

Semimembranosus is one muscle responsible for extension of the hip, and flexion of the knee.

Semimembranosus is a member of the Hamstring muscle group, located on the posterior thigh. Semimembranosus is the most medial of the Hamstring muscles.

Origin: Ischial Tuberosity
Insertion: Posterior Medial Condyle of Tibia
Action(s): Extension of Hip, Flexion of Knee
Innervation: Sciatic Nerve(Peroneal branch)
Synergist: Semitendinosus
Antagonist: Rectus Femoris

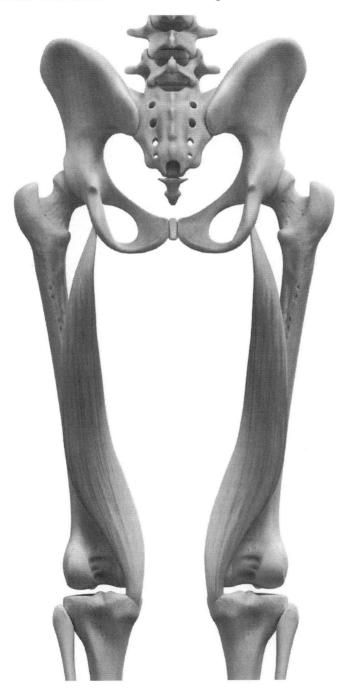

Semitendinosus

Semitendinosus is a muscle of the thigh, named for its appearance("semi" means "half", "tendinosus" refers to the Latin word "tendere", which means "to stretch").

Semitendinosus originates on the Ischial Tuberosity, and inserts onto the Pes Anserinus, located just medial to the Tibial Tuberosity.

Semitendinosus is one muscle responsible for extending the hip and flexing the knee, along with Semimembranosus and Biceps Femoris.

Semitendinosus is a member of the Hamstring muscle group, located on the posterior thigh.
Semimembranosus sits atop Semimembranosus, and is the intermediate Hamstring muscle.

Origin: Ischial Tuberosity
Insertion: Pes Anserinus
Action(s): Extension of Hip, Flexion of Knee
Innervation: Sciatic Nerve(Peroneal branch)
Synergist: Biceps Femoris
Antagonist: Rectus Femoris

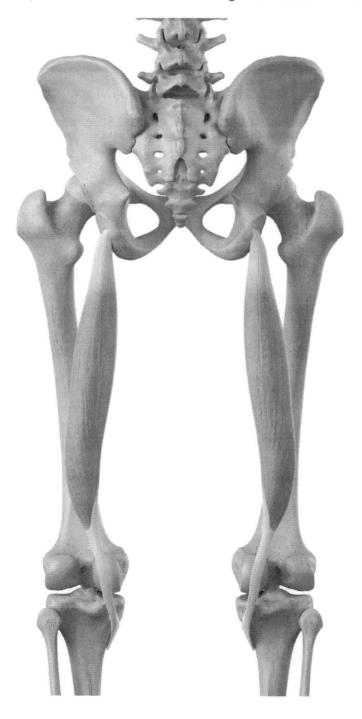

Tensor Fasciae Latae

Tensor Fasciae Latae is a muscle of the thigh, named after its appearance("tensor" comes from the Latin "tensere", which means "to stretch". "Fasciae" is Latin for "band". "Latae" is Latin for "side", such as the term "lateral").

Tensor Fasciae Latae originates on the Anterior Superior Iliac Spine(ASIS) and the Iliac Crest. Tensor Fasciae Latae inserts into the Iliotibial Tract(also known as the IT Band).

Tensor Fasciae Latae is a synergist in hip flexion.

Origin: Anterior Superior Iliac Spine, Iliac Crest
Insertion: Iliotibial Tract
Action(s): Flexion of Hip
Innervation: Superior Gluteal Nerve
Synergist: Rectus Femoris
Antagonist: Hamstrings

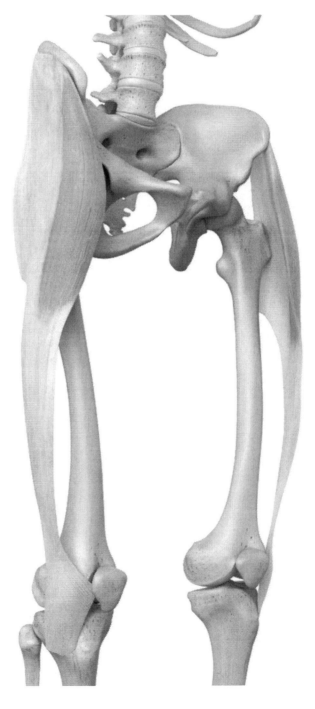

Muscles of the Leg

Muscles to Know:
Gastrocnemius
Peroneus Longus
Plantaris
Soleus
Tibialis Anterior
Tibialis Posterior

Terms to Know:
Gastr/o: Stomach
Kneme: Leg
Longus: Long

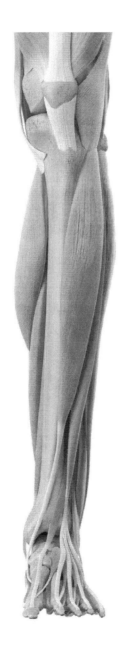
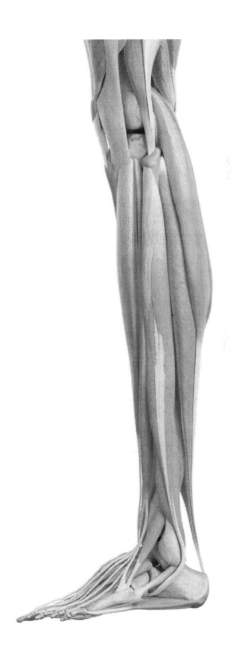

Gastrocnemius

Gastrocnemius is a muscle of the posterior leg. Its name means stomach(gastro) of the leg(kneme), from Greek origin.

Gastrocnemius originates on the Medial and Lateral Epicondyles of the Femur on the posterior side. The two muscle bellies join together at the Calcaneal Tendon, and insert at the Calcaneus. The Calcaneal Tendon is the strongest tendon in the body. Another name for the Calcaneal Tendon is "Achilles Tendon", so named after the Greek legend of Achilles.

Gastrocnemius, when contracted, assists the Hamstrings in performing flexion of the knee. Gastrocnemius is the prime mover of plantarflexion.

A primary synergist to Gastrocnemius is the Soleus, the muscle deep to the Gastrocnemius. Soleus joins with the Gastrocnemius at the Calcaneal Tendon, and assists in plantarflexion.

Origin: Medial and Lateral Epicondyles on Posterior Femur
Insertion: Calcaneus via Calcaneal Tendon
Action(s): Flexion of Knee, Plantarflexion
Innervation: Tibial Nerve
Synergist: Hamstrings, Soleus
Antagonist: Rectus Femoris, Tibialis Anterior

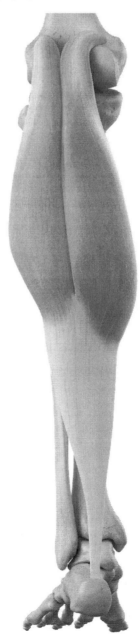

Peroneus Longus

Peroneus Longus is a muscle of the lateral leg, named after its origin("perone" means "fibula" and the two are interchangeable) and length.

Peroneus Longus originates on the Proximal Lateral Shaft of the Fibula, and the Head of the Fibula. It wraps beneath the Lateral Malleolus and onto the plantar surface of the foot, inserting onto the Base of the 1st Metatarsal and Cuneiform I(also known as the Medial Cuneiform).

When Peroneus Longus contracts, it is the prime mover of eversion/pronation of the foot. It also assists the Gastrocnemius and Soleus in performing plantarflexion.

Origin: Head of Fibula, Proximal Shaft of Fibula
Insertion: Base of 1st Metatarsal, Cuneiform I
Action(s): Plantarflexion, Eversion/Pronation of Foot
Innervation: Superficial Peroneal Nerve
Synergist: Peroneus Brevis
Antagonist: Tibialis Anterior

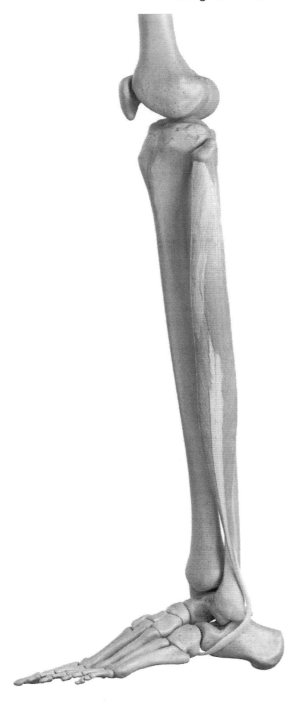

Plantaris

Plantaris is a muscle of the posterior leg, named after its action(plantarflexion).

Plantaris originates on the Lateral Supracondylar Ridge of the Femur, just above the Lateral Epicondyle. It crosses the knee and ankle, inserting onto the Calcaneus. The longest tendon in the body attaches the Plantaris to the Calcaneus.

Plantaris is a synergist in all of its actions. At the knee, it assists the Hamstrings and Gastrocnemius in flexion. At the ankle, it assists Gastrocnemius and Soleus in plantarflexion.

If a person injures the Plantaris, they may be diagnosed with a condition known as Tennis Leg, a straining of not just the Plantaris, but the other calf muscles.

Origin: Lateral Supracondylar Ridge of Femur
Insertion: Calcaneus
Action(s): Flexion of Knee, Plantarflexion
Innervation: Tibial Nerve
Synergist: Gastrocnemius
Antagonist: Tibialis Anterior

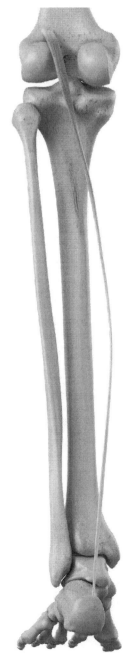

Soleus

Soleus is a muscle of the posterior leg, named after its appearance(resembles a sole fish in shape).

Soleus originates on the Soleal Line, a ridge located on the posterior proximal surface of the Tibia, and the Head of the Fibula. Soleus joins with the Gastrocnemius at the Calcaneal Tendon, inserting onto the Calcaneus.

Soleus is primarily a synergist to the Gastrocnemius, performing plantarflexion.

Origin: Soleal Line, Head of Fibula
Insertion: Calcaneus via Calcaneal Tendon
Action(s): Plantarflexion
Innervation: Tibial Nerve
Synergist: Gastrocnemius
Antagonist: Tibialis Anterior

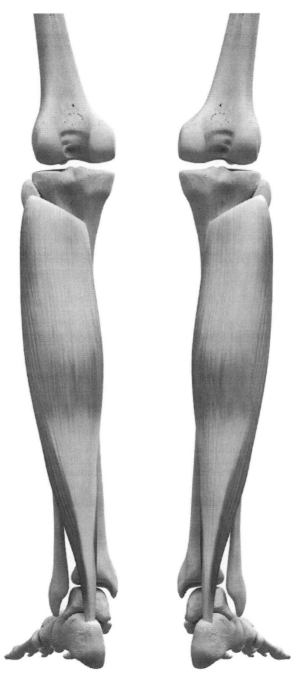

Tibialis Anterior

Tibialis Anterior is a muscle of the anterior leg, named after its origin(Tibia) and location(Anterior).

Tibialis Anterior originates on the Lateral Proximal Shaft of the Tibia, beside the Fibula. Tibialis Anterior wraps onto the medial plantar surface of the foot, inserting onto the Base of the 1st Metatarsal, and Cuneiform I(also known as the Medial Cuneiform). It shares its insertion with Peroneus Longus, its direct antagonist.

Tibialis Anterior is the prime mover of inversion/supination of the foot, pulling the soles of the feet in towards the midline when the muscle contracts. It is also the prime mover of dorsiflexion, pulling the foot up.

If a person is affected by paralysis in the Deep Peroneal Nerve, the Tibialis Anterior is severely weakened. This results in inability to dorsiflex, a condition known as Drop Foot.

Origin: Lateral Proximal Shaft of Tibia
Insertion: Base of 1st Metatarsal, Cuneiform I
Action(s): Dorsiflexion, Inversion/Supination of Foot
Innervation: Deep Peroneal Nerve
Synergist: Extensor Digitorum Longus, Tibialis Posterior
Antagonist: Peroneus Longus

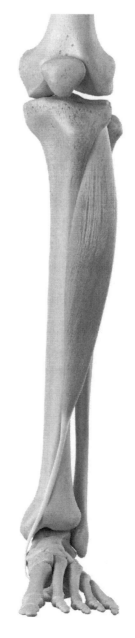

Tibialis Posterior

Tibialis Posterior is a muscle of the posterior leg, named after its location(on the posterior Tibia).

Tibialis Posterior originates on the Posterior Proximal Shaft of the Tibia and Fibula. It crosses the ankle and runs into the plantar surface of the foot, inserting onto the Navicular, Cuneiform I(also called the Medial Cuneiform), and Metatarsals 2-4.

Tibialis Anterior is primarily a synergist, assisting Tibialis Anterior in inversion/supination of the foot, and assisting Gastrocnemius and Soleus in plantarflexing the ankle.

Origin: Posterior Proximal Shaft of Tibia and Fibula
Insertion: Navicular, Cuneiform I, Metatarsals 2-4
Action(s): Inversion of Foot, Plantarflexion
Innervation: Tibial Nerve
Synergist: Tibialis Anterior, Gastrocnemius
Antagonist: Peroneus Longus, Extensor Digitorum Longus

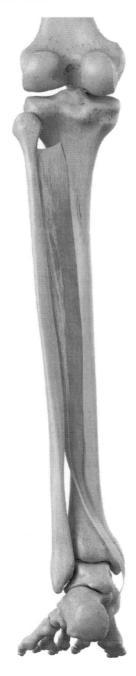

Kinesiology Matching

_____: Action performed by Brachialis

_____: Insertion of Brachioradialis

_____: Muscle that inserts on the Mastoid Process of the Temporal bone

_____: Insertion of Gracilis

_____: Origin of Temporalis

_____: Action shared by Tibialis Anterior and Tibialis Posterior

_____: Muscle inserting onto the Radial Tuberosity

_____: Prime mover of shoulder abduction

_____: Insertion of Rectus Abdominis

_____: Muscle inserting onto the Pes Anserinus

_____: Origin of Sartorius

_____: Muscles responsible for retracting/adducting the scapula

_____: Action performed by the Biceps Brachii, in which it is the prime mover

_____: Bipennate muscle that crosses the hip and knee on the anterior thigh

_____: Origin of the Infraspinatus

_____: Insertion of the Quadriceps

_____: Action performed by the Latissimus Dorsi

_____: Muscle originating in the Supraspinous Fossa

_____: Primary action performed by the Pectoralis Major

_____: Action of the Hamstrings and Gastrocnemius

A: Biceps Brachii

B: Anterior Superior Iliac Spine

C: Elbow Flexion

D: Supraspinatus

E: Deltoid

F: Pes Anserinus

G: Knee Flexion

H: Shoulder Adduction

I: Rectus Femoris

J: Tibial Tuberosity

K: Sartorius

L: Styloid Process of Radius

M: Temporal Fossa

N: Sternocleidomastoid

O: Horizontal Adduction of the Shoulder

P: Rhomboids

Q: Infraspinous Fossa

R: Xiphoid Process

S: Supination

T: Inversion

Kinesiology

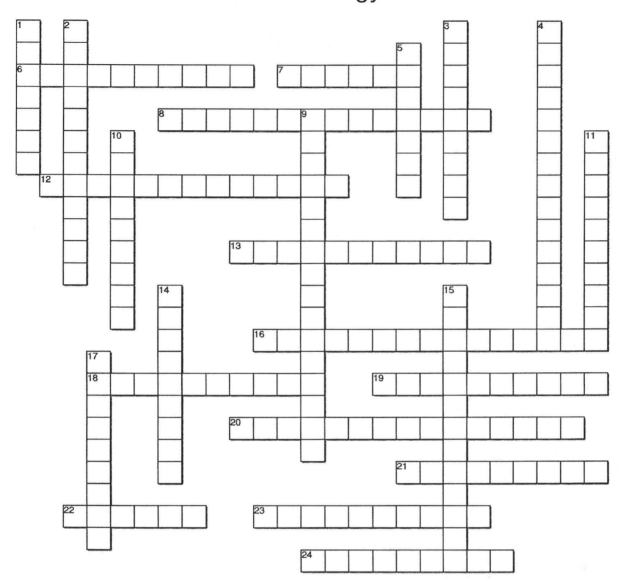

Across

6. Synergist to Latissimus Dorsi
7. Type of rotation Subscapularis performs on the shoulder
8. Action Gastrocnemius performs on the ankle
12. Muscle originating on the Anterior Inferior Iliac Spine
13. Action of the Pectoralis Minor on the scapula
16. Origin of Coracobrachialis
18. Strongest flexor of the elbow
19. Action of the Rhomboids on the scapula
20. Muscle primarily response for flexion of the trunk
21. The longest tendon in the body attaches to this muscle
22. Synergist to Gastrocnemius while moving the ankle
23. Antagonists to the Quadriceps
24. Strongest tendon in the body

Down

1. Type of rotation Infraspinatus performs on the shoulder
2. Action Tibialis Anterior performs on the ankle
3. Muscle originating on the Anterior Superior Iliac Spine
4. Insertion of Infraspinatus, Supraspinatus, and Teres Minor
5. Primary action of Iliopsoas on the hip
9. Insertion of Biceps Brachii
10. Action of Triceps Brachii on the elbow
11. Muscle group inserting onto the Tibial Tuberosity
14. Primary action of Gracilis on the hip
15. Insertion of Levator Scapulae
17. Primary action of the Deltoid

Muscle Actions Fill-In-The-Blank

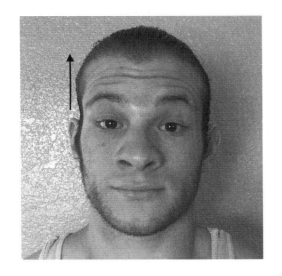
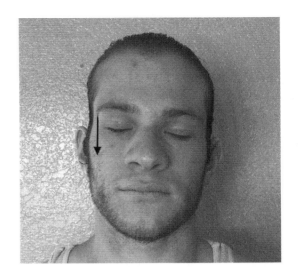
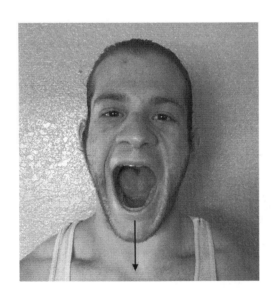
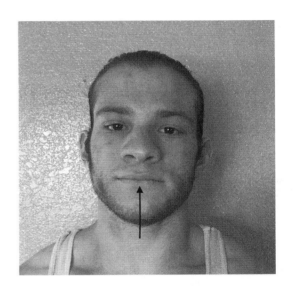
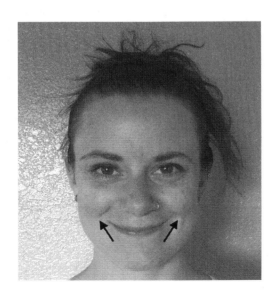
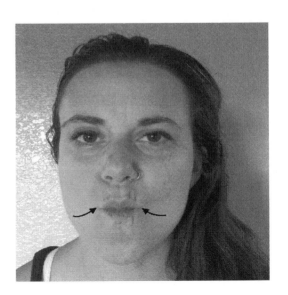

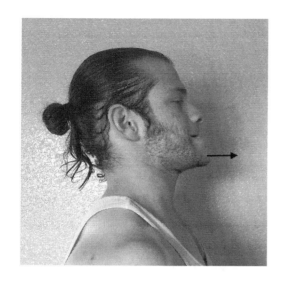

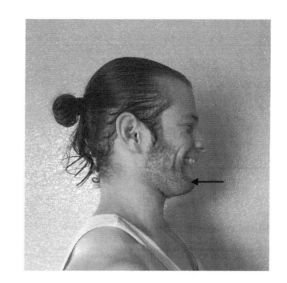

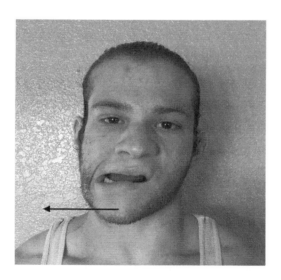

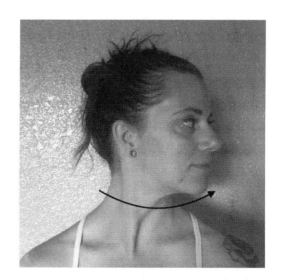

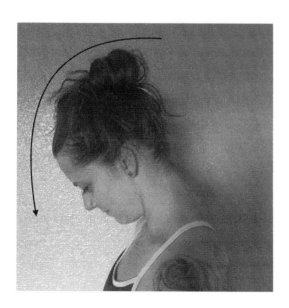

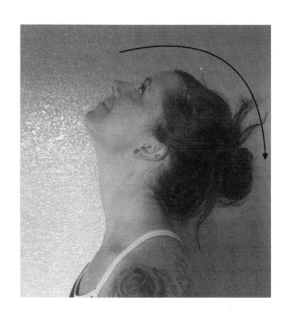

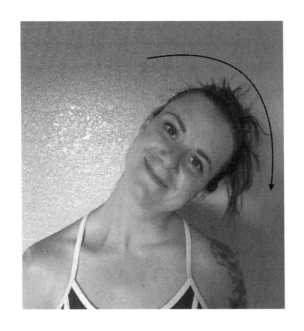
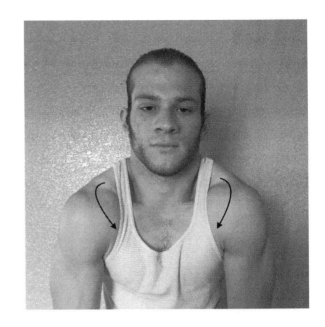
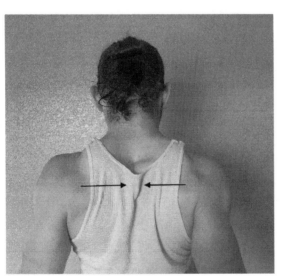
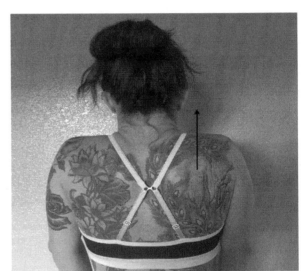
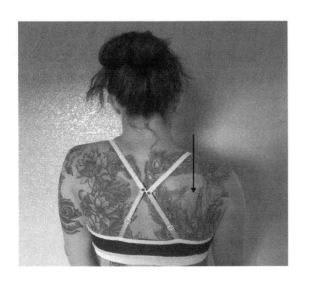
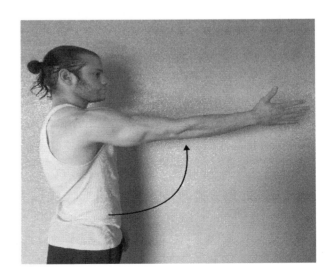

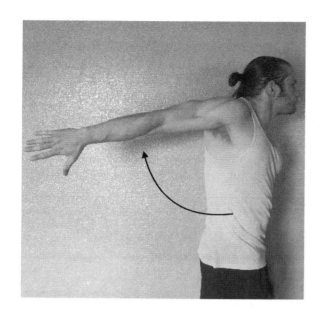 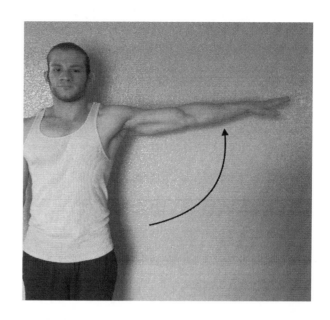

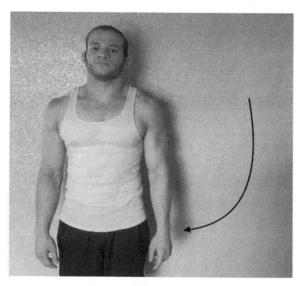 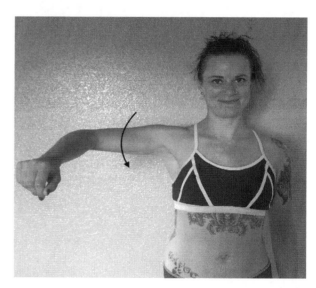

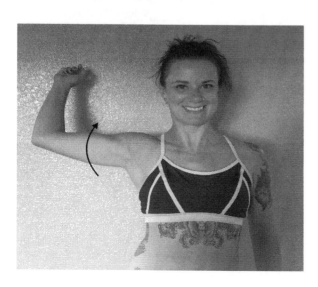 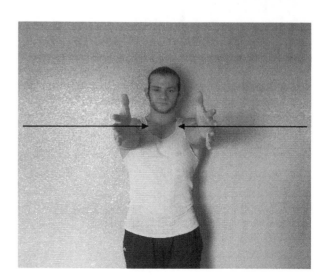

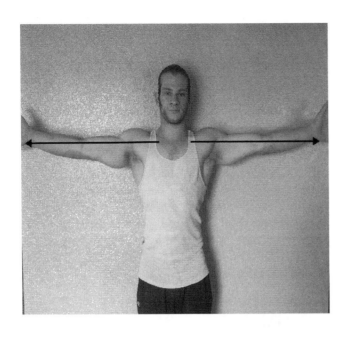

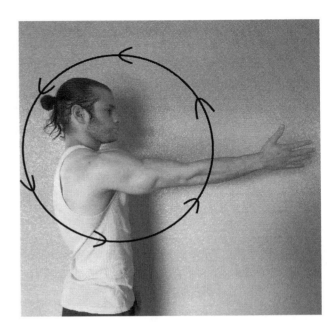

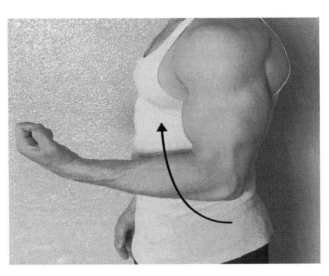

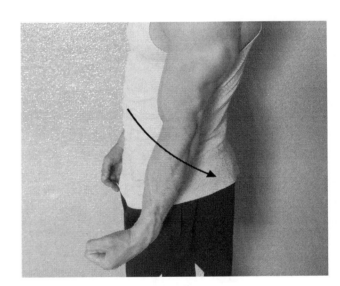

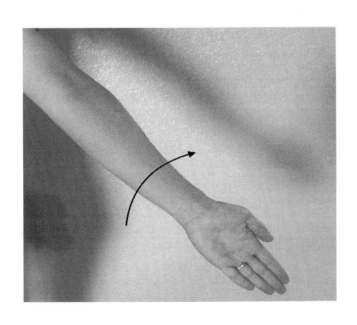

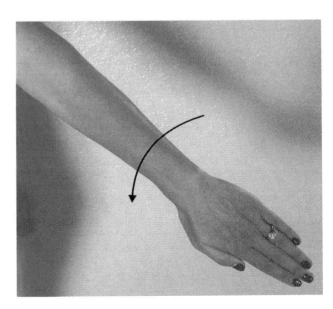

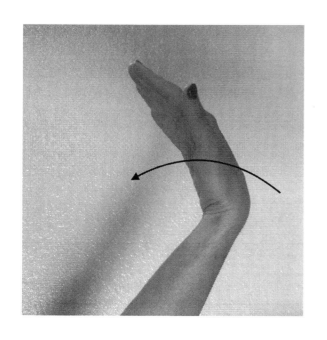
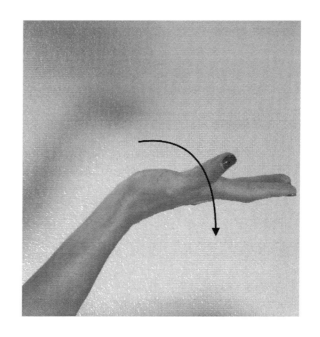
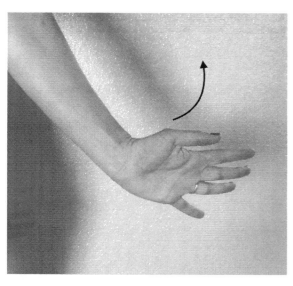
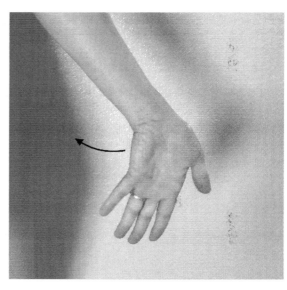
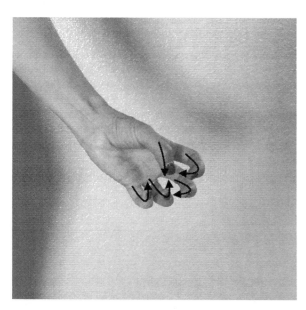
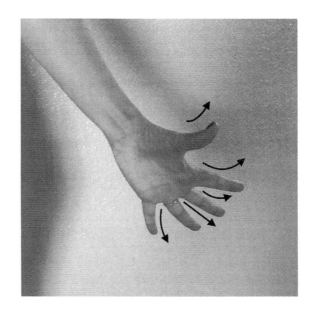

214

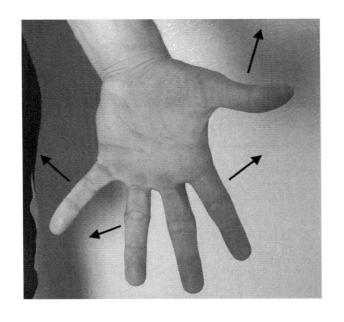
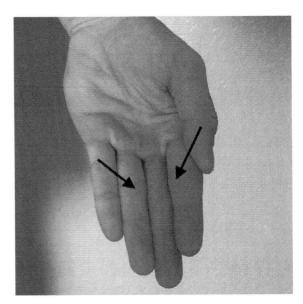
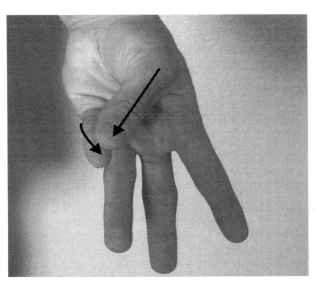
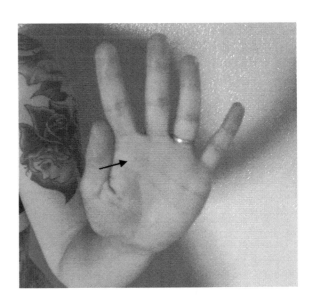
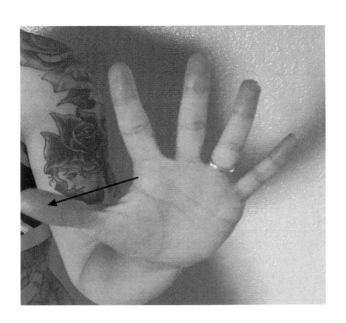
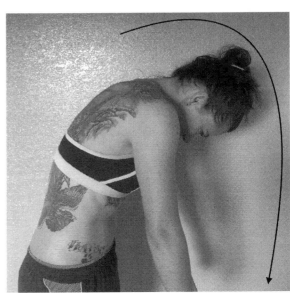

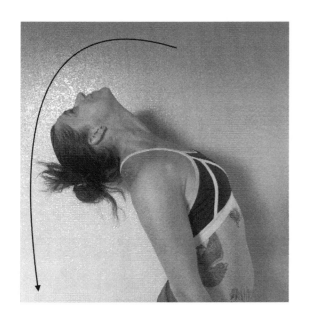 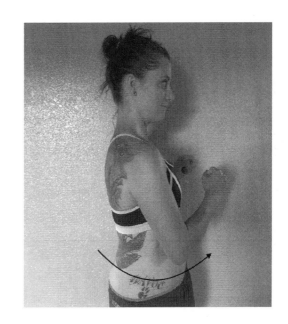

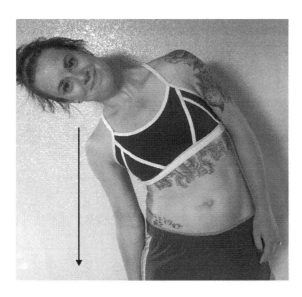 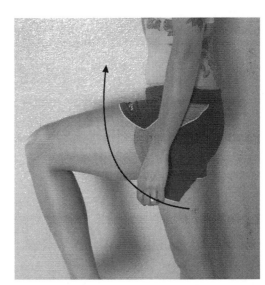

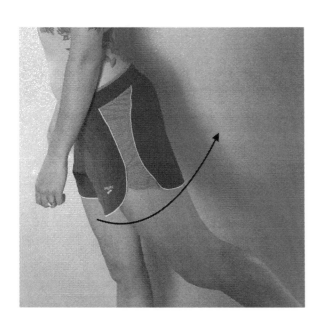 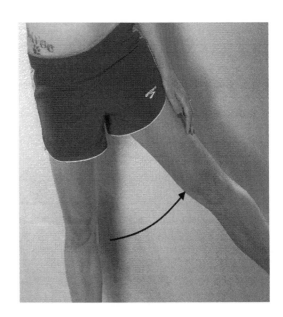

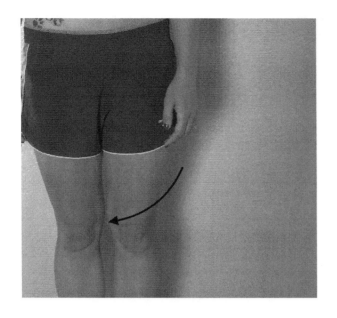

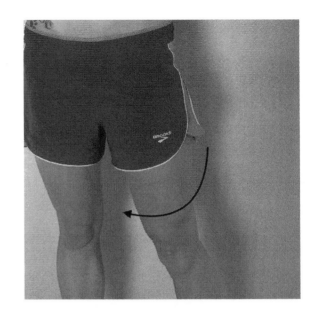

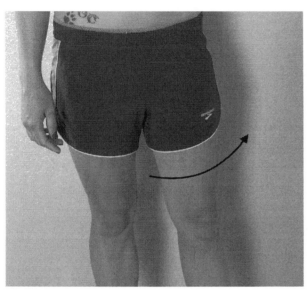

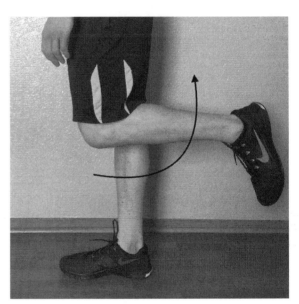

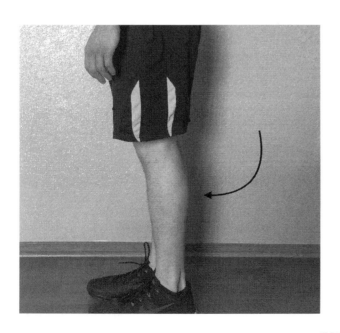

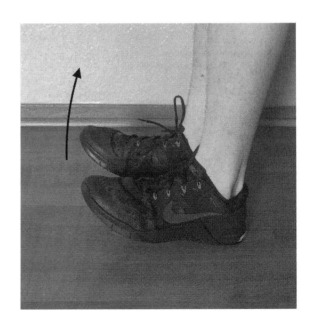

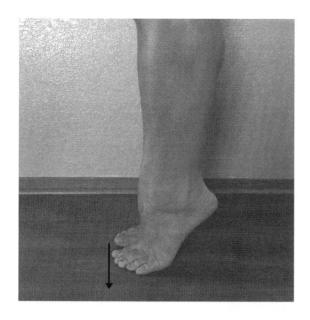 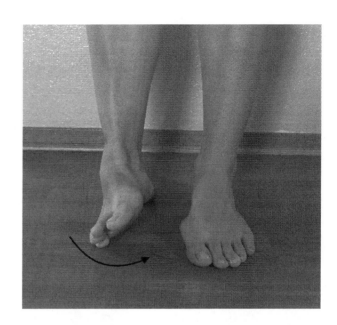

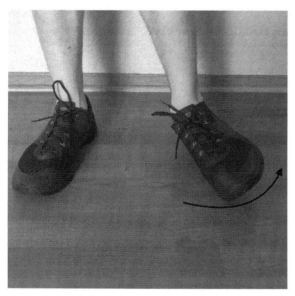 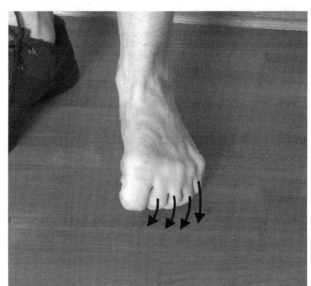

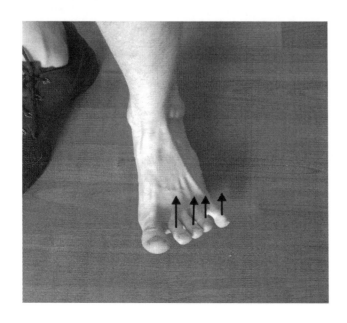

Bony Landmarks Fill-In-The-Blank

The bony landmarks are specific locations on bones where muscles attach to. There are many different kinds of landmarks, from tubercles and tuberosities, to condyles and epicondyles.

A condyle is a _____ projection coming off a bone at an articulation.
An epicondyle is the part of the bone located _____ to the condyle.
A crest is a thin _____ of a bone.
A facet is a smooth _____ surface of a bone.
A fissure is a narrow opening, resembling a _____.
A foramina(foramen) is a _____ or _____ in a bone.
A fossa is a shallow _____ in a bone.
A linea is a narrow _____, less pronounced than a crest.
A meatus is a _____-like passage.
A process is a prominent _____ on a bone.
A ramus is an _____, seemingly stretched-out part of a bone.
A sinus is a _____ created by bones.
A suture is a type of synarthrotic joint that doesn't allow _____.
A trochanter is a very large process, only found on the _____.
A tubercle is a small, _____ projection.
A tuberosity is a large, rounded, often _____ projection.

Bones have numerous different types of landmarks. Landmarks are not only named after their type(above), but often times what they look like(example, "coracoid" means "resembling a crow's beak"), what muscles attach to them(example, deltoid tuberosity), or even where they're located in the body(example, anterior superior iliac spine).

Head

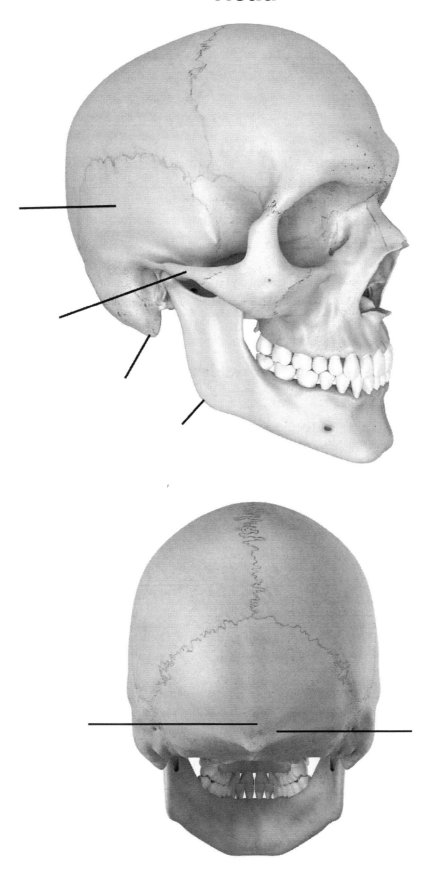

Vertebrae

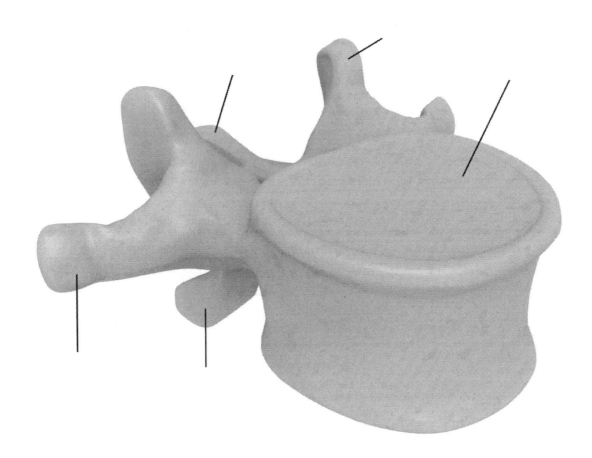

Back

Anterior Scapula

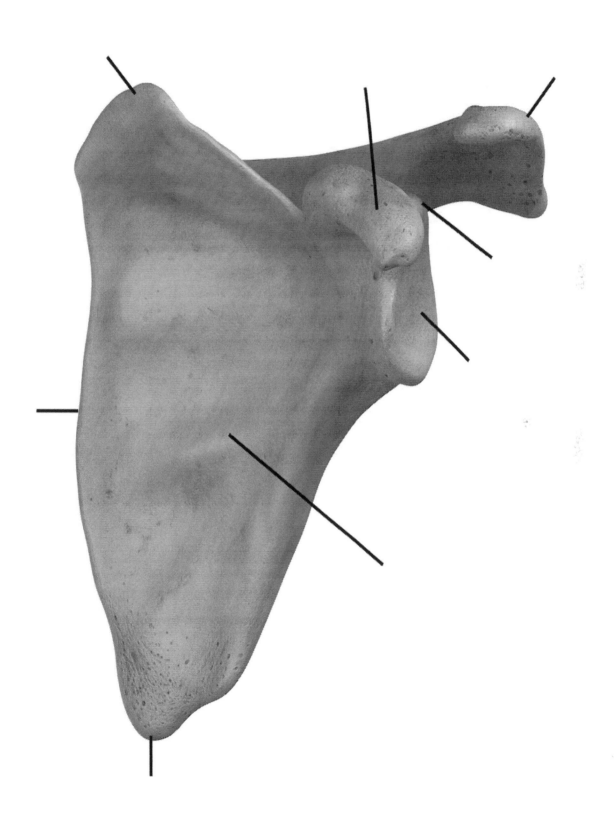

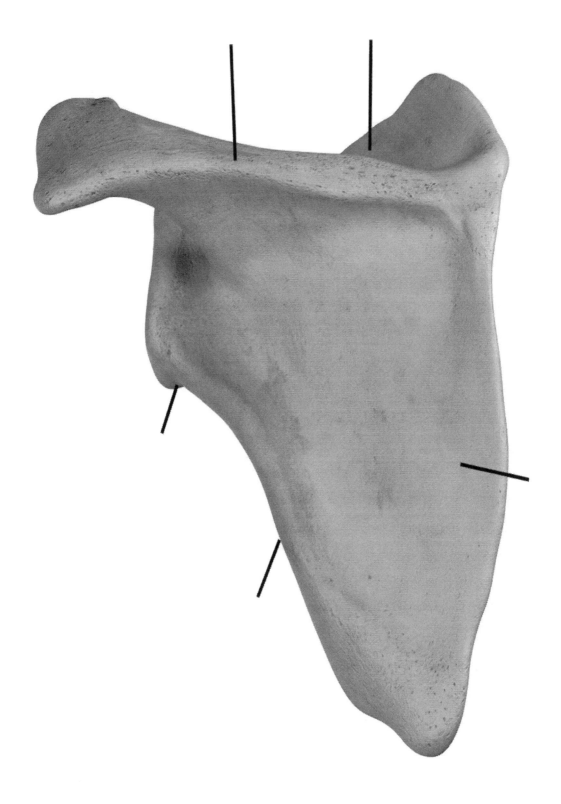

Chest

Clavicle

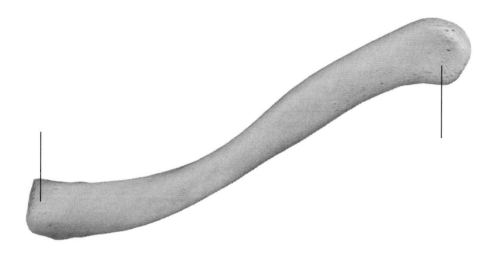

Sternum

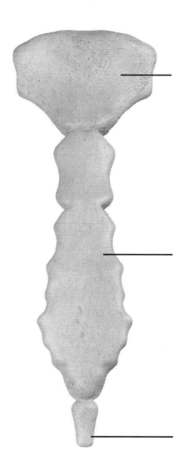

Arm

Anterior Humerus

Posterior Humerus

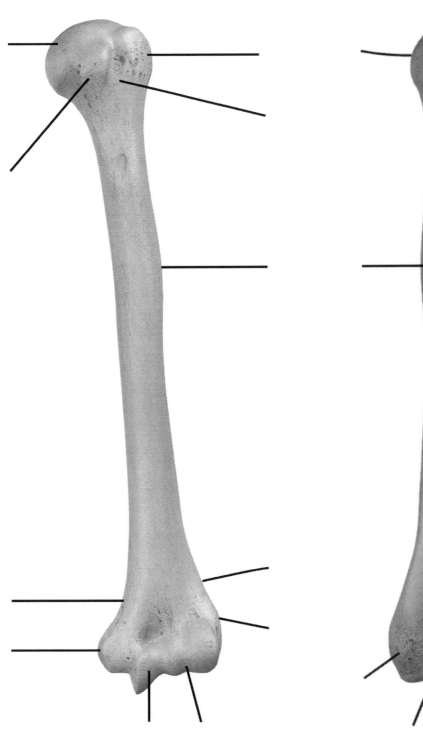
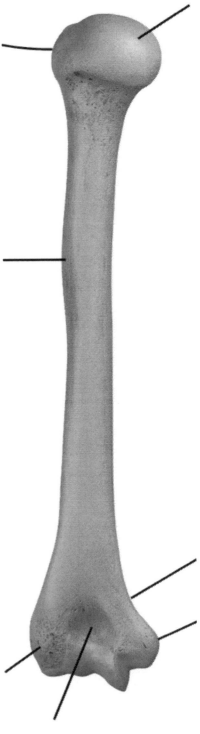

225

Forearm

Radius

Ulna

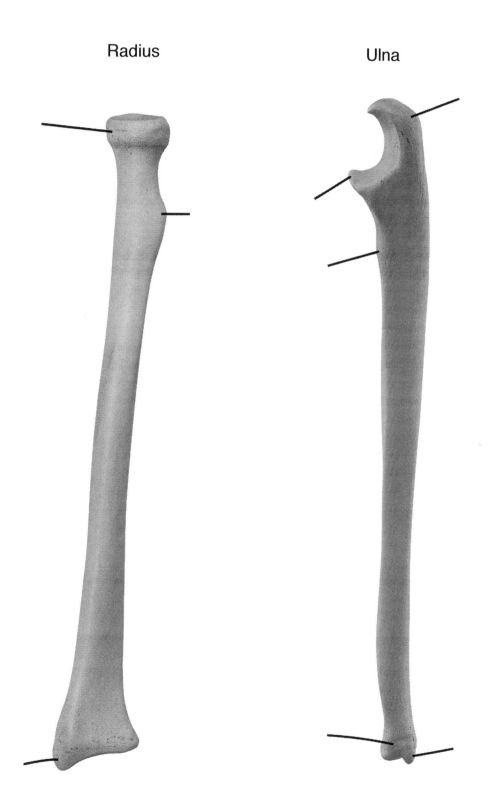

Wrist

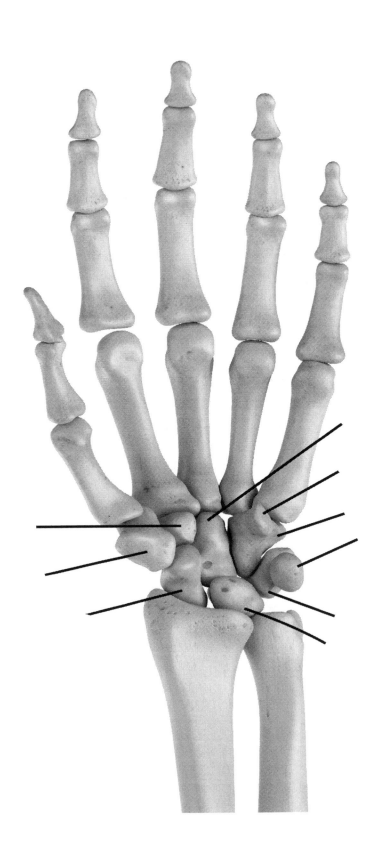

Pelvis

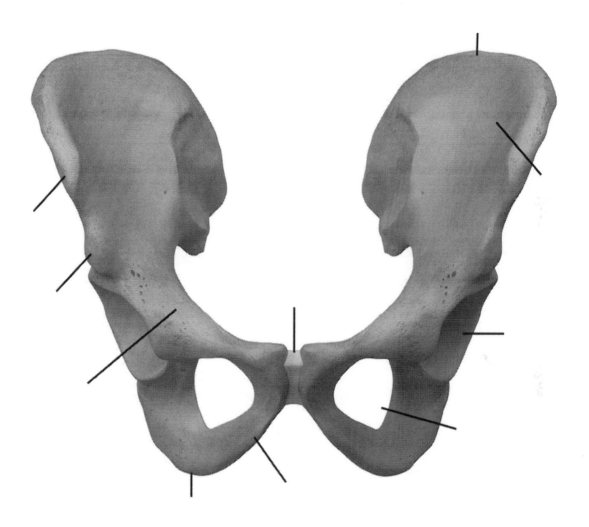

Thigh

Anterior Femur

Posterior Femur

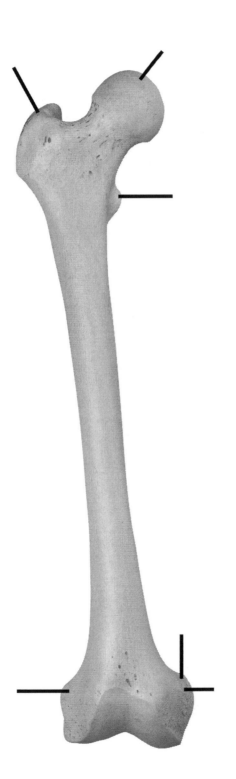
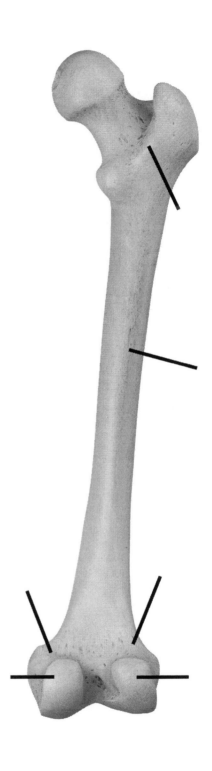

Leg

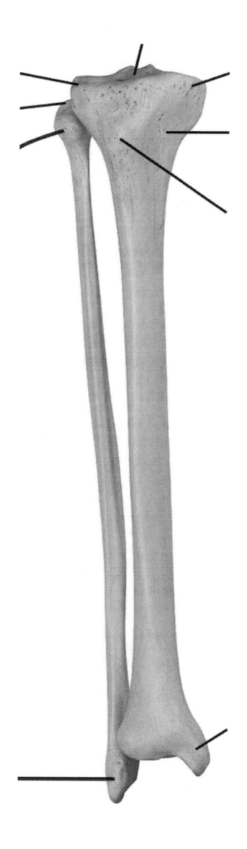

Ankle

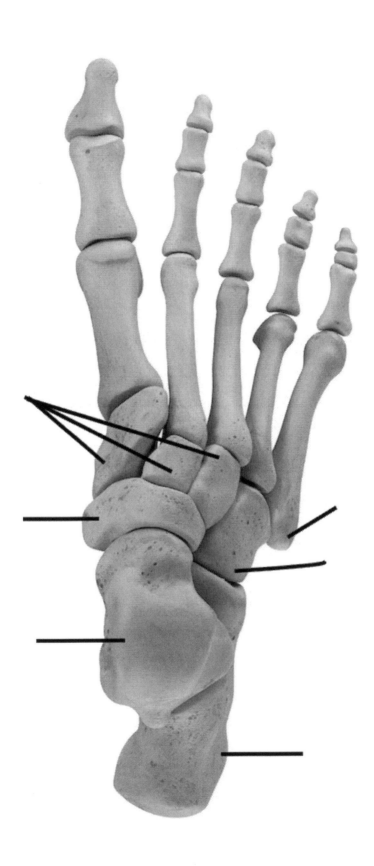

Muscle Fill-In-The-Blank

Head

Buccinator

Insertion:

Action(s):

Synergist:

Masseter

Origin:

Insertion:

Action(s):

Synergist:

Temporalis

Origin:

Insertion:

Action(s):

Synergist:

Neck

Levator Scapulae

Insertion:

Action(s):

Synergist:

Antagonist:

Scalenes

Origin:

Insertion:

Action(s):

Medical Condition:

Sternocleidomastoid

Origin:

Insertion:

Action(s):

Back

Infraspinatus

Origin:

Insertion:

Action(s):

Synergist:

Antagonist:

Latissimus Dorsi

Origin:

Insertion:

Action(s):

Synergist:

Antagonist:

Longissimus

Action(s):

Synergist:

Antagonist:

Multifidus

Origin:

Insertion:

Action(s):

Synergist:

Antagonist:

Quadratus Lumborum

Origin:

Insertion:

Action(s):

Synergist:

Antagonist:

Medical Condition:

Rhomboids

Origin:

Insertion:

Action(s):

Synergist:

Antagonist:

Medical Condition:

Rotatores

Origin:

Insertion:

Action(s):

Synergist:

Antagonist:

Spinalis

Origin:

Insertion:

Action(s):

Synergist:

Antagonist:

Subscapularis

Origin:

Insertion:

Action(s):

Synergist:

Antagonist:

Supraspinatus

Origin:

Insertion:

Action(s):

Synergist:

Antagonist:

Teres Major

Origin:

Insertion:

Action(s):

Synergist:

Antagonist:

Teres Minor

Origin:

Insertion:

Action(s):

Synergist:

Antagonist:

Trapezius

Origin:

Insertion:

Action(s):

Synergist:

Antagonist:

Chest

Pectoralis Major

Origin:

Insertion:

Action(s):

Synergist:

Antagonist:

Pectoralis Minor

Origin:

Insertion:

Action(s):

Synergist:

Antagonist:

Medical Conditions:

Serratus Anterior

Origin:

Insertion:

Action(s):

Synergist:

Antagonist:

Medical Condition:

Abdomen

Rectus Abdominis

Origin:

Insertion:

Action(s):

Medical Condition:

Arm

Biceps Brachii

Origin:

Insertion:

Action(s):

Synergist:

Antagonist:

Brachialis

Origin:

Insertion:

Action(s):

Synergist:

Antagonist:

Coracobrachialis

Origin:

Action(s):

Synergist:

Antagonist:

Deltoid

Origin:

Insertion:

Action(s):

Synergist:

Antagonist:

Triceps Brachii

Origin:

Insertion:

Action(s):

Synergist:

Antagonist:

Forearm

Anconeus

Origin:

Insertion:

Action(s):

Synergist:

Antagonist:

Medical Condition:

Brachioradialis

Origin:

Insertion:

Action(s):

Synergist:

Antagonist:

Pronator Teres

Origin:

Insertion:

Action(s):

Synergist:

Antagonist:

Pelvis

Gluteus Maximus

Origin:

Insertion:

Action(s):

Synergist:

Antagonist:

Iliacus

Origin:

Insertion:

Action(s):

Synergist:

Antagonist:

Medical Condition:

Piriformis

Origin:

Insertion:

Action(s):

Synergist:

Antagonist:

Medical Condition:

Psoas Major

Origin:

Insertion:

Action(s):

Synergist:

Antagonist:

Medical Condition:

Thigh

Adductor Magnus

Origin:

Insertion:

Action(s):

Synergist:

Antagonist:

Biceps Femoris

Origin:

Insertion:

Action(s):

Synergist:

Antagonist:

Gracilis

Origin:

Insertion:

Action(s):

Synergist:

Antagonist:

Rectus Femoris

Origin:

Insertion:

Action(s):

Synergist:

Antagonist:

Sartorius

Origin:

Insertion:

Action(s):

Synergist:

Antagonist:

Semimembranosus

Origin:

Action(s):

Synergist:

Antagonist:

Semitendinosus

Origin:

Insertion:

Action(s):

Synergist:

Antagonist:

Tensor Fasciae Latae

Origin:

Insertion:

Action(s):

Synergist:

Antagonist:

Leg

Gastrocnemius

Origin:

Insertion:

Action(s):

Synergist:

Antagonist:

Peroneus Longus

Origin:

Insertion:

Action(s):

Synergist:

Antagonist:

Plantaris

Origin:

Insertion:

Action(s):

Synergist:

Antagonist:

Soleus

Origin:

Insertion:

Action(s):

Synergist:

Antagonist:

Tibialis Anterior

Origin:

Insertion:

Action(s):

Synergist:

Antagonist:

Medical Condition:

Tibialis Posterior

Origin:

Insertion:

Action(s):

Synergist:

Antagonist:

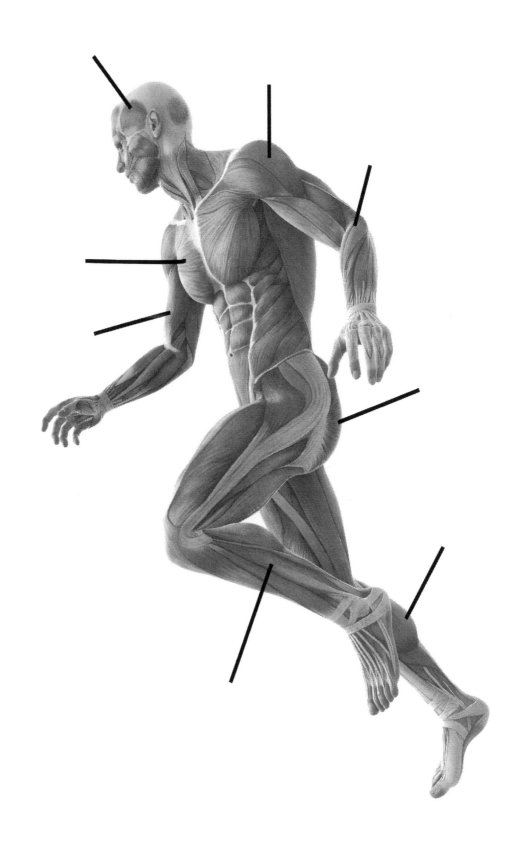

237

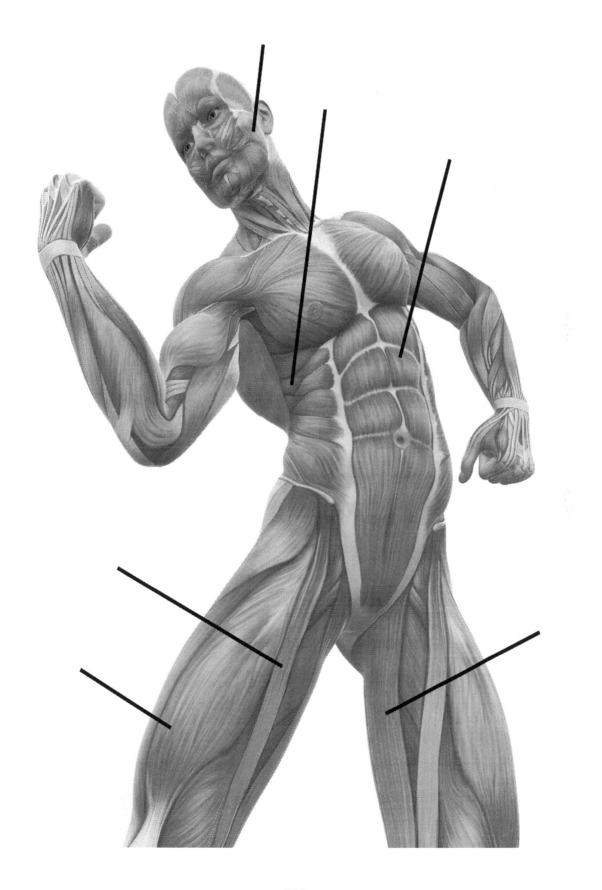

238

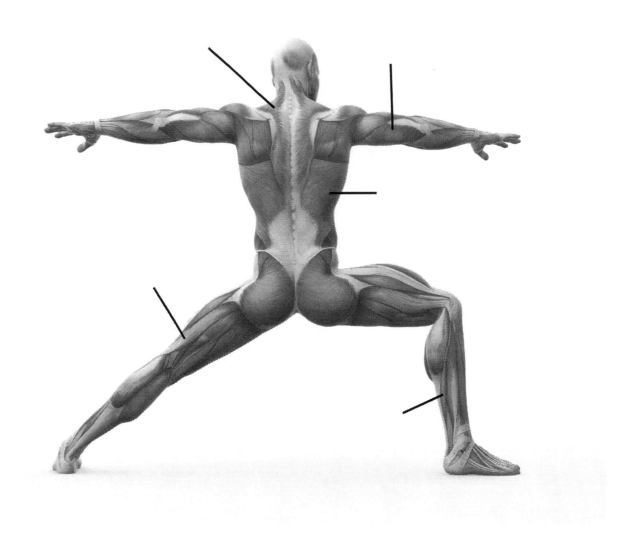

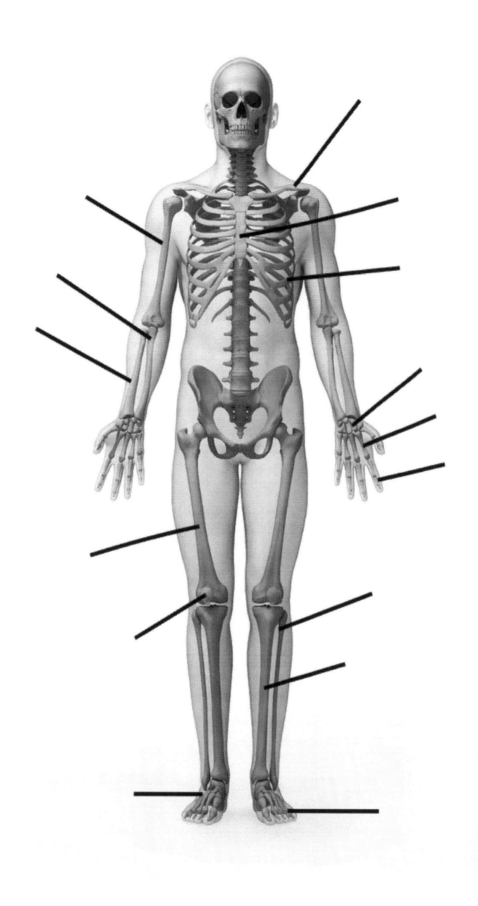

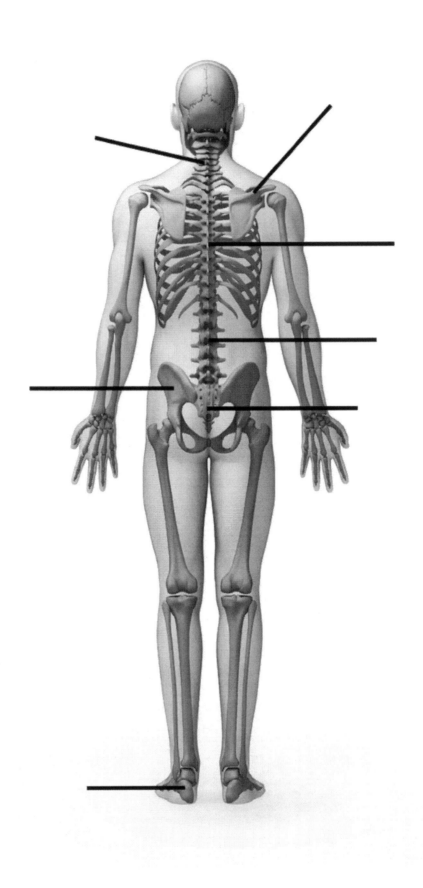

Kinesiology Matching

C   P
L   S
N   I
F   Q
M   J
T   H
A   D
E   O
R   G
K
B

Kinesiology Answers

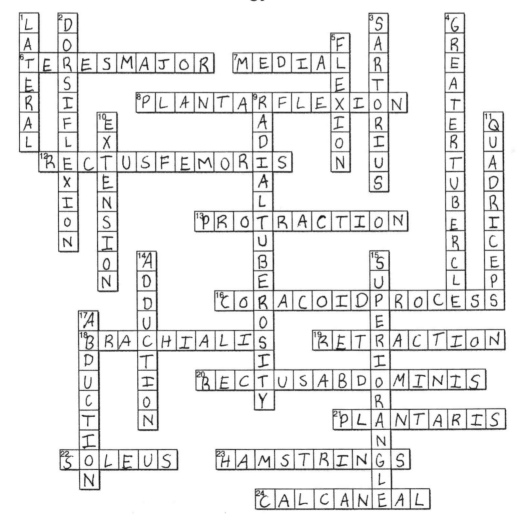

242

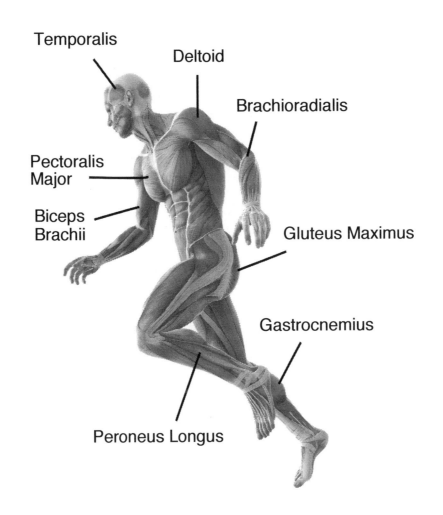

Temporalis

Deltoid

Brachioradialis

Pectoralis
Major

Biceps
Brachii

Gluteus Maximus

Gastrocnemius

Peroneus Longus

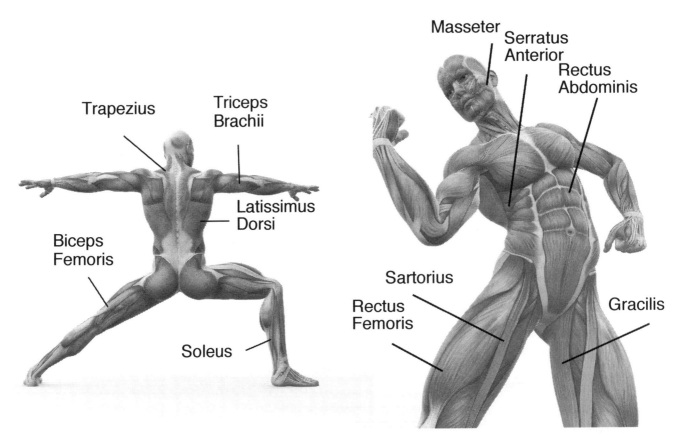

Trapezius

Triceps
Brachii

Latissimus
Dorsi

Biceps
Femoris

Soleus

Masseter

Serratus
Anterior

Rectus
Abdominis

Sartorius

Rectus
Femoris

Gracilis

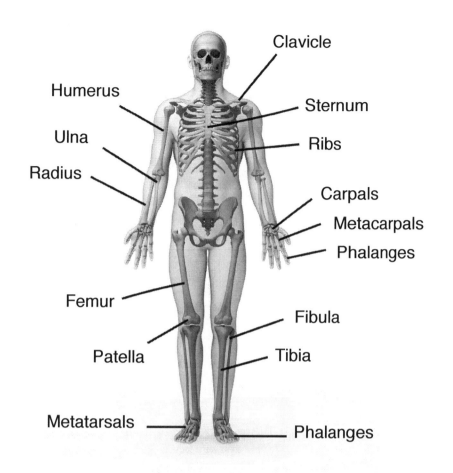

Clavicle

Humerus

Sternum

Ulna

Ribs

Radius

Carpals

Metacarpals

Phalanges

Femur

Fibula

Patella

Tibia

Metatarsals

Phalanges

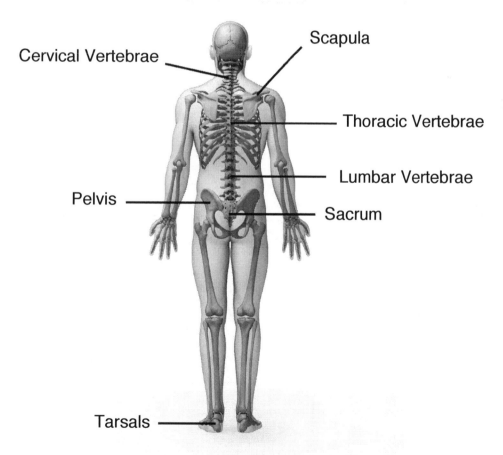

Scapula

Cervical Vertebrae

Thoracic Vertebrae

Lumbar Vertebrae

Pelvis

Sacrum

Tarsals

Kinesiology Practice Exam

1. Most medial muscle of the erector spinae muscle group
A. Longissimus
B. Semispinalis
C. Spinalis
D. Iliocostalis

2. Insertion of the adductor longus
A. Lesser trochanter
B. Pectineal line
C. Linea aspera
D. Greater trochanter

3. Elbow extension and shoulder extension is performed by the following muscle
A. Triceps brachii
B. Biceps brachii
C. Coracobrachialis
D. Anconeus

4. Part of the scapula serratus anterior inserts onto
A. Medial border
B. Lateral border
C. Spine
D. Inferior angle

5. Muscle originating in the subscapular fossa
A. Pectoralis Minor
B. Supraspinatus
C. Infraspinatus
D. Subscapularis

6. Large bony structures located at the proximal end of the humerus
A. Trochlea and capitulum
B. Medial and lateral epicondyles
C. Deltoid tuberosity and olecranon fossa
D. Greater and lesser tubercles

7. An antagonist to the biceps brachii is
A. Coracobrachialis
B. Brachialis
C. Pronator Teres
D. Supinator

8. Adductor magnus has a common origination site with which muscle group
A. Wrist flexors
B. Quadriceps
C. Rotator cuff
D. Hamstrings

9. All of the following are located on the femur except
A. Medial condyle
B. Greater trochanter
C. Linea alba
D. Adductor tubercle

10. The second cervical vertebrae is also known as
A. Atlas
B. Axis
C. Occiput
D. Temporal

11. Muscle originating on the spinous processes of T7-L5, the iliac crest, and lumbar aponeurosis
A. Quadratus lumborum
B. Latissimus dorsi
C. Spinalis
D. Psoas major

12. Which fiber of the deltoid originates on the acromion process of the scapula
A. Inferior deltoid
B. Anterior deltoid
C. Posterior deltoid
D. Middle deltoid

13. Shoulder flexion, elbow flexion, and forearm supination are all performed by which muscle
A. Brachialis
B. Coracobrachialis
C. Brachioradialis
D. Biceps Brachii

14. Which of the following is a hinge joint
A. Knee
B. Hip
C. Shoulder
D. Wrist

15. Muscle inserting onto the medial lip of the linea aspera and adductor tubercle of the femur
A. Adductor longus
B. Adductor magnus
C. Adductor brevis
D. Gracilis

16. The linea aspera is located on which side of the femur
A. Anterior
B. Posterior
C. Medial
D. Lateral

17. The following muscle inserts onto the lateral lip of the intertubercular groove
A. Pectoralis minor
B. Pectoralis major
C. Latissimus dorsi
D. Teres major

18. The origin of teres minor
A. Lateral border of the scapula
B. Medial border of the scapula
C. Spine of the scapula
D. Inferior angle of the scapula

19. Origin of the rectus femoris
A. Anterior Superior Iliac Spine
B. Anterior Inferior Iliac Spine
C. Ischial tuberosity
D. Body of the pubis

20. Which two structures form the hip joint
A. Head of femur and obturator foramen
B. Head of femur and acetabulum
C. Head of humerus and glenoid fossa
D. Head of humerus and acromion process

21. Contraction of the middle fibers of the trapezius result in
A. Retraction
B. Protraction
C. Elevation
D. Depression

22. The coronal suture connects the following bones of the cranium
A. Occipital and parietal
B. Parietal and parietal
C. Parietal and frontal
D. Temporal and parietal

23. The interphalangeal joints can perform which actions
A. Adduction and abduction
B. Rotation
C. Flexion and extension
D. Protraction and retraction

24. Brachioradialis inserts onto which part of the radius
A. Styloid process
B. Radial tuberosity
C. Head
D. Interosseous border

25. A massage therapist is working on the lateral side of the forearm. The bone they are working on top of is the
A. Radius
B. Ulna
C. Humerus
D. Fibula

26. Muscles originating on the spinous processes of C7-T5
A. Levator scapulae
B. Serratus anterior
C. Trapezius
D. Rhomboids

27. The socket of the hip is also called the
A. Ischial tuberosity
B. Obturator foramen
C. Acetabulum
D. Iliac crest

28. Primary muscle a massage therapist palpates on the lateral edge of the leg
A. Soleus
B. Tibialis anterior
C. Peroneus longus
D. Gastrocnemius

29. The ankle joint is comprised of which two bones
A. Tibia and talus
B. Tibia and fibula
C. Talus and calcaneus
D. Talus and fibula

30. Origin of pectoralis minor
A. Coracoid process
B. Ribs 3-5
C. Ribs 1-3
D. Sternum

31. Extension of the thumb can be accomplished by contraction of which muscle
A. Extensor pollicis longus
B. Flexor pollicis longus
C. Extensor hallucis longus
D. Flexor hallucis longus

32. The saddle joint is located where
A. Elbow
B. Thumb
C. Knee
D. Ankle

33. Structure located on the lateral distal end of the humerus
A. Medial epicondyle
B. Greater tubercle
C. Lateral epicondyle
D. Trochlea

34. Antagonist to the rhomboids, responsible for abduction of the scapula
A. Latissimus dorsi
B. Pectoralis major
C. Trapezius
D. Serratus anterior

35. Proximal attachment of coracobrachialis
A. Coracoid process
B. Coronoid process
C. Medial proximal shaft of humerus
D. Radial tuberosity

36. Joint located between the occiput and first cervical vertebrae, responsible for flexion and extension of the head
A. Atlantoaxial
B. Atlantooccipital
C. Occipitofrontalis
D. Occipitoaxial

37. Three of the four rotator cuff muscles insert onto the greater tubercle of the humerus. The only one that does not is
A. Teres Minor
B. Supraspinatus
C. Infraspinatus
D. Subscapularis

38. Which of the following muscles crosses the glenohumeral joint
A. Pectoralis minor
B. Trapezius
C. Coracobrachialis
D. Brachialis

39. Distal attachment of the peroneus longus
A. Head of the fibula
B. Tuberosity of the fifth metatarsal
C. Base of first metatarsal
D. Lateral condyle of the tibia

40. Synergist to the hamstrings while flexing the knee
A. Gastrocnemius
B. Soleus
C. Tibialis anterior
D. Rectus femoris

41. A concentric contraction of this muscle causes the hip to extend and the knee to flex
A. Gastrocnemius
B. Rectus femoris
C. Biceps brachii
D. Semitendinosus

42. Structure located immediately distal to the coronoid process of the ulna
A. Ulnar tuberosity
B. Coronoid fossa
C. Olecranon fossa
D. Styloid process

43. If a client were to resist the actions of the pectineus, how would they move their body
A. Adduction and flexion of the hip
B. Abduction and extension of the hip
C. Abduction and flexion of the hip
D. Adduction and extension of the hip

44. Muscle originating on the sternum and clavicle, responsible for neck flexion and unilateral head rotation to the opposite side
A. Levator scapulae
B. Sternocleidomastoid
C. Scalenes
D. Pectoralis major

45. The capitulum articulates with
A. Head of the radius
B. Tibial plateau
C. Coracoid process
D. Greater trochanter

46. Which muscle originates on the sternum, ribs, and medial half of the clavicle
A. Teres minor
B. Pectoralis minor
C. Anterior deltoid
D. Pectoralis major

47. What are the two actions performed by the rectus femoris
A. Hip flexion, knee flexion
B. Hip extension, knee extension
C. Hip flexion, knee extension
D. Hip extension, knee flexion

48. Where does the biceps brachii insert?
A. Ulnar Tuberosity
B. Radial Process
C. Coronoid Process
D. Radial Tuberosity

49. Muscle originating on the medial epicondyle of the humerus
A. Brachioradialis
B. Biceps brachii
C. Brachialis
D. Pronator teres

50. Triceps brachii is innervated by the following nerve
A. Ulnar
B. Radial
C. Musculocutaneous
D. Median

Kinesiology Practice Exam Answer Key

01. C	26. D
02. C	27. C
03. A	28. C
04. A	29. A
05. D	30. B
06. D	31. A
07. C	32. B
08. D	33. C
09. C	34. D
10. B	35. A
11. B	36. B
12. D	37. D
13. D	38. C
14. A	39. C
15. B	40. A
16. B	41. D
17. B	42. A
18. A	43. B
19. B	44. B
20. B	45. A
21. A	46. D
22. C	47. C
23. C	48. D
24. A	49. D
25. A	50. B

For detailed answer explanations, watch the video at mblextestprep.com/resources.html

Practice Exams

This is one of the most important parts of the book! Practice exams! This is where you can finally put your knowledge to use and see what you know, what you don't, what you need to work on, and using your test-taking techniques!

Just be aware: THESE ARE NOT THE EXACT SAME QUESTIONS YOU WILL SEE ON THE MBLEx. I DO NOT WORK FOR, NOR HAVE ANY ASSOCIATION WITH, THE FSMTB OR HAVE ANY INSIGHT INTO THE QUESTIONS ASKED ON THE EXAM. These questions were created by me, and only me.

These questions test you on the material you MAY see on the exam! There are even questions in these practice exams covering information not seen in this study guide. Just like the MBLEx, you will have questions on things you've never seen or learned before. This is where your test-taking techniques come in! Practice answering questions on things you've never learned before, and it can help you do the exact same thing on the MBLEx!

What I always recommend my students do while taking their exams is, if they have access to a piece of paper, write down as many test-taking techniques as they can remember. This way, while they're taking the MBLEx, they can look at their test-taking techniques and remind themselves to do them. Write down things like: Take your time, don't change answers, identify key words, eliminate answers, stay relaxed, and read the entire question.

On the MBLEx, you may have questions giving you scenarios involving clients, therapists, coworkers, etc, and it expects you to deconstruct the situation and give the appropriate answer. With regards to ethical questions like these, I've mostly left them out of the practice exams. I'd rather test you on more difficult information than something that should be common sense. The simplest way to approach any ethical question is simple: Just ask yourself, "If I wanted to keep my job, what would I do?" It can't get much easier than that!

For a reminder of your test-taking techniques, visit page 3.

For more practice exams, go online to: http://www.mblextestprep.com/resources.html

Practice Exam 1

1. Most proximal structure of the fibula
A. Lateral malleolus
B. Head
C. Neck
D. Styloid process

2. Antagonist to sartorius in regards to hip flexion
A. Iliacus
B. Rectus femoris
C. Gracilis
D. Semitendinosus

3. Connective tissue responsible for transport of leukocytes to areas of inflammation
A. Blood
B. Bone
C. Cartilage
D. Fascia

4. Excessive use of synthetic corticosteroids may result in the following condition
A. Addison's disease
B. Cushing's syndrome
C. Hepatitis
D. Grave's disease

5. Person responsible for developing Chair Massage
A. John Harvey Kellogg
B. Emil Vodder
C. James Cyriax
D. David Palmer

6. Stretch technique in which a muscle is stretched to resistance, followed by an isometric contraction by the client, then the muscle stretched further after the contraction
A. Active static stretch
B. Proprioceptive neuromuscular facilitation
C. Strain counter-strain
D. Myofascial release

7. Epidermis
A. Is located deep to the dermis and allows water to move in and out of the body
B. Is vascular and provides protection for the body from microorganisms and trauma
C. Is avascular and provides protection for the body from microorganisms and trauma
D. Contains sensory receptors that detect pressure, pain, and temperature

8. A boil is also known as a
A. Sebaceous Cyst
B. Furuncle
C. Ganglion Cyst
D. Hookworm

9. Name of the tendon that connects the quadriceps to the tibial tuberosity
A. Rectus femoris tendon
B. Vastus tendon
C. Patellar tendon
D. Tibial tendon

10. A set of guiding moral principles is known as
A. Regulations
B. Scope of practice
C. Ethics
D. Reputation

11. Stance used to perform massage strokes such as effleurage and nerve strokes
A. Bowler
B. Bow
C. Horse
D. Swimmer

12. Origin of pectoralis minor
A. Coracoid process
B. Ribs 3-5
C. Ribs 1-3
D. Sternum

13. Follicle-stimulating hormone stimulates production of
A. Milk
B. Oocytes
C. Epinephrine
D. Norepinephrine

14. The larynx is located between
A. Tongue and uvula
B. Trachea and bronchus
C. Epiglottis and pharynx
D. Pharynx and trachea

15. A client would be referred to a dermatologist for all of the following conditions except
A. Cellulitis
B. Lupus
C. Warts
D. Sebaceous cyst

16. The axilla is considered
A. A local contraindication
B. An absolute contraindication
C. An endangerment site
D. Not a contraindication

17. The first cervical vertebrae is also called the
A. Occiput
B. Axis
C. Atlas
D. Dens

18. Melanocytes produce
A. Hair
B. Skin pigment
C. Bone
D. Sweat glands

19. Diverticulosis
A. Autoimmune disorder resulting in inflammation of the inner linings of the small intestine and large intestine
B. Irritation of the stomach, resulting in inflammation of the stomach, forcing pepsin through the cardiac sphincter
C. Formation of pouches in the large intestine as a result of contractions of smooth muscle in the large intestine without substances to press against
D. Inflammation of diverticular pouches, resulting in abscesses and ulcerations, causing severe septicemia

20. Modern Chinese massage is known as
A. Amma
B. Tsubo
C. Shiatsu
D. Tuina

21. Suggestions for future treatments by the massage therapist would be documented under which section of SOAP notes
A. Subjective
B. Objective
C. Assessment
D. Plan

22. Form used to report income of a sole proprietor to the IRS
A. Schedule C
B. Schedule K-1
C. 1099
D. W2

23. Carpal tunnel syndrome affects which nerve of the brachial plexus
A. Median
B. Radial
C. Axillary
D. Femoral

24. Pus is formed by
A. Dead white blood cells
B. Dead red blood cells
C. Bacteria waste
D. Plasma

25. Which of the following is not a function of epithelial tissue
A. Absorption
B. Protection
C. Heat production
D. Secretion

26. Good body mechanics are important to
A. Perform a shorter massage
B. Prevent injuries to the therapist
C. Massage the head and neck
D. Prevent injuries to the client

27. The true ribs connect to which bone
A. Scapula
B. Humerus
C. Sternum
D. Clavicle

28. The salivary glands produce which substance, which is the first chemical to begin digestion
A. Amylase
B. Pepsin
C. Hydrochloric acid
D. Insulin

29. Movement of a joint through the entire extent of its action is known as
A. Stretching
B. Range-of-motion
C. Traction
D. Active movement

30. With a client lying supine, a bolster should be placed
A. Between the legs and arms, and under the head
B. Under the ankles and neck
C. Under the knees
D. Under the head only

31. An abnormal growth of tissue results in the formation of a
A. Tumor
B. Mole
C. Callus
D. Mucous membrane

32. Stimulation of the sartorius is provided by which nerve
A. Sciatic
B. Obturator
C. Femoral
D. Tibial

33. Muscle responsible for extension and support of the vertebrae
A. Spinalis
B. Rectus abdominis
C. Trapezius
D. Rhomboids

34. The thyroid produces which hormone
A. Epinephrine
B. Progesterone
C. Testosterone
D. Calcitonin

35. Eversion of the foot is also known as
A. Pronation
B. Supination
C. Plantarflexion
D. Dorsiflexion

36. The most distal structure on the tibia
A. Lateral condyle
B. Lateral malleolus
C. Medial condyle
D. Medial malleolus

37. How much may be reported per client per year as gift tax
A. $100
B. $75
C. $50
D. $25

38. Chris has recently recovered from a severe pneumonia infection. A massage technique that may aid in lung decongestion would be
A. Vibration
B. Effleurage
C. Tapotement
D. Friction

39.The longest tendon in the body connects to the
A. Plantaris
B. Biceps Brachii
C. Gracilis
D. Rectus Abdominis

40. All of the following are structures that pass through the diaphragm except
A. Inferior vena cava
B. Esophagus
C. Abdominal aorta
D. Stomach

41. Shirodhara is a therapy used in
A. Tuina
B. Shiatsu
C. Tsubo
D. Ayurveda

42. Pain felt at the tibiofemoral joint upon flexion may involve the following muscle
A. Rectus femoris
B. Gastrocnemius
C. Soleus
D. Tibialis anterior

43. The phalanges are classified as which type of bone
A. Short
B. Long
C. Flat
D. Irregular

44. Leukemia
A. Malignant cancer of white blood cells, resulting in a decrease in functioning leukocytes in the body
B. Cancer of lymph nodes and ducts causing tumors in and around the armpits and neck
C. Tumors arising from bone tissue, causing an increase in the susceptibility to fracture at the site of tumor growth
D. Cancer of melanocytes, spreading to other organs throughout the body via lymph ducts

45. The cerebellum
A. Responsible for emotions
B. Responsible for coordination and balance
C. Responsible for visual reflexes
D. Responsible for olfaction and memory input

46. Which is the only organ in the body that contains both endocrine and exocrine glands
A. Liver
B. Pancreas
C. Stomach
D. Lungs

47. Which of the following is a bone that does not fuse together with other bones to form the pelvis
A. Ischium
B. Ilium
C. Sacrum
D. Pubis

48. The flexors of the wrist are innervated by the following two nerves
A. Ulnar and median
B. Median and radial
C. Axillary and musculocutaneous
D. Radial and ulnar

49. The intertubercular groove is located on the proximal end of which bone
A. Tibia
B. Radius
C. Femur
D. Humerus

50. Laryngitis
A. Inflammation of the throat
B. Inflammation of the voice box
C. Inflammation of bronchial tubes
D. Inflammation of tonsils

51. The term "massage" became popularized in America by
A. Johann Mezger
B. The Taylor Brothers
C. Douglas Graham
D. Per Henrik Ling

52. A soft end feel is felt at the end of a range of motion due to
A. Tight muscle
B. Bone
C. Injuries
D. Resistance

53. Antagonist to supinator
A. Brachialis
B. Biceps brachii
C. Pronator teres
D. Coracobrachialis

54. Ligament holding teeth to the mandible or maxilla
A. Periodontal
B. Dental
C. Periodental
D. Molar ligament

55. Ability to perform services legally according to occupational standards and licensing
A. Certification
B. Scope of practice
C. Reciprocity
D. Regulations

56. Medical device implanted into patients with uncontrolled arrhythmia
A. Angioplasty
B. Electrocardiogram
C. Arterial stent
D. Pacemaker

57. Addison's Disease affects what portion of the kidney
A. Medulla
B. Cortex
C. Adrenal
D. Nephron

58. Sphincters in the digestive tract are responsible for
A. Preventing food from moving backwards
B. Secreting digestive enzymes
C. Absorbing nutrients
D. Preventing bloodflow into the organs

59. Which of the following is a structure located on the ulna
A. Olecranon fossa
B. Coronoid process
C. Radial tuberosity
D. Capitulum

60. The most distal structures on the femur that articulate with the condyles of the tibia
A. Medial and lateral epicondyles
B. Medial and lateral condyles
C. Lesser and greater trochanters
D. Adductor tubercle and medial epicondyle

61. Adipose is considered which type of connective tissue
A. Cartilage
B. Dense connective tissue
C. Loose connective tissue
D. Bone

62. There are how many pairs of cranial nerves in the peripheral nervous system
A. 12
B. 31
C. 24
D. 18

63. An independent contractor is responsible for filing which tax form
A. Schedule K1
B. W2
C. 1099
D. Gift Tax Form

64. Benign tumors
A. Spread to other parts of the body through lymph
B. Do not spread to other locations in the body
C. Spread to other parts of the body through blood
D. Spread to other parts of the body through interstitial fluid

65. Dermatomes are innervated by which type of nerve
A. Cranial nerve
B. Spinal nerve
C. Optic nerve
D. Accessory nerve

66. The humerus and scapula combine to form which joint
A. Humeroradial
B. Acromioclavicular
C. Sternoclavicular
D. Glenohumeral

67. Action resulting in the thumb moving toward the pinky
A. Opposition
B. Flexion
C. Abduction
D. Extension

68. Paraplegia
A. Paralysis of the legs due to an injury to the spinal cord below T1
B. Paralysis of the arms and legs due to an injury to the spinal cord between C5 and T1
C. Paralysis of one side of the body due to transient ischemic attack, resulting in brain damage
D. Paralysis of one side of the face due to an injury to cranial nerve VII

69. Hepatitis is a form of viral infection that causes inflammation of the
A. Brain
B. Liver
C. Kidneys
D. Bladder

70. Food that has been swallowed and entered the pharynx has become
A. Carbohydrates
B. Chyme
C. Feces
D. Bolus

71. Proximal attachment of semitendinosus
A. Linea aspera
B. Ischial tuberosity
C. Pes anserinus
D. Inferior ramus of pubis

72. Foramen located beneath the eye socket on the maxilla
A. Zygomatic foramen
B. Mental foramen
C. Infraorbital foramen
D. Temporal foramen

73. Production of egg cells and sperm is maintained by the following hormone, produced by the pituitary gland
A. Follicle-stimulating hormone
B. Prolactin
C. Lactogenic hormone
D. Epinephrine

74. Top cover draping
A. Towel or sheet used to cover the client
B. Wrapping a client in a cocoon-like structure
C. Uncovering a part of the body to massage
D. Only covering parts of the body not being worked on

75. Cryotherapy is used to reduce
A. Inflammation
B. Frostbite
C. Hypoxia
D. Edema

76. The peritoneum is a serous membrane found in the
A. Stomach
B. Abdomen
C. Intestines
D. Bladder

77. Blood clot formation in a vein, resulting in vein inflammation
A. Thrombophlebitis
B. Atherosclerosis
C. Iron-deficient anemia
D. Varicose veins

78. Massage produces what effect on blood vessels
A. Breaks down blood vessel walls
B. Decreases the size of blood vessel lumen
C. Develops new blood vessels
D. Increases the size of blood vessel lumen

79. Brain wave activity is recorded by using the following device
A. Electroencephalogram
B. Sphygmomanometer
C. Centrifuge
D. Mammogram

80. Most questions asked by the massage therapist towards the client during a massage session should be
A. Closed-ended
B. Open-ended
C. Informative
D. Assessment related

81. Largest muscle of the adductor muscle group
A. Gracilis
B. Adductor longus
C. Adductor brevis
D. Adductor magnus

82. Leukemia is a malignant form of cancer arising from
A. Bone marrow
B. Red blood cells
C. Plasma
D. White blood cells

83. Cephalosporin is a type of
A. Antigen
B. Antifungal
C. Antiviral
D. Antibiotic

84. Ligaments have no blood supply. This makes them
A. Avascular
B. Vascular
C. Serous
D. Elastic

85. The bone that comprises the upper jaw is also called
A. Mandible
B. Maxilla
C. Zygomatic
D. Vomer

86. The radius and ulna are positioned where in relation to the humerus
A. Distal
B. Proximal
C. Medial
D. Lateral

87. A wound resulting in jagged edges
A. Abrasion
B. Puncture
C. Avulsion
D. Laceration

88. A client experiences pain while abducting the shoulder. The muscle most likely involved would be
A. Pectoralis Major
B. Rhomboid Major
C. Deltoids
D. Infraspinatus

89. Ribs eleven and twelve are also known as
A. True ribs
B. Floating ribs
C. Superior ribs
D. Levitating ribs

90. A client presents with warts on the bottom of the foot. An appropriate response would be
A. Perform the massage, avoiding the affected area
B. Perform the massage, performing cross-fiber friction over the affected area
C. Reschedule the massage and refer the client to a dermatologist
D. Perform the massage and apply wart removing cream to the affected area

91. MET is also known as
A. Massage Elongation Trigger
B. Massage Extremity using Tapotement
C. Myofascial Elasticity Technique
D. Muscle Energy Technique

92. Muscle inserting onto the radial tuberosity and originating on the coracoid process and supraglenoid tubercle
A. Biceps brachii
B. Coracobrachialis
C. Triceps brachii
D. Brachioradialis

93. Muscle responsible for hip flexion, knee flexion, and lateral rotation of the hip
A. Sartorius
B. Gracilis
C. Pectineus
D. Rectus femoris

94. Medications that specifically control heart rhythm are known as
A. Antihistamines
B. Beta-blockers
C. Antiarrhythmics
D. Vasodilators

95. Mammary glands
A. Endocrine glands that produce and secrete milk
B. Exocrine glands that produce and secrete sebum
C. Exocrine glands that produce and secrete milk
D. Endocrine glands that produce and secrete sebum

96. Cartilaginous portion of an intervertebral disc
A. Annulus fibrosus
B. Nucleus pulposus
C. Dens
D. Vertebral facet

97. Chucking and wringing are forms of
A. Effleurage
B. Petrissage
C. Tapotement
D. Friction

98. A trigger point that causes pain without palpation
A. Acute
B. Latent
C. Active
D. Chronic

99. Muscle originating on the ischial tuberosity
A. Tensor fasciae latae
B. Semimembranosus
C. Rectus femoris
D. Pectineus

100. Part of the small intestine that attaches to the stomach via the pyloric sphincter
A. Cecum
B. Jejunum
C. Ileum
D. Duodenum

Practice Exam 1 Answer Key

1. D	26. B	51. C	76. B
2. D	27. C	52. A	77. A
3. A	28. A	53. C	78. D
4. B	29. B	54. A	79. A
5. D	30. C	55. B	80. B
6. B	31. A	56. D	81. D
7. C	32. C	57. B	82. D
8. B	33. A	58. A	83. D
9. C	34. D	59. B	84. A
10. C	35. A	60. B	85. B
11. B	36. D	61. C	86. A
12. B	37. D	62. A	87. D
13. B	38. C	63. C	88. C
14. D	39. A	64. B	89. B
15. B	40. D	65. B	90. A
16. C	41. D	66. D	91. D
17. C	42. B	67. A	92. A
18. B	43. B	68. A	93. A
19. C	44. A	69. B	94. C
20. D	45. B	70. D	95. C
21. D	46. B	71. B	96. A
22. A	47. C	72. C	97. D
23. A	48. A	73. A	98. C
24. A	49. D	74 A	99. B
25. C	50. B	75. A	100. D

Practice Exam 2

1. Which of the following massage strokes is best in aiding lung decongestion
A. Tapotement
B. Effleurage
C. Friction
D. Petrissage

2. A massage therapist bringing their own unresolved issues into the therapeutic relationship
A. Self-disclosure
B. Transference
C. Counter-transference
D. Ethics

3. Muscle located on the lateral side of the leg, responsible for pronation and plantarflexion of the foot
A. Tibialis anterior
B. Peroneus longus
C. Gastrocnemius
D. Soleus

4. A client with Raynaud's Syndrome comes in for a massage. What would be an appropriate modification to the treatment to help with this condition
A. Warm the massage room
B. Apply ice on the affected area
C. Position the client in a semi-reclined position
D. Diffuse eucalyptus oil to aid in lung decongestion

5. The gallbladder
A. Filters out dead or dying red blood cells from the blood stream
B. Stores bilirubin and supplies bilirubin to the liver
C. Secretes insulin and glucagon into the duodenum
D. Stores bile and empties bile into the duodenum

6. A high ankle sprain results in tearing of the
A. Interosseous ligament
B. Meniscus
C. Anterior cruciate ligament
D. Medial collateral ligament

7. Achilles tendonitis is especially common in people who perform the following action
A. Swimming
B. Jumping
C. Running
D. Walking

8. Periostitis
A. Infection of periosteum
B. Degeneration of periosteum
C. Overproduction of periosteum
D. Inflammation of periosteum

9. Reception, conduction, transmission, and response are all responses when the body produces a
A. Bone
B. Contraction
C. Thought
D. Reflex

10. A neuron is what type of cell
A. Nerve
B. Skin
C. Muscle
D. Bone

11. The adductor magnus performs all the following actions except
A. Adduction
B. Abduction
C. Flexion
D. Extension

12. The Thoracic Duct is the body's largest
A. Artery
B. Lymph vessel
C. Air passage
D. Heart chamber

13. Muscular dystrophy is
A. A genetic disorder
B. A sexually transmitted disease
C. A viral infection
D. Degeneration of bone after menopause

14. Centrifugal massage strokes are directed
A. Around the abdomen
B. Towards the heart
C. Away from the heart
D. On the scalp

15. All of the following are examples of short bones except
A. Cuboid
B. Scaphoid
C. Patella
D. Hamate

16. The deltoids originate on which bony landmarks
A. Acromion process, clavicle, spine of scapula
B. Acromion process, clavicle, lateral border of scapula
C. Deltoid tuberosity, clavicle, acromion process
D. Superior angle of scapula, acromion process, clavicle

17. Plan information is
A. Information the client shares about themselves
B. Measurable information visible to the massage therapist
C. Medical conditions the client has been assessed with
D. Recommendations for future massage sessions

18. Digestive enzyme produced by the liver, responsible for emulsification of lipids in the small intestine
A. Glucagon
B. Insulin
C. Bile
D. Amylase

19. Inflammation of a tendon and its protective sheath
A. Tennis Elbow
B. Tenosynovitis
C. Bursitis
D. Rheumatoid Arthritis

20. A diet high in iron is helpful in prevention of a specific form of
A. Varicose veins
B. Leukemia
C. Lymphedema
D. Anemia

21. Photoreceptors detect
A. Taste
B. Smell
C. Sight
D. Sound

22. An injury to the gracilis would partially inhibit which actions
A. Hip adduction, knee flexion
B. Hip flexion, knee extension
C. Hip abduction, knee flexion
D. Hip extension, knee extension

23. Muscles that cross the knee include all of the following except
A. Gastrocnemius
B. Gracilis
C. Adductor magnus
D. Biceps femoris

24. Lice, scabies, and ticks are all types of
A. Parasites
B. Bacterium
C. Fungi
D. Viruses

25. A bolster should be placed under the ankles when a client is laying in which position
A. Prone
B. Supine
C. Side-lying
D. Semi-reclining

26. Terms for the massage strokes were developed by
A. Ida Rolf
B. Randolph Stone
C. Per Henrik Ling
D. Johann Mezger

27. The facial nerve is also known as which number cranial nerve
A. V
B. VII
C. X
D. XII

28. Skeletal muscle is controlled
A. Voluntarily
B. Involuntarily
C. Autonomically
D. Sympathetically

29. Primary functions of nervous tissue include all of the following except
A. Mental activity
B. Sensory reception
C. Stimulating muscle
D. Pumping blood

30. Technique primarily used to work on trigger points
A. Wringing
B. Ischemic compression
C. Cross-fiber friction
D. Myofascial release

31. Stoppage of range of motion due to trauma to an area
A. Soft end feel
B. Hard end feel
C. Empty end feel
D. Nervous end feel

32. Inability of the blood to properly clot
A. Hemorrhage
B. Hemophilia
C. Hemopoiesis
D. Cystic fibrosis

33. In Parkinson's disease, what happens to dopamine
A. Dopamine converts to cortisol
B. Dopamine levels increase
C. Dopamine levels stay the same
D. Dopamine levels drop

34. Expectorants help in
A. Thinning mucous
B. Draining sinuses
C. Blocking histamines
D. Dilating respiratory passages

35. Which muscle inserts onto the ulnar tuberosity and the coronoid process
A. Coracobrachialis
B. Biceps brachii
C. Brachialis
D. Brachioradialis

36. Goals are
A. Measurable or attainable accomplishments
B. A generalized statement about the purpose of a business
C. The theme of a business
D. Business plans detailing projected income

37. A pregnant client complains of feeling dizzy and light-headed during a massage session. What would be an appropriate response
A. Ignore the complaint
B. Place the client into a semi-reclined position
C. Apply ginger essential oil
D. Perform circular effleurage on the abdomen

38. The more anterior point of the mandible, which the muscles of mastication attach to
A. Ramus of the mandible
B. Mandibular tubercle
C. Coronoid process
D. Coracoid process

39. Joint located at the lateral end of the clavicle
A. Coracoclavicular
B. Glenohumeral
C. Sternoclavicular
D. Acromioclavicular

40. The circadian rhythm is regulated by
A. Prolactin
B. Melatonin
C. Estrogen
D. Testosterone

41. An injury to a muscle or tendon
A. Infarct
B. Sprain
C. Burn
D. Strain

42. Diverticulosis is a condition that affects the
A. Ribs
B. Cartilage
C. Large intestine
D. Vertebrae

43. A certification is obtained via
A. Passing a jurisprudence exam
B. Paying a fee to a jurisdiction licensing agency
C. Obtaining liability insurance to protect against malpractice
D. Completing educational requirements in a school setting

44. Structural realignment therapy working on muscles and fascia over the course of ten sessions
A. Rolfing
B. Trager method
C. Feldenkrais
D. Myofascial release

45. Nerve innervating the wrist extensor muscle group
A. Median
B. Obturator
C. Radial
D. Ulnar

46. Turning the foot in towards the midline of the body
A. Pronation
B. Inversion
C. Eversion
D. Dorsiflexion

47. Massage results in increased production of
A. Cortisol
B. Blood cells
C. Pathogens
D. Water retention

48. Information the client shares about themselves is documented under which section of SOAP notes
A. Objective
B. Subjective
C. Assessment
D. Plan

49. Movement produced at the atlantoaxial joint
A. Extension
B. Flexion
C. Rotation
D. Adduction

50. In a herniated disc, the nucleus pulposus protrudes through the
A. Annulus fibrosus
B. Vertebral body
C. Intervertebral facet
D. Sacral foramina

51. Waste is filtered from the blood in which part of the kidney
A. Cortex
B. Adrenal glands
C. Nephron
D. Renal papilla

52. Melatonin is produced by the
A. Pineal gland
B. Pituitary gland
C. Adrenal gland
D. Thalamus

53. Pins and needles is a sensation known as
A. Parasthesia
B. Anaesthesia
C. Paralysis
D. Paraplegia

54. A massage therapist should wash their hands
A. Only after using the restroom
B. Before each massage
C. After each massage
D. Before and after each massage

55. Boil
A. Bacterial infection of hair follicles
B. Bacterial infection of mucous membranes
C. Viral infection of mucous membranes
D. Bacterial infection of bone

56. There are how many bones in the ankle
A. Eight
B. Two
C. Seven
D. Five

57. The largest part of the brain is also known as
A. Cerebellum
B. Cerebrum
C. Spinal cord
D. Diencephalon

58. Observable information the massage therapist can physically see is documented under what category in SOAP notes
A. Subjective
B. Objective
C. Assessment
D. Plan

59. Liabilities are
A. Large companies free to operate independently
B. Possessions owned by a business
C. Raising the price of a product for sale
D. Debts owed to a person or business

60. Muscle originating on the medial epicondyle of the humerus
A. Brachioradialis
B. Biceps brachii
C. Brachialis
D. Pronator teres

61. Medication that destroys bacteria or prevents further bacterial growth
A. Antipsychotic
B. Antibiotic
C. Expectorant
D. Antiviral

62. The most fatal form of tumor is
A. Cystic
B. Benign
C. Malignant
D. Gangrenous

63. Holes in the mandible, allowing a passageway for blood vessels into and out of the bone
A. Mental foramina
B. Ossobuco
C. Mandibular tunnels
D. Maxillary foramen

64. The ankle is considered which type of synovial joint
A. Pivot
B. Hinge
C. Ball and socket
D. Ellipsoid

65. Bacterial infection spreading upwards from the urethra results in
A. Cholecystitis
B. Nephritis
C. Prostatitis
D. Cystitis

66. Thickening of arterial walls, leading to conditions such as hypertension
A. Arteriosclerosis
B. Angina pectoris
C. Scleroderma
D. Phlebitis

67. Hemodialysis involves filtering of
A. Feces
B. Urine
C. Blood
D. Water

68. Stimulation of tsubo points to stimulate nerves and increase circulation
A. Shiatsu
B. Reflexology
C. Amma
D. Ayurveda

69. Father of Lymphatic Drainage
A. David Palmer
B. Per Henrik Ling
C. Emil Vodder
D. Charles Taylor

70. The Rule of 9's is used to determine
A. The amount of breaths a person should take to relax
B. The number of massage strokes that are used in western massage therapy
C. Total percentage of the body that has been burned
D. Total percentage of the massage price the therapist is paid

71. Blood passes from the right atrium into which chamber
A. Left ventricle
B. Left atrium
C. Right ventricle
D. Aorta

72. Treatment mainly used to exfoliate dead skin cells from the body
A. Body wrap
B. Salt scrub
C. Immersion bath
D. Vichy shower

73. Inflammation of a vein which may result from immobilization or trauma
A. Hepatitis
B. Arteriosclerosis
C. Phlebitis
D. Nephritis

74. Nerve innervating the diaphragm
A. Vagus
B. Phrenic
C. Trigeminal
D. Facial

75. Part of the ulna that wraps around the trochlea to make the elbow joint
A. Coronoid process
B. Ulnar tuberosity
C. Head of the radius
D. Radial tuberosity

76. A client moving a joint in the opposite direction that a massage therapist is moving it is an example of which joint movement
A. Active
B. Assistive
C. Passive
D. Resistive

77. Broadening of tendons, ligaments, and muscles which breaks down adhesions
A. Deep transverse friction
B. Sports massage
C. Passive joint mobilization
D. Bindegewebsmassage

78. Contraindications for hydrotherapy include all of the following except
A. Contagious conditions
B. Hypertension
C. Acne
D. Skin rash

79. Arrector pili muscles attach to
A. Walls of intestines
B. Hair follicles
C. Hair shafts
D. Bronchial tubes

80. Which of the following is a function of connective tissue
A. Protection
B. Secretion
C. Absorption
D. Contraction

81. Muscle surrounding the eye socket
A. Buccinator
B. Occipitofrontalis
C. Orbicularis oculi
D. Masseter

82. Insertion of triceps brachii
A. Olecranon process
B. Styloid process
C. Radial tuberosity
D. Coronoid process and ulnar tuberosity

83. Fossa located on the anterior surface of the scapula
A. Subscapular fossa
B. Glenoid fossa
C. Supraspinous fossa
D. Infraspinous fossa

84. Progesterone is produced by the
A. Uterus
B. Ovary
C. Fallopian tube
D. Eye

85. Rheumatoid arthritis is what type of disorder
A. Sarcoma
B. Viral
C. Bacterial
D. Autoimmune

86. Group of bones located distally to the metatarsals
A. Carpals
B. Metacarpals
C. Tarsals
D. Phalanges

87. Upon opening, the esophageal sphincter allows food to move between the
A. Small intestine and large intestine
B. Esophagus and stomach
C. Stomach and small intestine
D. Pharynx and esophagus

88. Ancient massage technique involving kneading, tapotement, friction, popping the fingers and toes, and the use of scented perfumes
A. Tshanpau
B. Tsubo
C. Amma
D. Shiatsu

89. Application of hot and cold on the skin results in the blood vessels
A. Breaking down and building up
B. Constricting and closing
C. Dilating and opening
D. Dilating and constricting

90. The radial tuberosity is located on which side of the radius
A. Posterior
B. Lateral
C. Medial
D. Distal

91. Structure found between the pubic body and ischial tuberosity
A. Ischial spine
B. Superior ramus of the pubis
C. Pubic crest
D. Inferior ramus of the pubis

92. The ACL, PCL, LCL, and MCL are all ligaments of the
A. Elbow
B. Ankle
C. Shoulder
D. Knee

93. Lack of sufficient water in feces may result in
A. Diarrhea
B. Constipation
C. Diverticulosis
D. Crohn's disease

94. The radiocarpal joint is comprised of the radius and which carpal bone
A. Hamate
B. Lunate
C. Trapezium
D. Scaphoid

95. Where do rhomboid major and rhomboid minor originate
A. Lateral border of the scapula
B. Medial border of the scapula
C. Superior angle of the scapula
D. Spinous processes of C7-T5

96. The most superior layer of the skin is known as the
A. Dermis
B. Epidermis
C. Subcutaneous Layer
D. Superficial Fascia

97. Intentionally popping the joint of a client without proper credentials is a violation of
A. Communication
B. Scope of Practice
C. Boundaries
D. HIPAA

98. ABMP and AMTA offer
A. Business plans
B. Massage licensure
C. Massage certification
D. Liability insurance

99. Stimulating massage strokes include all of the following except
A. Friction
B. Effleurage
C. Tapotement
D. Vibration

100. The first cervical vertebrae is also known as
A. Atlas
B. Axis
C. Occiput
D. Temporal

Practice Exam 2 Answer Key

1. A	26. D	51. C	76. D
2. C	27. B	52. A	77. A
3. B	28. A	53. A	78. C
4. A	29. D	54. D	79. B
5. D	30. B	55. A	80. A
6. A	31. C	56. C	81. C
7. C	32. B	57. B	82. A
8. D	33. D	58. B	83. A
9. D	34. A	59. D	84. B
10. A	35. C	60. D	85. D
11. B	36. A	61. B	86. D
12. B	37. B	62. C	87. D
13. A	38. C	63. A	88. A
14. C	39. D	64. B	89. D
15. C	40. B	65. D	90. C
16. A	41. D	66. A	91. D
17. D	42. C	67. C	92. D
18. C	43. D	68. A	93. B
19. B	44. A	69. C	94. D
20. D	45. C	70. C	95. D
21. C	46. B	71. C	96. B
22. A	47. B	72. B	97. B
23. C	48. B	73. C	98. D
24. A	49. C	74. B	99. B
25. A	50. A	75. A	100. A

Practice Exam 3

1. Ligament connecting teeth to the mandible and maxilla
A. Periodontal
B. Cementum
C. Maxillary
D. Gingiva

2. Erythrocytes are also called
A. White blood cells
B. Red blood cells
C. Platelets
D. Plasma

3. Reciprocity
A. A license from one jurisdiction being valid in a second jurisdiction
B. A massage therapist and client both benefiting from a session
C. A certification allowing for licensure to take place
D. Massage therapist obtaining more than one certification

4. Massage developed by Elizabeth Dicke which focuses on subcutaneous connective tissue
A. Myofascial release
B. Lymphatic drainage
C. Rolfing
D. Bindegewebsmassage

5. Gradual destruction of synovial membranes surrounding joints with an increase in formation of fibrous tissue
A. Gouty arthritis
B. Osteoarthritis
C. Ankylosing spondylitis
D. Rheumatoid arthritis

6. Highly contagious bacterial infection of mucous membranes, most common in children
A. Impetigo
B. Herpes simplex
C. Psoriasis
D. Boil

7. A lateral ankle sprain is the result of the ankle being forced into which position
A. Plantarflexion
B. Eversion
C. Dorsiflexion
D. Inversion

8. Distal attachment of the supinator
A. Lateral and proximal surface of the radius
B. Radial tuberosity
C. Posterior lateral epicondyle of the humerus
D. Styloid process of the ulna

9. Antagonist of levator scapulae
A. Lower fibers of trapezius
B. Pectoralis minor
C. Upper fibers of trapezius
D. Rhomboids

10. Hair is made of which type of tissue
A. Muscular
B. Connective
C. Epithelial
D. Nervous

11. Contraction of Hepatitis A is most likely due to exposure to
A. Blood
B. Feces
C. Saliva
D. Semen

12. Points of manipulation similar to Amma, developed in Japan
A. Shiatsu
B. Tsubo
C. Ayurveda
D. Tshanpau

13. Keeping a client's information private and protected
A. Ethics
B. Confidentiality
C. Self-disclosure
D. Transference

14. Cranial nerve VII is also known as
A. Trigeminal nerve
B. Facial nerve
C. Olfactory nerve
D. Optic nerve

15. Another term for a blood clot within a blood vessel
A. Thrombus
B. Embolus
C. Aneurysm
D. Fibrin

16. Cranial nerve responsible for sending visual inputs to the brain
A. Optic
B. Oculomotor
C. Trigeminal
D. Olfactory

17. Temporary obstruction of a blood vessel leading to the brain results in
A. Myocardial infarction
B. Transient ischemic attack
C. Cerebral aneurysm
D. Pulmonary embolism

18. The most common form of malignancy in children
A. Leukemia
B. Anemia
C. Melanoma
D. Non-Hodgkins Lymphoma

19. Stoppage of a range of motion due to certain factors is known as
A. Static stretch
B. Resistance
C. End feel
D. Proprioceptive neuromuscular facilitation

20. Hypersensitivity of the body to substances that normally have no effect on others
A. Lupus Erythamatosus
B. Malignancy
C. Infection
D. Allergy

21. The scientific name of the knee is
A. Tibiofibular joint
B. Talocrural joint
C. Tibiofemoral joint
D. Iliofemoral joint

22. The wrist extensor group is innervated by the following nerve
A. Median
B. Radial
C. Ulnar
D. Femoral

23. Universal precautions
A. Controlling infectious agents to prevent the spread of disease
B. Understanding contraindications for massage therapy
C. Preventing injuries to the client due to faulty equipment
D. Being aware of any faulty body mechanics

24. The long head of the triceps brachii originates where
A. Supraglenoid tubercle
B. Infraglenoid tubercle
C. Olecranon process
D. Coracoid process

25. Hyperthyroidism leads to an increased sensitivity to
A. Heat
B. Cold
C. Light touch
D. Deep pressure

26. Localized ischemia can be produced by application of which massage stroke
A. Friction
B. Effleurage
C. Petrissage
D. Vibration

27. All of the following are formed by nervous tissue except
A. Brain
B. Spine
C. Spinal cord
D. Cerebellum

28. Muscle originating on the inferior angle of the scapula
A. Teres minor
B. Infraspinatus
C. Teres major
D. Levator scapulae

29. Carbon monoxide attaches to red blood cells and prevents the transport of oxygen throughout the body, resulting in
A. Hypothermia
B. Hypoxia
C. Raynaud's syndrome
D. Frostbite

30. Acute Tennis Elbow results in inflammation at the
A. Medial epicondyle of the humerus
B. Olecranon process
C. Lateral epicondyle of the humerus
D. Trochlea

31. Lomi Lomi is a massage which originated in
A. Thailand
B. Hawaii
C. Japan
D. China

32. Proximal attachment of the psoas major muscle
A. Anterior surface of lumbar vertebrae
B. Posterior surface of lumbar vertebrae
C. Greater trochanter
D. Lesser trochanter

33. Thermoreceptors detect
A. Changes in chemical concentration
B. Pressure in blood vessels
C. Changes in temperature
D. Pain

34. An audiometer measures a person's ability to
A. Feel
B. Hear
C. Taste
D. See

35. Cross-fiber friction is also known as
A. Longitudinal friction
B. Transverse friction
C. Compression
D. Circular friction

36. The knee joint is made of which two bones
A. Femur and fibula
B. Tibia and femur
C. Tibia and fibula
D. Humerus and ulna

37. Migraine headaches are also known as
A. Trigeminal headaches
B. Muscular tension headaches
C. Glycemic headaches
D. Vascular headaches

38. Each of the following are contagious conditions except
A. Mononucleosis
B. Impetigo
C. Meningitis
D. Lupus

39. Stance used to perform massage strokes such as petrissage, friction, and tapotement
A. Bow
B. Archer
C. Warrior
D. Swimmer

40. Muscle inserting onto the pectineal line of the femur
A. Psoas major
B. Adductor magnus
C. Gracilis
D. Pectineus

41. Stimulation of the parasympathetic nervous response has what action on the digestive tract
A. Increases peristalsis
B. Shuts down peristalsis
C. Decreases absorption
D. Increases lymph circulation

42. A ganglion cyst is primarily located
A. On the legs and thighs
B. On the hands, wrists, and feet
C. On the back and neck
D. On the chest, abdomen, and pelvis

43. The lateral supracondylar ridge of the humerus is the origination site of which muscle
A. Brachioradialis
B. Biceps brachii
C. Biceps femoris
D. Coracobrachialis

44. The adductor tubercle is located directly superior to which bony marking on the femur
A. Medial epicondyle
B. Lateral epicondyle
C. Greater trochanter
D. Lesser trochanter

45. HIPAA ensures client information remains
A. With the client's spouse
B. Unimportant
C. Confidential
D. In the government's possession

46. The outer portion of a kidney is known as its
A. Medulla
B. Cortex
C. Cavity
D. Adrenal

47. The "S" of "SOAP" stands for
A. Standard
B. Sustained
C. Superficial
D. Subjective

48. Massage therapy increases the production of
A. Cortisol
B. Urine
C. Hypertension
D. Bacteria

49. Influenza is considered
A. A local contraindication
B. An absolute contraindication
C. An endangerment site
D. Not a contraindication

50. Exocrine glands secrete their substances where
A. Onto a surface
B. Into plasma
C. Inside the blood stream
D. Between bone cells

51. The father of orthopedic medicine
A. Per Henrik Ling
B. David Palmer
C. James Cyriax
D. Lawrence Jones

52. Skeletal muscle is responsible for which actions
A. Protection and secretion
B. Beating the heart and transporting nutrients
C. Peristalsis and absorption
D. Moving the limbs and creating heat

53. Which of these muscles does not insert onto the medial border of the scapula
A. Rhomboid major
B. Serratus anterior
C. Pectoralis minor
D. Rhomboid minor

54. A dermatologist is a doctor who specializes in the
A. Heart
B. Kidneys
C. Skin
D. Brain

55. The widest muscle in the body is
A. Rectus abdominis
B. Trapezius
C. Latissimus dorsi
D. Pectoralis major

56. The head of the radius enters into the following fossa when the elbow is placed into flexion
A. Coronoid fossa
B. Radial fossa
C. Olecranon fossa
D. Glenoid fossa

57. Wear and tear arthritis, resulting in destruction of hyaline cartilage between articulating bones, increasing friction
A. Osteoarthritis
B. Rheumatoid arthritis
C. Gouty arthritis
D. Arthralgia

58. A client with Bell's palsy would be referred to which doctor
A. Cardiologist
B. Neurologist
C. Rheumatologist
D. Dermatologist

59. The subclavian vein arises from the
A. Superior vena cava
B. Brachial vein
C. Aorta
D. Axillary vein

60. The anterior cruciate ligament connects the following bones
A. Ulna and humerus
B. Femur and fibula
C. Humerus and radius
D. Tibia and femur

61. The tibia sits on top of which bone to produce the ankle joint
A. Cuboid
B. Calcaneus
C. Navicular
D. Talus

62. Hyper-curvature in the thoracic region, forcing the vertebrae laterally
A. Lordosis
B. Kyphosis
C. Scoliosis
D. Spondylitis

63. Realignment of muscle and connective tissue to return the body to a vertical axis
A. Reiki
B. Myofascial release
C. Thai massage
D. Rolfing

64. Massage stroke best utilized to break up adhesions in tissue
A. Petrissage
B. Effleurage
C. Friction
D. Tapotement

65. Connective tissue surrounding substances in the body, such as an infection
A. Pleurisy
B. Serous membrane
C. Peritoneal membrane
D. Cyst

66. The sclera is found in which part of the body
A. Eye
B. Ear
C. Oral cavity
D. Appendix

67. Blood exposure requires which of the following for proper cleaning
A. Paper towels
B. Personal protective equipment
C. An autoclave
D. Linen service

68. Client files should be kept for IRS purposes for up to
A. Two years
B. Six years
C. One year
D. Five years

69. The proper temperature to keep a massage room should be around
A. 65 degrees
B. 75 degrees
C. 80 degrees
D. 60 degrees

70. Nerve passing through the popliteal region on its way to the plantar surface of the foot
A. Obturator
B. Common peroneal
C. Femoral
D. Tibial

71. Influenza
A. Viral infection affecting the respiratory tract
B. Viral infection affecting the endocrine system
C. Bacterial infection affecting the respiratory tract
D. Bacterial infection affecting the digestive system

72. Innervation of the brachioradialis is provided by which nerve
A. Radial
B. Median
C. Ulnar
D. Musculocutaneous

73. Digestive enzyme responsible for increasing glucose levels in the blood
A. Bile
B. Insulin
C. Glucagon
D. Pepsin

74. The thymus produces which type of cell
A. Natural killer cell
B. T cell
C. Erythrocyte
D. Thrombocyte

75. All of the following are structures on the humerus except
A. Greater tubercle
B. Greater trochanter
C. Intertubercular groove
D. Coronoid fossa

76. A massage therapist moving a part of the body without the client's help
A. Assistive joint mobilization
B. Active joint mobilization
C. Passive joint mobilization
D. Resistive joint mobilization

77. Phlebitis is inflammation of a/an
A. Artery
B. Blood
C. Lung
D. Vein

78. Very light form of effleurage performed at the end of a massage session
A. Petrissage
B. Friction
C. Nerve stroke
D. Tapotement

79. Proprioceptive Neuromuscular Facilitation may also be known as
A. Positional release
B. Myofascial Release
C. Strain-counter strain
D. Muscle Energy Technique

80. Which of the following movements is trapezius not responsible for
A. Elevation of the scapula
B. Medial rotation of the shoulder
C. Retraction of the scapula
D. Depression of the scapula

81. Large bony projection on the proximal end of the radius
A. Radial tuberosity
B. Styloid process
C. Radial fossa
D. Olecranon process

82. Shortening of the tibialis anterior can be achieved with the following actions
A. Dorsiflexion and eversion
B. Dorsiflexion and inversion
C. Plantarflexion and inversion
D. Plantarflexion and eversion

83. Water, telephone, and linen service are all
A. Business assets
B. Business expenses
C. Business arrangements
D. Business property

84. Confidentiality
A. Protecting client information
B. Allowing only a client's spouse to view information
C. Disregarding a client's right to privacy
D. Allowing a client to discuss other client's treatments

85. Intermediate portion of the sternum, directly inferior to the manubrium
A. Body
B. Xiphoid process
C. Jugular notch
D. Costal cartilage

86. The medulla oblongata controls heart rate, blood vessel diameter, and
A. Release of growth hormone
B. Balance
C. Coordination
D. Sneezing

87. A massage therapist is unable to diagnose any medical condition. Performing a diagnosis is not within the massage therapist's
A. Scope of practice
B. Liability
C. Certification
D. Capabilities

88. Muscle inserting into the iliotibial tract and gluteal tuberosity
A. Gluteus medius
B. Gluteus minimus
C. Gluteus maximus
D. Piriformis

89. Hyper-curvature in the lumbar region
A. Kyphosis
B. Lordosis
C. Scoliosis
D. Spondylitis

90. Type of cell that typically does not regenerate
A. Stratum germinativum
B. Epithelial
C. Nervous
D. Muscular

91. Glucagon is a digestive enzyme produced in the pancreas by
A. Alpha cells
B. Beta cells
C. Lymphatic tissue
D. Erythrocytes

92. Pressure felt in walls of arteries as blood passes through them
A. Arteriole
B. Diastolic
C. Systolic
D. Veinous

93. There are twelve bones in which region of the vertebral column
A. Sacral
B. Lumbar
C. Cervical
D. Thoracic

94. A client stretching themselves into resistance with the assistance of a massage therapist
A. Passive stretch
B. Active stretch
C. Active assistive stretch
D. Resistive stretch

95. An example of a superficial lesion is
A. Birthmark
B. Abscess
C. Pimple
D. Wart

96. Cessation of breathing during sleep
A. Narcolepsy
B. Dyspnea
C. Sleep apnea
D. Insomnia

97. Involuntary reaction in response to a stimulus
A. Withdrawal
B. Contraction
C. Reflex
D. Regeneration

98. The heart contains how many chambers
A. Four
B. Two
C. Three
D. Five

99. Multiple sclerosis is caused by destruction of the
A. Cerebellum
B. Dendrites
C. Axons
D. Myelin sheaths

100. Insertion of the Tibialis Anterior and Peroneus Longus
A. Calcaneus
B. Navicular
C. Base of the first metatarsal
D. Tuberosity of the fifth metatarsal

Practice Exam 3 Answer Key

01. A	26. A	51. C	76. C
02. B	27. B	52. D	77. D
03. A	28. C	53. C	78. C
04. D	29. B	54. C	79. D
05. D	30. C	55. C	80. B
06. A	31. B	56. B	81. A
07. D	32. A	57. A	82. B
08. A	33. C	58. B	83. B
09. A	34. B	59. D	84. A
10. C	35. B	60. D	85. A
11. B	36. B	61. D	86. D
12. B	37. D	62. C	87. A
13. B	38. D	63. D	88. C
14. B	39. C	64. C	89. B
15. A	40. D	65. D	90. C
16. A	41. A	66. A	91. A
17. B	42. B	67. B	92. C
18. A	43. A	68. B	93. D
19. C	44. A	69. B	94. C
20. D	45. C	70. D	95. A
21. C	46. B	71. A	96. C
22. B	47. D	72. A	97. C
23. A	48. B	73. C	98. A
24. B	49. B	74. B	99. D
25. A	50. A	75. B	100. C

Practice Exam 4

1. If a client suffers from menopause, an ideal essential oil to use during treatment is
A. Lemon
B. Peppermint
C. Ginger
D. Lavender

2. Proximal attachment of pectineus
A. Body of pubis
B. Inferior ramus of pubis
C. Superior ramus of pubis
D. Ischial tuberosity

3. The trigeminal nerve is which numbered cranial nerve
A. X
B. VII
C. V
D. III

4. Telling a client that they have a specific medical condition is an example of
A. Inquiry
B. Assessment
C. Prognosis
D. Diagnosis

5. Which of the following is not a bone of the cranium
A. Mandible
B. Parietal
C. Occipital
D. Frontal

6. Satisfying an impulse, often negative, by substitution
A. Displacement
B. Denial
C. Projection
D. Assimilation

7. Idiopathic condition resulting in pain in muscles
A. Bell's palsy
B. Muscular dystrophy
C. Tendonitis
D. Fibromyalgia

8. Medical history may be filled out by the client as part of the
A. Assessment form
B. Intake form
C. SOAP notes
D. PPALM form

9. Gross income minus expenses deducted results in
A. Net worth
B. Net income
C. State income
D. Federal income

10. The Art of Massage was written by
A. Celsus
B. John Harvey Kellogg
C. Per Henrik Ling
D. James Cyriax

11. A bolster placed under the knees is used in which position
A. Prone
B. Supine
C. Side-lying
D. Chair

12. Inflammation of the gums
A. Tonsilitis
B. Gastritis
C. Stomatitis
D. Gingivitis

13. Gradual degeneration of parts of the adrenal glands
A. Grave's disease
B. Addison's disease
C. Cushing's syndrome
D. Adrenal hyperplasia

14. Muscle group primarily responsible for extension of the hip and flexion of the knee
A. Glutes
B. Quadriceps
C. Adductors
D. Hamstrings

15. The lesser trochanter is positioned where in relation to the greater trochanter
A. Lateral
B. Medial
C. Anterior
D. Posterior

16. If a massage therapist advertises products not related to a massage treatment, it may be a
A. Networking
B. Opportunistic marketing
C. Outside scope of practice
D. Violation of ethics

17. Inflammation of a tendon and its protective sheath, affecting the thumb
A. Carpal Tunnel Syndrome
B. Dupuytren's Contracture
C. De Quervain's Tenosynovitis
D. Osteoarthritis

18. Cryotherapy is the use of
A. Cold
B. Heat
C. Water
D. Body wraps

19. The radiocarpal joint is considered which type of synovial joint
A. Hinge
B. Ball and socket
C. Condyloid
D. Pivot

20. A metastasis is also known as
A. A secondary tumor
B. A primary tumor
C. Chewing
D. Epiphyseal plate

21. Cupping, hacking, and tapping all are forms of
A. Petrissage
B. Effleurage
C. Friction
D. Tapotement

22. The Thoracic Duct empties lymph into the
A. Right brachiocephalic vein
B. Brachial artery
C. Aorta
D. Left subclavian vein

23. Prolactin, produced by the anterior pituitary, produces
A. Insulin
B. Milk
C. Glucagon
D. Estrogen

24. The cerebellum is formed by which type of tissue
A. Connective
B. Nervous
C. Epithelial
D. Muscular

25. A fracture that breaks through the skin
A. Simple
B. Bilateral
C. Compound
D. Compression

26. Thoracic outlet syndrome may be caused by
A. Trapezius
B. Serratus anterior
C. Rhomboids
D. Pectoralis minor

27. Muscle group primarily responsible for flexion of the hip and extension of the knee
A. Glutes
B. Hamstrings
C. Adductors
D. Quadriceps

28. Reiki and Therapeutic Touch are both forms of
A. Manipulative techniques
B. Energy techniques
C. Movement techniques
D. Stretching techniques

29. Ankylosing spondylitis
A. Protrusion of the gelatinous center of an intervertebral disc through the cartilaginous portion
B. Vertebrae moving out of place, resulting in pinching of spinal nerves
C. Degeneration of intervertebral discs, resulting in fusion of vertebrae and loss of natural curvature of the spine
D. Hyper-curvature of the vertebrae, forcing the vertebrae laterally

30. Connective tissue holding bones together
A. Tendon
B. Ligament
C. Cartilage
D. Periosteum

31. Melanin
A. Provides pigmentation to the skin
B. Allows protection by producing a thickened area of skin
C. Waterproofs the skin
D. Allows absorption of water into the skin

32. Abduction of the scapula can be accomplished by contraction of which muscle
A. Serratus anterior
B. Rhomboids
C. Latissimus dorsi
D. Trapezius

33. Percussion strokes, used to loosen phlegm in the respiratory tract and activate muscle spindle cells
A. Petrissage
B. Effleurage
C. Friction
D. Tapotement

272

34. The atlantooccipital joint is responsible for producing which two actions on the head
A. Lateral deviation
B. Rotation
C. Flexion and extension
D. Adduction and abduction

35. Angina pectoris, hypertension, and migraines may all be treated with
A. Vasodilators
B. Antihistamines
C. Beta-blockers
D. Corticosteroids

36. Resistance to insulin in the blood stream leads to
A. Diabetes type II
B. Diabetes type I
C. Juvenile diabetes
D. Hypoglycemia

37. Gastritis, often caused by bacteria, is
A. Inflammation of the liver
B. Inflammation of the gallbladder
C. Inflammation of the small intestine
D. Inflammation of the stomach

38. Plane joint connecting the scapula to the clavicle
A. Sternoclavicular
B. Acromioclavicular
C. Atlantooccipital
D. Atlantoaxial

39. Controlling infectious agents to prevent the spread of disease
A. Universal precautions
B. Sanitization
C. Contraindications
D. Disinfection

40. Primary action of the pronator teres
A. Elbow extension
B. Supination
C. Elbow flexion
D. Pronation

41. Muscle inserting on the pes anserinus, responsible for flexing and externally rotating the hip, and flexing the knee
A. Gracilis
B. Sartorius
C. Semitendinosus
D. Biceps femoris

42. The outer most membrane of a serous membrane is called
A. Peritoneal membrane
B. Visceral serous membrane
C. Temporal serous membrane
D. Parietal serous membrane

43. James Cyriax is responsible for popularizing
A. Deep transverse friction
B. Lymphatic drainage
C. Sports massage
D. Osteosymmetry

44. The "C" in PRICE stands for
A. Compensation
B. Compression
C. Contraction
D. Concentric

45. A contrast bath should always end with emersion in
A. Cold water
B. Hot water
C. Lukewarm water
D. Salt water

46. Stasis dermatitis
A. Inflammation of the skin caused by irritants coming in contact with the epidermis
B. Inflammation of the skin caused by blockages of the sebaceous glands
C. Inflammation of the skin caused by fluid buildup beneath the skin due to lack of mobility
D. Inflammation of the skin caused by exposure to cold

47. The suture connecting the frontal and parietal bones is called
A. Coronal suture
B. Lambdoid suture
C. Sagittal suture
D. Squamous suture

48. Adhesions forming between the head of the humerus and glenoid fossa, severely restricting range of motion in the shoulder
A. Multiple sclerosis
B. Adhesive capsulitis
C. Osteoarthritis
D. Synovitis

49. The definition of physiology is
A. Studying movement
B. Studying the structure of the body
C. Studying the cause of disease
D. Studying the function of the body

50. Structure bringing air into the lungs
A. Epiglottis
B. Pleural membrane
C. Trachea
D. Uvula

51. Muscle primarily responsible for elevation of the scapula
A. Middle fibers of trapezius
B. Supraspinatus
C. Levator scapulae
D. Sternocleidomastoid

52. A tumor that does not spread throughout the body
A. Malignant
B. Benign
C. Melanoma
D. Basal

53. PRICE is used to treat injuries to
A. Bone
B. Hard tissue
C. Soft tissue
D. Lungs

54. Stance in which the feet run perpendicular to the massage table
A. Archer
B. Warrior
C. Bow
D. Swimmer

55. A primary tumor
A. Is the site of lymphatic drainage into a tumor
B. Is the site of spreading tumors in malignant cancer
C. Is the site of the original tumor in malignant cancer
D. Is derived from a secondary tumor

56. The ovaries produce
A. Luteinizing hormone
B. Testosterone
C. Progesterone
D. Melatonin

57. The inferior five pairs of ribs are also called
A. True ribs
B. False ribs
C. Superior ribs
D. Inferior ribs

58. Book-keeping and taxes for a massage business may be handled by a massage therapist or
A. Client
B. Insurer
C. Practitioner
D. Accountant

59. Areas of the body in which caution is advised during massage of a pregnant client include all of the following except
A. Face
B. Abdomen
C. Ankles
D. Lumbar

60. Hookworm, ascariasis, and pinworm are all forms of
A. Parasite
B. Virus
C. Bacteria
D. Fungus

61. Which part of a long bone is the diaphysis
A. Shaft
B. End
C. Articular surface
D. Growth plate

62. Flexion is
A. Moving a structure towards the midline
B. Increasing the angle of a joint
C. Decreasing the angle of a joint
D. Taking a structure away from the midline

63. Which of the following is a hinge joint
A. Wrist
B. Shoulder
C. Hip
D. Elbow

64. Inflammation of the brain
A. Meningitis
B. Encephalitis
C. Endocarditis
D. Osteomyelitis

65. A partnership is a business owned by
A. One person
B. Two or more people
C. No people
D. The government

66. The lumbar region contains how many vertebrae
A. Seven
B. Twelve
C. Five
D. One

67. Of the following, which is not a fossa located on the scapula
A. Supraspinous fossa
B. Glenoid fossa
C. Subscapular fossa
D. Coronoid fossa

68. Equipment featuring seven shower heads, which can pin-point specific areas on a client's body
A. Contrast Bath
B. Vichy Shower
C. Shirodhara
D. Swiss Shower

69. Proximal attachment of the biceps femoris
A. Supraglenoid tubercle
B. Head of the fibula
C. Coracoid process
D. Ischial tuberosity

70. Phlebitis
A. Bulge in an artery wall, usually caused by a weakened artery due to a condition such as hypertension
B. Inflammation of a vein due to trauma, resulting in blood clot formation
C. Blood clot in the blood stream becoming lodged in the heart, lungs, or brain, resulting in death of tissue
D. Ischemia in the myocardium due to a blockage in the coronary arteries, resulting in myocardial infarction

71. The urinary bladder is found in which body cavity
A. Cranial
B. Abdominal
C. Thoracic
D. Pelvic

72. Proximal attachment of the tibialis anterior
A. Lateral two thirds of the proximal tibia
B. Base of the first metatarsal
C. Head of the fibula
D. Medial condyle of the tibia

73. Spinous processes extend which direction
A. Laterally
B. Dorsally
C. Medially
D. Ventrally

74. Pressing of tsubo points to increase the flow of Ki
A. Amma
B. Shiatsu
C. Ayurveda
D. Tshanpau

75. A wage and tax statement detailing income and withheld taxes from the previous year for an employee
A. W-2
B. Schedule C
C. Schedule K1
D. 1099

76. A client stretching themselves into resistance without the assistance of a massage therapist
A. Passive stretch
B. Active stretch
C. Active assistive stretch
D. Resistive stretch

77. An accumulation of infectious fluid in the alveoli
A. Influenza
B. Pneumonia
C. Emphysema
D. Bronchitis

78. The hip joint is considered which type of synovial joint
A. Ball and socket
B. Pivot
C. Ellipsoid
D. Hinge

79. Insertion of pectoralis minor
A. Sternum
B. Ribs 3-5
C. Coracoid process
D. Intertubercular groove

80. Peristalsis takes place in all of the following organs except
A. Esophagus
B. Liver
C. Stomach
D. Large intestine

81. Form most commonly used to document work performed during a massage session
A. Intake form
B. SOAP notes
C. Assessment form
D. Massage notes

82. Insertion of infraspinatus
A. Greater Tubercle
B. Infraspinous Fossa
C. Lesser Tubercle
D. Intertubercular Groove

83. Diarrhea is most often caused by
A. Consumption of spicy foods
B. Lack of water in feces
C. Bacterial infection of the large intestine
D. Overabundance of water in feces

84. Effects of massage that produce involuntary responses of the body
A. Mechanical effects
B. Emotional effects
C. Reflex effects
D. Sensory effects

85. The phrenic nerve
A. Originates in the chest and innervates the digestive tract to allow peristalsis
B. Originates in the neck and innervates the heart to reduce heart rhythm
C. Originates in the neck and innervates the diaphragm to allow breathing
D. Originates in the head and innervates the tongue to allow speech

86. Most internal layer of a serous membrane
A. Deep serous membrane
B. Parietal serous membrane
C. Elastic serous membrane
D. Visceral serous membrane

87. Trauma to the skin may result in
A. Urticaria
B. Edema
C. Bruising
D. Melanoma

88. The groin is also known as which body region
A. Thorax
B. Popliteal
C. Antecubital
D. Inguinal

89. All of the following are end feels except
A. Soft end feel
B. Hard end feel
C. Empty end feel
D. Nervous end feel

90. Lymphatic drainage massage stimulates increased lymph circulation directed
A. Medially
B. Distally
C. Proximally
D. Laterally

91. Eversion of the foot turns the foot which way
A. Toes pointed down
B. In towards the midline
C. Toes pointed up
D. Out away from the midline

92. Stimulation of specific points on the hands, feet, and ears that may correspond to tissues and organs throughout the body
A. Reflexology
B. Reiki
C. Rolfing
D. Polarity

93. The diaphragm descending produces
A. External pressure
B. Exhalation
C. Force
D. Inhalation

94. Of the following, which condition is contagious
A. Impetigo
B. Bradycardia
C. Tendonitis
D. Lordosis

95. Pleurisy
A. Inflammation of pleural membrane resulting in chest pain
B. Inflammation of bronchial tubes with increased mucous production
C. Spasm of smooth muscle surrounding bronchial tubes, reducing oxygen intake
D. Bacterial infection resulting in increased fluid in the lungs

96. Study of the function of the human body
A. Anatomy
B. Physiology
C. Pathology
D. Etiology

97. Amylase is located in the
A. Saliva
B. Stomach
C. Small intestine
D. Pancreas

98. "Would you like your neck massaged?" is an example of
A. Listening question
B. Open-ended question
C. Feedback question
D. Closed-ended question

99. Nerve found running along the zygomatic bone, partially responsible for taste reception and facial movement
A. Hypoglossal
B. Trigeminal
C. Facial
D. Accessory

100. To take pressure off the lower back of a client lying prone, a bolster should be placed
A. Under the knees
B. Under the ankles
C. Between the legs
D. Under the hips

Practice Exam 4 Answer Key

1. D	26. D	51. C	76. B
2. C	27. D	52. B	77. B
3. C	28. B	53. C	78. A
4. D	29. C	54. B	79. C
5. A	30. B	55. C	80. B
6. A	31. A	56. C	81. B
7. D	32. A	57. B	82. A
8. B	33. D	58. D	83. D
9. B	34. C	59. A	84. C
10. B	35. C	60. A	85. C
11. B	36. A	61. A	86. D
12. D	37. D	62. C	87. C
13. B	38. B	63. D	88. D
14. D	39. A	64. B	89. D
15. B	40. D	65. B	90. C
16. D	41. B	66. C	91. D
17. C	42. D	67. D	92. A
18. A	43. A	68. B	93. D
19. C	44. B	69. D	94. A
20. A	45. A	70. B	95. A
21. D	46. C	71. D	96. B
22. D	47. A	72. A	97. A
23. B	48. B	73. B	98. D
24. B	49. D	74. B	99. C
25. C	50. C	75. A	100. B

Practice Exam 5

1. All of the following are regulated by the temporal lobe except
A. Hearing
B. Smell
C. Vision
D. Memory

2. The long head of the biceps brachii originates where
A. Supraglenoid tubercle
B. Infraglenoid tubercle
C. Coracoid process
D. Radial tuberosity

3. Decreasing the angle of a joint
A. Extension
B. Flexion
C. Rotation
D. Abduction

4. Keeping client information private and protected
A. Self-disclosure
B. Assurance
C. Confidentiality
D. Closed-ended

5. The Art of Massage details
A. The use of herbs for healing
B. Exercise as part of personal hygiene
C. Physiological effects of massage
D. The use of contrast baths for inflammation relief

6. Medical procedure used to remove waste products and toxic substances from the blood when the kidneys are unable to function properly
A. Dialysis
B. Electrolysis
C. Paracentesis
D. Transfusion

7. Structure located immediately proximal to the styloid process of the ulna
A. Ulnar tuberosity
B. Olecranon process
C. Head of the ulna
D. Coronoid process

8. Form of friction in which the massage therapist presses tissue down against deeper tissue to broaden or flatten the tissue
A. Circular friction
B. Cross-fiber friction
C. Compression
D. Superficial friction

9. Vein found in the region of the arm
A. Femoral vein
B. Brachial vein
C. Great saphenous vein
D. Axillary vein

10. The shaft of a long bone is also called
A. Periosteum
B. Epiphysis
C. Metaphysis
D. Diaphysis

11. A pregnant client experiencing dizziness while supine may be due to the fetus placing pressure on the
A. Renal artery
B. Abdominal aorta
C. External iliac artery
D. Urinary bladder

12. Licensing regulations detail the activities a massage therapist may engage in for their practice. These are known as
A. Scope of practice
B. Business standards
C. Regulations
D. Liabilities

13. Endangerment sites
A. Structures that may be massaged freely
B. Areas of the body that must not be massaged
C. Areas of the body that warrant caution
D. Areas of the body the massage therapist may only massage with gloves

14. The knee is considered which type of synovial joint
A. Ellipsoid
B. Pivot
C. Ball and socket
D. Hinge

15. Substance found in erythrocytes which attaches to oxygen and carbon dioxide, allowing transport of these molecules to parts of the body
A. Platelets
B. Leukocyte
C. Anemia
D. Hemoglobin

16. Contrast baths should always end with immersion in cold to reduce
A. Exfoliation
B. Bacterial growth
C. Hypoxia
D. Inflammation

17. Tinea pedis and ringworm are both caused by
A. Fungus
B. Bacteria
C. Virus
D. Parasite

18. Effleurage, petrissage, friction, and tapotement are all strokes found in the following type of massage
A. Trager
B. Lymphatic drainage
C. Shiatsu
D. Swedish

19. The intake form should detail all of the following information except
A. Health history
B. Hobbies
C. Occupation
D. Income

20. Modality consisting of stretching, performed on a mat on the floor, with the client clothed
A. Reiki
B. Thai massage
C. Craniosacral therapy
D. Therapeutic Touch

21. The frontal lobe is responsible for controlling and interpreting
A. Motivation
B. Vision
C. Balance
D. Memory

22. The deltoid is an antagonist to itself. This means
A. It has actions that aren't connected
B. It has two of the same actions
C. It has actions that are similar
D. It has two opposing actions

23. Tendon attaching the gastrocnemius to the calcaneus
A. Tibial
B. Calcaneal
C. Gastroc
D. Patellar

24. High fever and malaise may be a sign of
A. Arrhythmia
B. Septicemia
C. Anemia
D. Myocardial ischemia

25. A person who signs a contract to work for a person or company is known as
A. Partner
B. Employee
C. Sole proprietor
D. Independent contractor

26. Muscle found in the skin is also known as
A. Interdermal muscle
B. Epidermal muscle
C. Arrector pili
D. Papillary muscle

27. Blockages in the following arteries may result in myocardial infarction
A. Coronary
B. Carotid
C. Brachial
D. Subclavian

28. During the course of a massage, a massage therapist discovers a client's right scapula is slightly elevated in relation to the left scapula. This information would be documented under which section of SOAP notes
A. Subjective
B. Objective
C. Assessment
D. Plan

29. Another term for inversion of the foot is
A. Supination
B. Pronation
C. Dorsiflexion
D. Plantarflexion

30. The quadriceps are located on which side of the body
A. Anterior
B. Posterior
C. Medial
D. Lateral

31. Function of non-striated muscle in the digestive tract
A. Contracting skeletal muscle
B. Absorbing nutrients
C. Transporting blood
D. Peristalsis

32. Blood flowing backwards in the heart between chambers due to decrease in function of valves
A. Arrhythmia
B. Heart murmur
C. Bradycardia
D. Ventricular septal defect

33. Muscle inserting onto the calcaneus via the calcaneal tendon
A. Tibialis anterior
B. Soleus
C. Extensor hallucis longus
D. Extensor digitorum

34. John Barnes developed the following technique
A. Lymphatic Drainage
B. Myofascial Release
C. Rolfing
D. Craniosacral Therapy

35. The antecubital region is located on the anterior portion of which joint
A. Elbow
B. Knee
C. Wrist
D. Ankle

36. A common area used to assess a client with jaundice is
A. Teeth
B. Tongue
C. Eyes
D. Hair

37. Melanoma tumors are usually
A. The same size throughout
B. Symmetrical
C. Brown in color
D. Raised off the skin

38. Ureters connect which two structures together
A. Liver and gallbladder
B. Bladder and urethra
C. Small intestine and pancreas
D. Kidneys and bladder

39. Reddening and increased heat of the skin as the result of a massage is known as
A. Varicose veins
B. Anemia
C. Hyperemia
D. Phlebitis

40. A hernia is
A. A strained muscle
B. A fracture in the vertebrae
C. A swollen vein in the anus
D. A protrusion of an organ through its protective membrane

41. Muscle located deep to the Tensor Fasciae Latae
A. Semimembranosus
B. Gluteus Maximus
C. Gracilis
D. Vastus Lateralis

42. Muscle group originating on the lateral epicondyle of the humerus
A. Flexors of the wrist
B. Extensors of the wrist
C. Abductors of the wrist
D. Adductors of the wrist

43. The sympathetic nervous response causes an increase in heart rate, which is caused by an increase in which hormone in the body
A. Calcitonin
B. Norepinephrine
C. Melatonin
D. Prolactin

44. Distal attachment of the soleus
A. Head of the fibula
B. Talus
C. Calcaneus
D. Soleal line

45. The ridge of the ilium is also known as the
A. Anterior superior iliac spine
B. Iliac spine
C. Ischial spine
D. Iliac crest

46. Cerebral palsy
A. Impairment of motor functions due to damage to specific areas of the brain
B. Paralysis of one side of the face due to stimulation of the Herpes Simplex virus
C. Loss of function of part of the face due to an injury to the facial nerve
D. Pain in the face due to compression placed on cranial nerve V

47. Fungal infection affecting the scalp
A. Tinea cruris
B. Tinea corporis
C. Tinea capitis
D. Tinea pedis

48. The ankle joint produces which of the following movement
A. Abduction
B. Rotation
C. Adduction
D. Dorsiflexion

49. All of the following are contagious conditions except
A. Ringworm
B. Rheumatoid arthritis
C. Influenza
D. Mononucleosis

50. A 1099 may be filed how often
A. Monthly
B. Bi-annually
C. Bi-monthly
D. Quarterly

51. Lifting and squeezing tissue is a part of
A. Friction
B. Effleurage
C. Tapotement
D. Petrissage

52. Pain resulting from a trigger point being felt in a different region of the body is known as
A. Latent pain
B. Contagious pain
C. Contracted pain
D. Referred pain

53. Lentigo
A. Benign skin lesion with increased production of melanin
B. Rapid formation of melanocytes resulting in a cancerous tumor
C. Form of skin cancer that grows slowly and is easily detectable
D. Also known as sun spots, usually form during senescence

54. A wound causing a hole in the skin
A. Laceration
B. Abrasion
C. Avulsion
D. Puncture

55. Cranial nerve which branches into the ophthalmic, maxillary, and mandibular divisions
A. Vagus
B. Facial
C. Vestibulocochlear
D. Trigeminal

56. Massage stroke designed to stimulate muscle spindle activity, especially useful in pre-event sports massage
A. Tapotement
B. Friction
C. Effleurage
D. Petrissage

57. The inner portion of a kidney is called
A. Medulla
B. Cortex
C. Oblongata
D. Adrenal

58. Mesentery is part of which serous membrane
A. Pleural
B. Pericardium
C. Peritoneal
D. Meninges

59. The four signs of inflammation
A. Pain, swelling, redness, heat
B. Pain, swelling, inflammation, heat
C. Pain, inflammation, cyanosis, heat
D. Pain, inflammation, redness, sweat

60. The joints found between the vertebrae are categorized as which type of synovial joint
A. Gliding
B. Hinge
C. Pivot
D. Ellipsoid

61. TIA is also known as
A. Transient ischemic attack
B. Temporoinguinal angle
C. Tubercular interosseous attachment
D. Thyroid immunity ailment

62. Essential oils are mainly used in which type of treatment
A. Hydrotherapy
B. Aromatherapy
C. Body wraps
D. Body scrubs

63. All of the following are local contraindications except
A. Wart
B. Sprain
C. Bruise
D. Head lice

64. Gelatinous center of an intervertebral disc
A. Dens
B. Annulus fibrosus
C. Nucleus pulposus
D. Vertebral canal

65. Person who introduced Medical Gymnastics to America
A. Per Henrik Ling
B. Charles Taylor
C. Emil Vodder
D. David Palmer

66. Which of the following is not a hinge joint
A. Knee
B. Shoulder
C. Elbow
D. Ankle

67. The radiocarpal joint can perform all of the following actions except
A. Circumduction
B. Rotation
C. Adduction
D. Flexion

68. Type of tissue that forms exocrine glands
A. Connective
B. Epithelial
C. Nervous
D. Muscular

69. A client accidentally rolls off the table and injures themselves. The type of liability insurance that covers these instances is
A. Malpractice insurance
B. Professional liability insurance
C. Privacy Rule
D. General liability insurance

70. Decreased absorption of iron into the body may result in
A. Scurvy
B. Anemia
C. Scabies
D. Atherosclerosis

71. A massage therapist should wash their hands before and after each massage using
A. Cold water
B. Bleach
C. Rubbing alcohol
D. Anti-bacterial soap

72. Edematic tissue is composed primarily of
A. Synovial fluid
B. Blood
C. Lymph
D. Serous fluid

73. Lipoma
A. Tumor formed by melanocyte production
B. Tumor formed by sebaceous glands
C. Tumor of fatty tissue
D. Malignant tumor on the lips

74. The interphalangeal joints are which type of synovial joints
A. Hinge
B. Pivot
C. Ball and socket
D. Ellipsoid

75. A neutrophil is what type of cell
A. Leukocyte
B. Osteocyte
C. Squamous cell
D. Epithelium

76. Meissner's corpuscles detect
A. Smell
B. Deep pressure
C. Pain
D. Light pressure

77. The definition of "scoli/o" is
A. Crooked
B. Spine
C. Lumbar
D. Swayback

78. A thrombus in the cerebrum restricting circulation may result in
A. Angina pectoris
B. Heart attack
C. Arrhythmia
D. Stroke

79. Shiatsu involves
A. Stimulating tsubo points to increase Ki flow
B. Pulling of limbs to increase range of motion
C. Channeling universal energy throughout the client's body without touching
D. Cupping movements to stimulate circulation

80. A feather stroke is also known as
A. Aura stroke
B. Nerve stroke
C. Deep gliding stroke
D. Vibration

81. Nerve responsible for stimulation of the smooth muscle in the digestive tract, allowing peristalsis to take place
A. Gastrointestinal
B. Trigeminal
C. Vagus
D. Hypoglossal

82. Urea and ammonia are filtered from the blood by the
A. Large intestine
B. Bladder
C. Kidneys
D. Spleen

83. Which of the following is not regulated by the frontal lobe
A. Aggression
B. Olfactory reception
C. Visual input
D. Language

84. Fever is considered
A. A local contraindication
B. An absolute contraindication
C. An endangerment site
D. Not a contraindication

85. Which of the following conditions would a client be referred to a nephrologist for
A. Pitting edema
B. Cellulitis
C. Hepatitis
D. Neuralgia

86. A short general statement detailing the goal of a business
A. Public image
B. Purpose
C. Mission statement
D. Business plan

87. The two bones that comprise the elbow joint are
A. Ulna and lunate
B. Radius and scaphoid
C. Scapula and humerus
D. Ulna and humerus

88. Massage stroke directed toward the heart used to increase circulation, transition between strokes, and apply massage lubricant
A. Friction
B. Petrissage
C. Effleurage
D. Vibration

89. Muscle group located on the posterior thigh
A. Hamstrings
B. Quadriceps
C. Adductors
D. Gluteals

90. Synergist to the gastrocnemius in performing plantarflexion of the ankle
A. Tibialis anterior
B. Peroneus longus
C. Biceps femoris
D. Rectus femoris

91. If a massage therapist becomes sexually attracted to a client, the proper course of action is
A. Act on these urges
B. Refer the client to another therapist
C. Tell the client
D. Document these feelings in SOAP notes

92. A client with thoracic outlet syndrome would be referred to which doctor
A. Neurologist
B. Cardiologist
C. Rheumatologist
D. Dermatologist

93. Generalized myalgia, localized muscle pain, and trouble sleeping could be the result of
A. Carpal tunnel syndrome
B. Fibromyalgia
C. Muscular dystrophy
D. Tendonitis

94. CPR stands for
A. Cerebroparietal Resonance
B. Carpal Protection Resist
C. Cardiopulmonary Resuscitation
D. Cerebellum Posture Realization

95. Reiki originated in
A. Japan
B. China
C. India
D. America

96. Calcitonin, which lowers calcium levels in the blood, is secreted by the
A. Testes
B. Thyroid
C. Thymus
D. Pituitary

97. Bile is produced by the
A. Gallbladder
B. Liver
C. Stomach
D. Pancreas

98. Function of the kidneys
A. Regulation of electrolytes
B. Absorption of nutrients from food
C. Preventing bacterial infection
D. Excretion of carbon dioxide

99. Sebaceous cyst
A. Formation of connective tissue surrounding oil gland
B. Formation of connective tissue containing fatty tissue
C. Formation of connective tissue attached to tendon sheaths
D. Formation of connective tissue spreading to other parts of the body

100. Oxygen, upon entering the bloodstream, attaches to an iron compound known as
A. Leukocyte
B. Plasma
C. Thrombocyte
D. Hemoglobin

Practice Exam 5 Answer Key

1. C	26. C	51. D	76. D
2. A	27. A	52. D	77. A
3. B	28. B	53. D	78. D
4. C	29. A	54. D	79. A
5. C	30. A	55. D	80. B
6. A	31. D	56. A	81. C
7. C	32. B	57. A	82. C
8. C	33. B	58. C	83. C
9. B	34. B	59. A	84. B
10. D	35. A	60. A	85. A
11. B	36. C	61. A	86. C
12. A	37. D	62. B	87. D
13. C	38. D	63. D	88. C
14. D	39. C	64. C	89. A
15. D	40. D	65. B	90. B
16. D	41. D	66. B	91. B
17. A	42. B	67. B	92. A
18. D	43. B	68. B	93. B
19. D	44. C	69. D	94. C
20. B	45. D	70. B	95. A
21. A	46. A	71. D	96. B
22. D	47. C	72. C	97. B
23. B	48. D	73. C	98. A
24. B	49. B	74. A	99. A
25. D	50. D	75. A	100. D

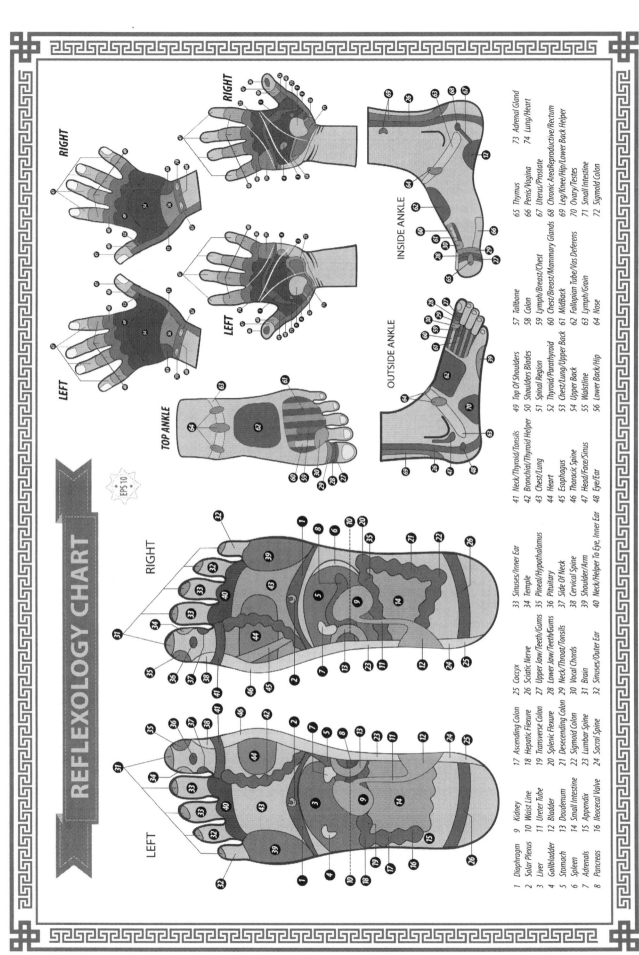

REFLEXOLOGY CHART

RIGHT

LEFT

TOP ANKLE

INSIDE ANKLE

OUTSIDE ANKLE

RIGHT

LEFT

1 Diaphragm
2 Solar Plexus
3 Liver
4 Gallbladder
5 Stomach
6 Spleen
7 Adrenals
8 Pancreas
9 Kidney
10 Waist Line
11 Ureter Tube
12 Bladder
13 Duodenum
14 Small Intestine
15 Appendix
16 Ileocecal Valve
17 Ascending Colon
18 Hepatic Flexure
19 Transverse Colon
20 Splenic Flexure
21 Desecending Colon
22 Sigmoid Colon
23 Lumbar Spine
24 Sacral Spine
25 Coccyx
26 Sciatic Nerve
27 Upper Jaw/Teeth/Gums
28 Lower Jaw/Teeth/Gums
29 Neck/Throat/Tonsils
30 Vocal Chords
31 Brain
32 Sinuses/Outer Ear
33 Sinuses/Inner Ear
34 Temple
35 Pineal/Hypothalamus
36 Pituitary
37 Side Of Neck
38 Cervical Spine
39 Shoulder/Arm
40 Neck/Helper To Eye, Inner Ear
41 Neck/Thyroid/Tonsils
42 Bronchial/Thyroid Helper
43 Chest/Lung
44 Heart
45 Esophagus
46 Thoracic Spine
47 Head/Face/Sinus
48 Eye/Ear
49 Top Of Shoulders
50 Shoulders Blades
51 Spinal Region
52 Thyroid/Parathyroid
53 Chest/Lung/Upper Back
54 Upper Back
55 Waistline
56 Lower Back/Hip
57 Tailbone
58 Colon
59 Lymph/Breast/Chest
60 Chest/Breast/Mammary Glands
61 MidBack
62 Fallopian Tube/Vas Deferens
63 Lymph/Groin
64 Nose
65 Thymus
66 Penis/Vagina
67 Uterus/Prostate
68 Chronic Area Reproductive/Rectum
69 Leg/Knee/Hip/Lower Back Helper
70 Ovary/Testes
71 Small Intestine
72 Sigmoid Colon
73 Adrenal Gland
74 Lung/Heart

EPS 10

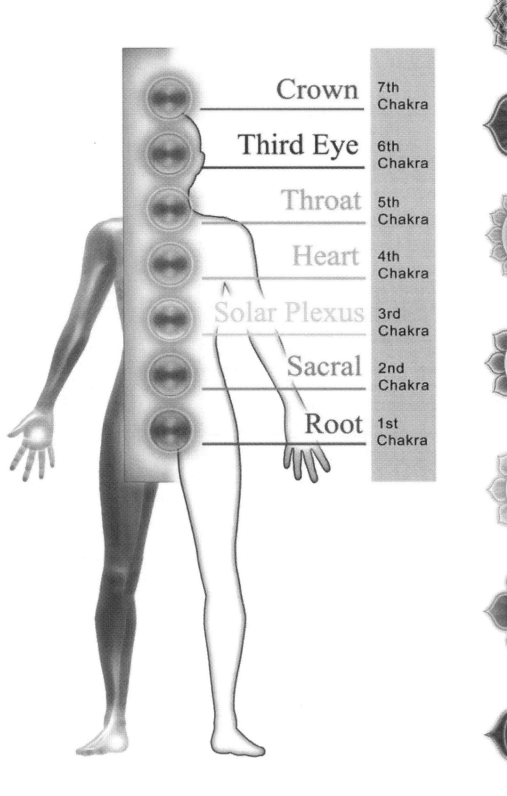

Crown — 7th Chakra

Third Eye — 6th Chakra

Throat — 5th Chakra

Heart — 4th Chakra

Solar Plexus — 3rd Chakra

Sacral — 2nd Chakra

Root — 1st Chakra

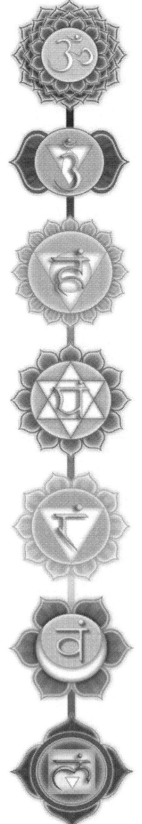

The Body Meridians

Two Centerline Meridians:

Conception Vessel
Governing Vessel

Twelve Principal Meridians:

Stomach Meridian
Spleen Meridian

Small Intestine Meridian
Heart Meridian

Bladder Meridian
Kidney Meridian

Pericardium Meridian
Triple Warmer Meridian

Gall Bladder Meridian
Liver Meridian

Lung Meridian
Large Intestine Meridian

posterior view

anterior view

References

This book was created with the assistance of the following resources:

- *Tappan's Handbook of Massage Therapy: Blending Art with Science(6th Edition), 2015* – Patricia J. Benjamin, PhD

- *30 Second Anatomy: The 50 Most Important Structures and Systems in the Human Body, Each Explained in Half a Minute, 2013* – Gabrielle M. Finn, Judith Barbaro-Brown

- *Anatomica: The Complete Home Medical Reference, 2010* – Ken Ashwell

- *Mosby's Pathology for Massage Therapists(3rd Edition) 2013* – Susan Salvo

- *The Four Hour Chef : The Simple Path to Cooking Like a Pro, Learning Anything, and Living the Good Life, 2013* – Timothy Ferriss

- *Gray's Anatomy* – Henry Gray

- *Essentials of Anatomy and Physiology(4th Edition) 2002* – Rod Seeley, Trent Stephens, Philip Tate

- *Introducing Medical Terminology Specialties: A Medical Specialties Approach with Patient Records, 2003* – Regina Masters, Barbara Gylys

- *Exploring Medical Language: A Student-Directed Approach(5th Edition), 2002* – Myrna LaFleur Brooks

- *Basic Clinical Massage Therapy: Integrating Anatomy and Treatment, 2003* – James H. Clay, David M. Pounds

- *Milady's Theory and Practice of Therapeutic Massage, 1999* – Mark F. Beck

Recommended Reading

- *The Obstacle is the Way: The Timeless Art of Turning Trials into Triumph, 2014* – Ryan Holiday

- *Ego is the Enemy, 2016* – Ryan Holiday

- *Outliers: The Story of Success, 2008* – Malcolm Gladwell

Index

Copyright Information

MBLEx Test Prep – Comprehensive Study Guide and Workbook is the copyrighted work of David Merlino, LMT. Any unauthorized reproduction or distribution is strictly prohibited.

Bulk pricing is available for schools and instructors. Email david@massagetestprep.com for more information.

Acknowledgements and Credits

I'd like to extend a thank you to my family for supporting me in all my endeavors. I'd like to thank my friends for putting up with my ability to never shut up about the progress of this and other works I've done. Thank you to every person who has purchased this study guide. Thank you to every student I've had, and continue to have, for making me the best teacher I can be. Thank you to everyone who has thanked me for helping them pass the exam. These words of encouragement and kindness keep me focused and inspired to continue helping in any way I can. Thank you to Tim Ferriss, without whom none of this would have been possible. Thank you to Christina Taylor, for helping me begin my career in teaching, and believing in me. Thank you to my wife, Amanda, and my son, Owen, for giving me a reason to work as hard as I do.

Image Credits: Sebastian Kaulitzki, Amanda Merlino, Chara Lawson, Spencer Wyman, Ashley Capone, Kayla Madsen

Editing and Proof-Reading: Chara Lawson

Cover: Ilian Georgiev

If this book has helped in any way, please consider leaving a review of it on Amazon.com. Reviews go a long way towards helping this study guide become more well-known. I sincerely appreciate it.

Thank you again.

44639146R00167

Made in the USA
San Bernardino, CA
19 January 2017